Current Research in Emergency Surgery

Current Research in Emergency Surgery

Edited by Gideon Allen

AMERICAN
MEDICAL PUBLISHERS
www.americanmedicalpublishers.com

American Medical Publishers,
41 Flatbush Avenue,
1st Floor, New York,
NY 11217, USA

Visit us on the World Wide Web at:
www.americanmedicalpublishers.com

ISBN: 978-1-63927-487-1

Cataloging-in-Publication Data

Current research in emergency surgery / edited by Gideon Allen.
p. cm.
Includes bibliographical references and index.
ISBN 978-1-63927-487-1
1. Surgical emergencies. 2. Medical emergencies. 3. Surgery. I. Allen, Gideon.
RD93 .C87 2022
617.026--dc23

Table of Contents

Preface

Emergency surgery is the surgery which is aimed at the management of an acute threat to organ, limb or tissue. It may also include threat to life caused due to extreme trauma, acute exacerbation of a disease, acute disease condition or complications arising due to a surgical or interventional procedure. The field of emergency surgery involves knowledge of surgical anatomy, and applied pathology and physiology. The understanding of the physiology of the condition or disease, pre-existing comorbidities and their influence on the current condition, and assessment of the condition including the need for surgery are vital to emergency surgery. Emergency surgical procedures include thoracic, abdominal, vascular and soft tissue procedures. This book is compiled in such a manner, that it will provide in-depth knowledge about the theory and practice of emergency surgery. The topics covered herein outline various medical emergencies, and their therapeutic interventions. In this book, using case studies and examples, constant effort has been made to make the understanding of the difficult concepts as easy and informative as possible, for the readers.

The researches compiled throughout the book are authentic and of high quality, combining several disciplines and from very diverse regions from around the world. Drawing on the contributions of many researchers from diverse countries, the book's objective is to provide the readers with the latest achievements in the area of research. This book will surely be a source of knowledge to all interested and researching the field.

In the end, I would like to express my deep sense of gratitude to all the authors for meeting the set deadlines in completing and submitting their research chapters. I would also like to thank the publisher for the support offered to us throughout the course of the book. Finally, I extend my sincere thanks to my family for being a constant source of inspiration and encouragement.

Editor

1

An audit of secondary peritonitis at a tertiary care university hospital of Sindh, Pakistan

Ahmer A Memon[1*], Faisal G Siddiqui[1], Arshad H Abro[1], Ahmed H Agha[1], Shahzadi Lubna[2] and Abdul S Memon[1]

Abstract

Objective: Peritonitis is the most common life threatening surgical emergency, which requires urgent surgical intervention and is a significant cause of morbidity and mortality. The objective of this study was to highlight the frequency of secondary peritonitis and to analyze the site and causes of perforation, in our tertiary care setup.

Methods: A retrospective analysis of 311 patients of secondary peritonitis was done from July 2008 to June 2010 at Liaquat University Hospital Jamshoro, Hyderabad, Sindh, Pakistan. All cases found to have peritonitis as a result of perforation of any part of gastrointestinal tract at the time of surgery were included in the study. All cases with either primary peritonitis or that due to anastomotic dehiscence were excluded.

Results: A total of 311 patients were studied. Most of the patients were males (77%) and (89%) were in the third and fourth decades of life. Majority of the patients presented with pain (97%) associated with bowel symptoms. Most common site of perforation was small bowel (ileal 59%, jujenal 2%). In this series, most common risk factor of perforation was typhoid (43%). Ileostomy was the most commonly performed procedure. Overall morbidity was 48.5% and mortality was 17%.

Conclusion: Considering the relatively higher rate of typhoid perforation quoted in this study, it is vital that typhoid fever ought to be eliminated by improved sanitation and immunizing programmes, otherwise surgeons will be confronted with its complications.

Keywords: Ileostomy, Typhoid, Peritonitis

Introduction

Generalized peritonitis is a common surgical emergency in developing countries [1]. Despite advances in surgical techniques, good antimicrobial therapy and intensive care support, it carries high morbidity and mortality while its management remains difficult and complex [2]. Peritonitis can be classified as primary, secondary or tertiary, depending upon the source of microbial contamination. Primary peritonitis is secondary to extra-peritoneal sources, the infection spreading mainly through haematogenous dissemination without visceral perforation. Secondary peritonitis, on the other hand, is caused by resident flora of the gastrointestinal or urogenital tracts, the organisms reaching peritoneum secondary to a mechanical break. Non-responding secondary peritonitis either due to failure of the host inflammatory response or overwhelming super infection leads to tertiary peritonitis [3].

Peritonitis, if not treated promptly, can lead to multi-system organ failure and death [4,5].

Current surgical treatment options include primary double-layered closure [6], segmental resection and anastomosis [7] and primary ileostomy [8,9].

This study aims to identify the causes, bacteriology and outcomes of different surgical methods for secondary peritonitis at Liaquat University Hospital.

Material and methods

This retrospective study was conducted in Surgical Emergency Unit-I, Liaquat University Hospital, Hyderabad, Sindh, Pakistan over a period of two years from July 2008 to June 2010. Three hundred and eleven patients with acute abdomen, admitted through Accident and Emergency (A&E) Department were included

* Correspondence: ahmer_akbar@hotmail.com
[1]Department of Surgery, Liaquat University of Medical & Health Sciences, Jamshoro, 71000, Pakistan
Full list of author information is available at the end of the article

in this study. The symptoms included abdominal pain, distension, vomiting and absolute constipation, dehydration and shock with an average of 3.5 days elapsing between onset of first symptom and admission to hospital. Based on history and physical examination, a provisional diagnosis of intestinal perforation was made which was confirmed by investigations including X-ray chest for pneumoperitoneum and abdominal X-ray for air fluid levels. All patients were resuscitated after passage of two 16-gauge cannulas, nasogastric tube and Foley's catheter. All patients received 2-3 l of Ringer's lactate and third generation cephalosporins (ceftriaxone) and quinolones (moxifloxacin), the later given in the last one year of study. With the confirmation of the initial diagnosis of intestinal perforation, emergency laparotomy was performed in all 311 patients. Perforations in the gastrointestinal tract were treated either with primary double-layered closure, segmental resection and anastomosis or loop ileostomy, depending upon the operative findings and general status of the patients. Peritoneal fluid was sent for culture and sensitivity in all patients. The peritoneal cavity was irrigated with an average of 2 l of warm normal saline and drains were left in abdomen and wound was closed either as mass closure or in layers depending upon the operator's choice. Patients were monitored post-operatively for recovery and early detection and management of complications.

Alvarado scoring was routinely done in our series in patients suspected to have peritonitis secondary to perforated appendicitis.

The study was given an approval by the institutional Ethical Review Committee (ERC).

Results

Three hundred and eleven patients with diagnosis of acute abdomen were included in this study. There were 239 (77%) males and 72 (23%) females. The age ranged from 18 to 75 years with the maximum incidence (89%) in the third decade. Presenting symptoms included abdominal pain (97%), abdominal distension (91%), absolute constipation (80%) and vomiting (58%). All patients (100%) presented with dehydration and shock. Abdominal tenderness and rigidity were present 85 and 83% of the patients respectively. Various investigative findings are depicted in Table 1.

All 311 patients underwent emergency laparotomy. In 182 (58%) cases, ileal perforation was the underlying cause for peritonitis. The second most common site of perforation was gastroduodenum, found in 56 (18%) patients. Other sites of perforation are shown in Table 2. The aetiology of perforations in 311 patients is depicted in Table 3.

Table 1 Abnormalities on the initial investigations

Investigations	n = 311
Hyponatraemia(Na < 130 mEq/L)	173 (56%)
Hypokalemia(K < 2.7 mEq/L)	139 (45%)
Blood Urea Nitrogen(> 167 mg/dl)	104 (33%)
Serum Creatinine(< 1.7 mg/dl)	82 (26%)
Pneumoperitoneum on Chest X-Ray	164 (53%)
Air fluid levels on abdominal X-Ray	90 (29%)

Two hundred and three (65%) cases were found to have generalized peritonitis while the remaining (35%) had localized peritonitis. Faecal exudate was seen in 243 (78%) patients while 68 (22%) cases had either clear or purulent exudate. The most commonly performed procedure in our series was ileostomy which was carried out in 81 (26%) patients, followed by simple closure in 73 (23%) patients. Other surgical procedures performed are depicted in Table 4. Postoperative complications were encountered in 143 (46%), cases (Table 5) especially in patients presenting late. The mean hospital stay ranged from 14 to 56 days. The morbidity and mortality in this series were 48.5 and 16.7%, respectively.

Discussion

Generalized peritonitis is a frequently encountered emergency and remains a significant cause of morbidity and mortality which usually requires emergency surgery [10]. Worldwide there is a predominance of males presenting with this life-threatening disease [11,12]; our series also shows a similar trend, with a male to female ratio of 3.3:1.

Early diagnosis and treatment leads to improved results in terms of mortality. Majority of patients in our series presented late with the time interval between the onset of symptoms and admission varying from 12 hours to up to 6 days with an average of 3.5 days. Delay in seeking treatment associated with other factors such as malnourishment and impaired immunity was one of the major reasons for high mortality and morbidity in our series. Kaur N et al., in their study also attribute

Table 2 Site of perforation

Site of perforation	n = 311
Gastroduodenal	56 (18%)
- Duodenal	37 (11.9%)
- Gastic	19 (6.1%)
Jejunal	07 (2%)
Ileal	182 (59%)
Appendicular	47 (15%)
Colonic	19 (6%)

Table 3 Aetiology of perforation

Aetiology	(n = 311)
Typhoid	134 (43%)
Acid peptic disease	56 (18%)
Appendicular	47 (15%)
Tuberculosis	43 (13.8%)
Trauma	20 (6.4%)
Malignancy	11 (3.53%)
Ileocaecal	02 (0.64%)
Large bowel	09 (2.9%)

delay seeking surgical treatment as an important cause for high morbidity [13].

The diagnosis of the patients with peritonitis is clinical; all patients in our series presented with abdominal pain. The pain was sharp, insidious, constant and intense, and was aggravated with movements. Other symptoms included anorexia, nausea, vomiting, absolute constipation and abdominal distension. Langell JT and Mulvihill SJ report similar symptoms in their study [10].

Investigations in patients with peritonitis have dubious reliability. Only 164 (52.7%) patients in this series had evidence of pneumoperitoneum on x-ray chest. This corresponds well with another study, which reports pneumoperitoneum in 50% of cases with peritonitis [14]. Similarly, only 28.9% cases showed air fluid levels on x-ray abdomen.

In our study, distal gastrointestinal tract was the common site of perforation and was seen in 182 (58.5%) patients. This is corroborated by similar study by Quereshi AM [15] and Dorairajan LN [2] who report majority of perforations involving distal gastrointestinal tract such as ileum.

In our study, the most common cause of secondary peritonitis due to gastrointestinal tract perforation was typhoid which was found in 134(43%) cases; this was followed by peptic ulcer disease in 56(18%) cases. Duodenal perforation was more common (11.9%) compared to gastric perforation (6.1%). Chaterjee H too reported typhoid as the commonest cause of perforations in two separate studies [16,17].

We performed primary closure of the perforation in patients with typhoid peritonitis who were clinically

Table 4 Surgical procedure performed

Surgical procedure	(n = 311)
Ileostomy	81 (26%)
Simple closure	73 (24%)
Closure with Graham's patch (Omentopexy)	56 (18%)
Appendicectomy	47 (15%)
Resection and anastomosis	28 (9%)
Stricturoplasty	9 (3%)
Colostomy	17 (5%)

Table 5 Post operative complications

Complications	(n = 311)
Abdominal collection	13 (4.1%)
Wound infection	32 (10.2%)
Electrolyte imbalance	21 (6.7%)
Septicemia	33 (10.6%)
Burst abdomen	14 (4.5%)
Faecal fistula	19 (6.1%)
Ileostomy related complications	11 (3.5%)
Overall morbidity	151 (48.5%)
Mortality	52 (16.7%)

stable and had minimal soling of the abdominal cavity. We selectively performed primary closure with proximal ileostomy in all other patients who presented late and had faecal contamination of peritoneal cavity, friable and gut and/or poor clinical condition, this is also supported by other studies [18-22].

Acid peptic disease was the second commonest cause of secondary peritonitis in our study being found in 56 (18%) cases. These perforations were found either along the first part of the duodenum anteriorly (11.9%) or in the pylorus of the stomach (6.1%). These patients presented with the classical signs and symptoms of peritonitis, and required early surgery for a favourable outcome. We found that in such cases, closure of the perforation using a Graham's omental patch was a simple and safe procedure with low mortality, as supported by Subramanyam SG [23].

Dandpat MC studied 340 cases of Gastrointestinal perforations and found that 22(6.4%) patients developed secondary peritonitis secondary to perforated appendix [24]. However, in our series, secondary peritonitis due to appendicular perforations was the underlying cause in 47 (15%) of patients. Afridi SP had reported that the patients who developed secondary peritonitis due to perforated appendix present with the typical history of pain starting in the periumbilical region than shift to the right iliac fossa, or originated directly in the right iliac fossa and then spread to all over the abdomen [25]. We also observed that most of the patients with appendicular perforation presented in the similar manner. The patients with perforated appendix belonged to young age group.

Primary intestinal tuberculosis is uncommon in the west [26] but is still common in developing countries like Pakistan [27]. In our study, the clinical picture of the patients presenting with tuberculous perforation included symptoms such as abdominal pain, fever with night sweats and weight loss. Eighteen (5%) patients had history of subacute intestinal obstruction. Radiologic images revealed evidence of tuberculosis in 11(3.5%) patients. 19 (6%) of patients presented with peritonitis during the course of anti tuberculosis treatment. The commonest sites of involvement were terminal ileum and ileocaecal region though, multiple sites were also commonly found. Management of these patients included resection anastomosis of small gut, repair of perforation with ileoileal or ileo-transverse bypass, primary repair of perforation, stricturoplasty and right hemicolectomy. Biopsies were taken for histopathological examination from the edge of the perforation, omentum and mesenteric lymph nodes which proved the diagnosis of tuberculosis. Similar observations are reported by Akgun Y [28] and Serf R [29]. 11 cases of malignancy were found in our study. The majority of malignancies (9 cases) involved the large bowel, while 2 cases showed involvement of ileocaecal junction. All carcinomas were identified as adenocarcinomas on histopathology.

Surgical treatment of secondary peritonitis is highly demanding. Some authors have adopted laparoscopy as preferred surgical approach for the management of secondary peritonitis [30]. Laparoscopy is an emerging facility and in emergency setup, it is still in its infancy, being performed in only a few medical institutions of Pakistan. Due to the non-availability of laparoscopy in our emergency setup during the study period, no patient was treated laparoscopically.

In our study, postoperative complications included wound infection (28%), septicaemia (20%) and electrolyte imbalance (7%). However, postoperative complication in secondary peritonitis reported by Jhobta RS [10] are respiratory tract infections (28%), wound infection (25%), septicaemia (18%) and dyselectrolaemia (17%). Kim et al. [31] in their study report mortality rate of 9.9%. This is related to the delayed presentation of the patient to a definitive care hospital. In our study mortality rate was 16.7%. The high mortality in our setup could be attributed to the fact that this hospital caters to patients from far flung rural areas of the province. Illiteracy, low socioeconomic status, improper infrastructure including inadequate transport and delayed referral to tertiary care hospital by the general practitioners are some of the reasons for these patients coming late to our medical facility.

Conclusion

The presentation of secondary peritonitis in Pakistan continues to be different from its western counterpart. The In majority of cases the presentation to the hospital was late with well established generalized peritonitis with purulent/fecal contamination and varying degree of septicemia. Good pre-operation assessment and early management will decrease the morbidity, mortality and complications of secondary peritonitis.

Author details

[1]Department of Surgery, Liaquat University of Medical & Health Sciences, Jamshoro, 71000, Pakistan. [2]Department of Gynea & Obs, Liaquat University of Medical & Health Sciences, Jamshoro, 71000, Pakistan.

Authors' contributions

AAM carried out acquisition, analysis, interpretation of the data and drafting of the manuscript. FGS was involved interpretation of the data, drafting of the manuscript, and revised it critically for the intellectual content till the final version was reached. AHA, AHA, SL and ASM have read, edited and approved the final manuscript. All authors read and approved the final manuscript.

Competing interests

The authors declare that they have no competing interests.

References

1. Adesunkanmi ARK, Badmus TA, Fadiora FO, Agbakwuru EA: **Generalized peritonitis secondary to typhoid ileal perforation: Assessment of severity using modified APACHE II score.** *Indian J Surg* 2005, **67**:29-33.
2. Dorairajan LN, Gupta S, Deo SV, Chumber S, Sharma L: **Peritonitis in India-a decade's experience.** *Trop Gastroenterol* 1995, **16(1)**:33-38.
3. Ordonez CA, Puyana JC: **Management of peritonitis in the critically ill patient.** *Surg Clin North Am* 2006, **86(6)**:1323-1349.
4. Gupta S, Kaushik R: **Peritonitis–the Eastern experience.** *World J Emerg Surg* 2006, **1**:13.
5. Eid HO, Hefny AF, Joshi S, Abu-Zidan FM: **Non-traumatic perforation of the small bowel.** *Afr Health Sci* 2008, **8(1)**:36-39.
6. Athie CG, Guizar CB, Alcantara AV, Alcaraz GH, Montalvo EJ: **Twenty-five years of experience in the surgical treatment of perforation of the ileum caused by Salmonella typhi at the General Hospital of Mexico City, Mexico.** *Surgery* 1998, **123(6)**:632-636.
7. Kaul BK: **Operative management of typhoid perforation in children.** *Int Surg* 1975, **60(8)**:407-410.
8. Singh KP, Singh K, Kohli JS: **Choice of surgical procedure in typhoid perforation: experience in 42 cases.** *J Indian Med Assoc* 1991, **89(9)**:255-256.
9. Khalid S, Irfan A: **Outcome of ileostomy in cases of typhoid perforation presenting after 48 hours.** *J Rawal Med Coll* 2000, **4**:17-19.
10. Langell JT, Mulvihill SJ: **Gastrointestinal perforation and the acute abdomen.** *Med Clin North Am* 2008, **92(3)**:599-625.
11. Jhobta RS, Attri AK, Kaushik R, Sharma R, Jhobta A: **Spectrum of perforation peritonitis in India-review of 504 consecutive cases.** *World J Emerg Surg* 2006, **1**:26.
12. Wani RA, Parray FQ, Bhat NA, Wani MA, Bhat TH, Farzana F: **Nontraumatic terminal ileal perforation.** *World J Emerg Surg* 2006, **1**:7.
13. Kaur N, Gupta MK, Minocha VR: **Early enteral feeding by nasoenteric tubes in patients with perforation peritonitis.** *World J Surg* 2005, **29(8)**:1023-1027, discussion 7-8.
14. Conroy JV: **Acute ileitis with ulceration and perforation due to paratyphoid fever; report of eighty-five cases.** *Mil Med* 1957, **120(2)**:79-92.
15. Qureshi AM, Zafar A, Saeed K, Quddus A: **Predictive power of Mannheim Peritonitis Index.** *J Coll Physicians Surg Pak* 2005, **15(11)**:693-696.
16. Chatterjee H, Jagdish S, Pai D, Satish N, Jayadev D, Reddy PS: **Changing trends in outcome of typhoid ileal perforations over three decades in Pondicherry.** *Trop Gastroenterol* 2001, **22(3)**:155-158.
17. Chatterjee H, Pai D, Jagdish S, Satish N, Jayadev D, Srikanthreddy P: **Pattern of nontyphoid ileal perforation over three decades in Pondicherry.** *Trop Gastroenterol* 2003, **24(3)**:144-147.
18. Adesunkanmi AR, Ajao OG: **The prognostic factors in typhoid ileal perforation: a prospective study of 50 patients.** *J R Coll Surg Edinb* 1997, **42(6)**:395-399.
19. Maurya SD, Gupta HC, Tiwari A, Sharma BD: **Typhoid bowel perforation: a review of 264 cases.** *Int Surg* 1984, **69(2)**:155-158.
20. Meier DE, Imediegwu OO, Tarpley JL: **Perforated typhoid enteritis: operative experience with 108 cases.** *Am J Surg* 1989, **157(4)**:423-427.
21. Archampong EQ: **Tropical diseases of the small bowel.** *World J Surg* 1985, **9(6)**:887-896.
22. Eustache JM, Kreis DJ Jr: **Typhoid perforation of the intestine.** *Arch Surg* 1983, **118(11)**:1269-1271.
23. Subramanyam SG, Sunder N, Saleem KM, Kilpadi AB: **Peritonitis in patients over the age of 50 years: 98 cases managed surgically.** *Trop Doct* 2005, **35(4)**:247-250.

24. Dandapat MC, Mukherjee LM, Mishra SB, Howlader PC: **Gastrointestinal perforations.** *Indian J Surg* 1991, **53**:189-193.
25. Afridi SP, Malik F, Ur-Rahman S, Shamim S, Samo KA: **Spectrum of perforation peritonitis in Pakistan: 300 cases Eastern experience.** *World J Emerg Surg* 2008, **3**:31.
26. Michalopoulos A, Papadopoulos VN, Panidis S, Papavramidis TS, Chiotis A, Basdanis G: **Cecal obstruction due to primary intestinal tuberculosis: a case series.** *J Med Case Reports* 2011, **5**:128.
27. Jamal S, Khan Z, Ahmed I, Shabbir S, Khaliq T: **Presentation and Outcome of Abdominal Tuberculosis in a Tertiary Care Unit.** *Ann Pak Inst Med Sci* 2011, **7(1)**:33-36.
28. Akgun Y: **Intestinal and peritoneal tuberculosis: changing trends over 10 years and a review of 80 patients.** *Can J Surg* 2005, **48(2)**:131-136.
29. Sefr R, Rotterova P, Konecny J: **Perforation peritonitis in primary intestinal tuberculosis.** *Dig Surg* 2001, **18(6)**:475-479.
30. Ramachandran CS, Agarwal S, Dip DG, Arora V: **Laparoscopic surgical management of perforative peritonitis in enteric fever: a preliminary study.** *Surg Laparosc Endosc Percutan Tech* 2004, **14(3)**:122-124.
31. Kim JP, Oh SK, Jarrett F: **Management of ileal perforation due to typhoid fever.** *Ann Surg* 1975, **181(1)**:88-91.

2

Damage control operations in non-trauma patients: defining criteria for the staged rapid source control laparotomy in emergency general surgery

Robert D. Becher[1*], Andrew B. Peitzman[2], Jason L. Sperry[2], Jared R. Gallaher[3], Lucas P. Neff[4], Yankai Sun[5], Preston R. Miller[5] and Michael C. Chang[5]

Abstract

Background: The staged laparotomy in the operative management of emergency general surgery (EGS) patients is an extension of trauma surgeons operating on this population. Indications for its application, however, are not well defined, and are currently based on the lethal triad used in physiologically-decompensated trauma patients. This study sought to determine the acute indications for the staged, rapid source control laparotomy (RSCL) in EGS patients.

Methods: All EGS patients undergoing emergent staged RSCL and non-RSCL over 3 years were studied. Demographics, physiologic parameters, perioperative variables, outcomes, and survival were compared. Logistic regression models determined the influence of physiologic parameters on mortality and postoperative complications. EGS-RSCL indications were defined.

Results: 215 EGS patients underwent emergent laparotomy; 53 (25 %) were staged RSCL. In the 53 patients who underwent a staged RSCL based on the lethal triad, adjusted multivariable regression analysis shows that when used alone, no component of the lethal triad independently improved survival. Staged RSCL may decrease mortality in patients with preoperative severe sepsis / septic shock, and an elevated lactate (≥3); acidosis (pH ≤ 7.25); elderly (≥70); male gender; and multiple comorbidities (≥3). Of the 162 non-RSCL emergent laparotomies, 27 (17 %) required unplanned re-explorations; of these, 17 (63 %) had sepsis preoperatively and 9 (33 %) died.

Conclusions: The acute physiologic indicators that help guide operative decisions in trauma may not confer a similar survival advantage in EGS. To replace the lethal triad, criteria for application of the staged RSCL in EGS need to be defined. Based on these results, the indications should include severe sepsis / septic shock, lactate, acidosis, gender, age, and pre-existing comorbidities. When correctly applied, the staged RSCL may help to improve survival in decompensated EGS patients.

Keywords: Damage control, Emergency general surgery, EGS, Rapid source control laparotomy, Physiologically decompensated

* Correspondence: robert.becher@yale.edu
[1]Section of General Surgery, Trauma, and Surgical Critical Care, Department of Surgery, Yale School of Medicine, 330 Cedar Street, BB 310, New Haven, CT 06510, USA
Full list of author information is available at the end of the article

Background

The staged laparotomy in the operative management of select trauma patients is designed to ensure their immediate survival [1–6]. The damage control (DC) laparotomy is therefore not an operation of last resort; rather, it is a well thought-out stage on a continuum of care which prioritizes the restoration of physiologic normality and homeostasis above definitive organ repair and anatomic reconstruction.

Application of DC principles are based on the clinical recognition of a trauma patient who is physiologically decompensated as defined by the lethal triad seen with hemorrhagic shock: acidosis, coagulopathy, and hypothermia. Decompensated trauma patients must be rescued to avoid progression to irreversible physiologic exhaustion and death; abbreviated operations allow stabilization, correction, and reevaluation of physiologic derangements in an intensive care unit setting [6–13].

Similarly, a select group of emergency general surgery (EGS) patients also present decompensated, near irreversible physiologic exhaustion and death, but for different reasons, often driven by severe sepsis or septic shock [14]. As a natural extension of trauma surgeons operating on the EGS patient-population, DC principles have been widely applied to the operative management of EGS patients.

Indications for DC application in EGS patients, however, are not well defined, and are currently based on the lethal triad used in trauma patients. Because the lethal triad in trauma is founded on patients presenting with hemorrhagic shock – something less commonly seen in EGS patients – its use to guide operative decision making in EGS patients may not be appropriate.

This study sought to determine the acute physiologic indications for the staged, rapid source control laparotomy (RSCL) in EGS patients. Our hypothesis was that application of the lethal triad to EGS patients as criteria for implementation of abbreviated laparotomy would not improve outcomes, and that the definition of a physiologically decompensated EGS patient would be unique from that used in trauma patients.

Methods

This is a retrospective review of consecutive EGS patients undergoing emergent, non-trauma related laparotomies over 3 years, from March 1, 2007 to March 1, 2010, at a tertiary medical center. Emergent operations were defined in accordance with the National Surgical Quality Improvement Program's (NSQIP) definition of an emergency case: one performed as soon as possible and no later than 12 h after the patient has been admitted to the hospital or after the onset of related preoperative symptomatology [15].

Variables were collected through electronic chart review. Data included demographics, physiologic parameters, perioperative variables, outcomes, and survival. Magnitude of the inflammatory response (four categories: no inflammation, SIRS, sepsis, or severe sepsis/septic shock) was classified based on the NSQIP definition; this definition is in concert with standardized definitions outlined by the American College of Chest Physicians (ACCP), the Society of Critical Care Medicine (SCCM), and the Surgical Infection Society (SIS) [16].

Patients were identified as undergoing a rapid source control laparotomy (RSCL; i.e., damage control laparotomy; planned re-laparotomy) if there was a deliberate, preemptive plan to perform an immediate, limited, staged operation as part of an ongoing continuum of resuscitation. The decision to proceed with staged RSCL was based on the lethal triad used in trauma patients; such RSCL intentions were identified in the operative note, which had to address the planned attempt to reverse the preterminal effects of pre-operative physiologic derangements, and/or intra-abdominal hypertension, by means of an abbreviated laparotomy. These patients were left with an open abdomen with a negative pressure dressing at the end of the initial operation, and transferred to the intensive care unit for stabilization. The second operation was then governed by a planned re-laparotomy, once resuscitation and stabilization had been achieved.

Non-RSCL patients were those who underwent non-staged operations, and had their fascia closed at the completion of the initial operation. If these patients subsequently required a re-laparotomy, this would be considered an unplanned re-laparotomy, or an "on-demand re-laparotomy" [17, 18]. For the current analyses, only patients who underwent open operations with colon or small bowel resections were included, based on their high degree of postoperative morbidity and mortality, comparable source for sepsis, and the increased power of the analyses [19–21].

Patient characteristics, physiologic parameters, perioperative variables, outcome metrics, and survival were first compared using univariate techniques. Chi-squared analysis ($\chi 2$) or Fisher's exact test were used to compare differences in proportions of categorical variables; such data were summarized by percentages. Student's t-tests were used to compare normally distributed continuous variables; such data were summarized by mean values with standard deviations (±SD). Wilcoxon rank sum tests were used to compare non-normally distributed continuous variables; such data were summarized by median values with interquartile ranges.

In hospital mortality was the primary outcome measure. Logistic regression models determined the influence of acute physiologic parameters and other patient characteristics on in-hospital mortality; analyses assessing determinants of postoperative complications were additionally completed. All candidate covariates for multivariable regression were included in a full selection model; variables were not excluded based on their statistical significance. Significance was defined as *p*-value < 0.05 throughout. EGS-based RSCL indications were defined.

All statistical analyses were conducting using a commercially available statistics software program (SAS 9.2; SAS Institute Inc., Cary, NC). Approval was obtained from the Wake Forest University Baptist Medical Center Institutional Review Board.

Results

215 EGS patients underwent emergent laparotomy during the study period, 162 (75 %) were non-rapid source control laparotomy (non-RSCL) operations and 53 (25 %) were staged rapid source control laparotomy (RSCL; damage control; planned re-laparotomy). Comparing the two operative groups, there were no significant differences in patient characteristics, including gender, race, age, or comorbidities (Table 1).

Peri-operative physiologic scores and metrics, however, did significantly differ (Table 1). Compared with emergent patients in the RSCL cohort, the non-RSCL group was overall healthier, with a significantly higher percentage of patients with no preoperative inflammation and with lower ASA scores (1, 2, or 3). The two groups did not differ significantly with regard to patients with severe sepsis / septic shock, hypothermia, coagulopathy, or acidosis. No patients in either group fit only into the SIRS only classification of preoperative inflammation, indicating that all had a presumed source of infection.

Table 1 Patient characteristics and peri-operative physiologic scores & metrics, by operation type

Variable[a]	non-RSCL (*n* = 162)	RSCL (*n* = 53)	*p*-value[b]
Male gender	94 (58.0 %)	29 (54.7 %)	0.6727
Race & Ethnicity:			
White	128 (79.0 %)	46 (86.8 %)	0.2107
Black	27 (16.7 %)	6 (11.2 %)	0.3486
Age, years	61 (17)	64 (13)	0.2336
Age (≥70)	55 (34.0 %)	19 (35.9 %)	0.8006
Comorbidities:			
Number comorbidities, average	1.9 (2.2)	2.2 (2.8)	0.4641
No comorbidities	71 (43.8 %)	23 (43.4 %)	0.9562
1 comorbidity	19 (11.7 %)	2 (3.8 %)	0.0904
2 comorbidities	14 (8.6 %)	7 (13.2 %)	0.3311
≥3 comorbidities	58 (35.8 %)	21 (39.6 %)	0.6166
Inflammatory status preoperatively:			
No inflammation	75 (46.3 %)	10 (18.9 %)	0.0004
Sepsis	59 (36.4 %)	28 (52.8 %)	0.0346
Severe sepsis/septic shock	28 (17.3 %)	15 (28.3 %)	0.0817
Lethal Triad:			
Hypothermia (temp ≤ 35C)	24 (16.8 %)	7 (14.9 %)	0.7610
Coagulopathy (INR ≥ 1.7)	13 (11.1 %)	9 (18.4 %)	0.2085
Acidosis (pH ≤ 7.25)	24 (22.2 %)	18 (35.3 %)	0.0810
Patient characteristics:			
ASA score, average	3 (1)	4 (1)	<0.0001
ASA score, 1 or 2	23 (14.2 %)	0 (0.0 %)	0.0015
ASA score, 3	65 (40.1 %)	8 (15.1 %)	0.0008
ASA score, 4 or 5	74 (45.7 %)	45 (84.9 %)	<0.0001
Lactate (≥3)	32 (33.3 %)	26 (51.0 %)	0.0372

RSCL rapid source control laparotomy, *PRBC* packed red blood cells, *C* Celsius, *INR* international normalized ratio, *ASA* American Society of Anesthesiologists, *L* liters
[a]Categorical variables are presented as number (%); continuous data are presented as mean (± standard deviation); and non-normally distributed continuous variables as median (interquartile range)
[b]*p*-values for overall tests of differences between the groups from $\chi 2$ or Fisher's Exact Test for categorical variables and one-way analysis of variance or Kruskal-Wallis test for continuous variables; *p*-value of <0.05 significant

Overall mortality in the RSCL group was significantly higher than in the non-RSCL population (45 % vs 20 %) (Table 2). Specifically, mortality was higher in RSCL compared to non-RSCL patients who were female, white, and without comorbidities. Interestingly, however, mortality between the two operative approaches was no different for patients with sepsis or severe sepsis / septic shock; males; elderly (age ≥70); patients with multiple comorbidities (≥3); patients with hypothermia (temperature ≤35C), coagulopathy (INR ≥1.7), and acidosis (pH ≤ 7.25) (the lethal triad criteria); for all ASA scoring levels; and for elevated lactate levels.

The application of the lethal triad to guide the use of RSCL did not discriminate between survivors and non-survivors in our multivariable logistic regression models (Table 3). Patients with hypothermia, coagulopathy, and acidosis who underwent damage control procedures had similar rates of mortality compared with the non-RSCL group.

In emergent operative patients undergoing non-RSCL (Table 4), multiple variables increased the chances of mortality in the univariate analyses, including severe sepsis/septic shock, male gender, elderly, acidosis, elevated lactate, and ASA score of 4 or 5. Two variables in this group portended an increased likelihood of survival: patients without inflammation and those with an ASA score of 3. The adjusted multivariable logistic regression model confirmed that four variables significantly and independently increased the chances of mortality for non-RSCL operations: patients with severe sepsis / septic shock, male gender, elderly, and acidosis.

In contrast to the non-RSCL group, there were no variables in the unadjusted univariate analyses for the RSCL cohort (Table 5) that increased the odds of mortality. In the adjusted multivariable regression, patients had significantly improved chances of survival when undergoing RSCL with two existing factors: elevated preoperative lactate levels or multiple comorbidities. Patients with

Table 2 Rates of in-hospital mortality for patient characteristics and peri-operative physiologic metrics, by operation type

Variable[a]	non-RSCL ($n = 162$)	RSCL ($n = 53$)	p-value[b]
All patients:	33 (20.4 %)	24 (45.3 %)	0.0004
Inflammatory status preoperatively:			
No inflammation	8 (10.7 %)	5 (50.0 %)	0.0012
Sepsis	10 (19.9 %)	10 (35.7 %)	0.0520
Severe sepsis/septic shock	15 (53.6 %)	9 (60.0 %)	0.6858
Patient Characteristics:			
Male Gender	25 (26.6 %)	13 (44.8 %)	0.0632
Female Gender	8 (11.7 %)	11 (45.8 %)	0.0004
Race, White	27 (21.1 %)	20 (43.5 %)	0.0034
Age (≥70)	20 (36.4 %)	10 (52.6 %)	0.2131
No comorbidities	17 (23.9 %)	11 (47.8 %)	0.0295
1 comorbidity	0 (0.0 %)	1 (50.0 %)	0.0016
2 comorbidities	3 (21.4 %)	3 (42.9 %)	0.3055
≥3 comorbidities	13 (22.4 %)	9 (42.9 %)	0.0733
Lethal Triad:			
Hypothermia (temp ≤ 35C)	8 (33.3 %)	3 (42.9 %)	0.6431
Coagulopathy (INR ≥ 1.7)	5 (38.5 %)	5 (55.6 %)	0.4285
Acidosis (pH ≤ 7.25)	12 (50.0 %)	10 (55.6 %)	0.7213
Patient characteristics:			
ASA score, 1 or 2	0 (0.0 %)	0 (0.0 %)	-
ASA score, 3	5 (7.7 %)	1 (12.5 %)	0.6404
ASA score, 4 or 5	28 (37.8 %)	23 (51.1 %)	0.1559
Lactate (≥3)	13 (40.6 %)	11 (42.3 %)	0.8970

RSCL rapid source control laparotomy, *PRBC* packed red blood cells, *C* Celsius, *INR* international normalized ratio, *ASA* American Society of Anesthesiologists, *L* liters
[a]Categorical variables are presented as number (%); continuous data are presented as mean (± standard deviation); and non-normally distributed continuous variables as median (interquartile range)
[b]*P*-values for overall tests of differences between the groups from $\chi 2$ or Fisher's Exact Test for categorical variables and one-way analysis of variance or Kruskal-Wallis test for continuous variables; *p*-value of <0.05 significant

Table 3 Logistic regression analyses predicting in-hospital mortality for RSCL patients, based only on the lethal triad

Variable[a]	Unadjusted model[a]		Adjusted multivariable model[b]	
	OR (95 % CI)	*p*-value[c]	OR (95 % CI)	*p*-value[c]
Lethal Triad:				
Hypothermia (temp ≤ 35C)	0.83 (0.16–4.19)	0.8205	0.70 (0.13–3.74)	0.5330
Coagulopathy (INR ≥ 1.7)	1.53 (0.36–6.55)	0.5680	1.52 (0.34–6.87)	0.5884
Acidosis (pH ≤ 7.25)	1.92 (0.60–6.15)	0.2703	1.70 (0.47–6.09)	0.4167

RSCL rapid source control laparotomy, *C* Celsius, *INR* international normalized ratio
[a]Unadjusted univariate analyses were used to test an independent variables's predictive ability on in-hospital mortality
[b]Model covariates for mortality were chosen by full selection
[c]*P*-value of <0.05 significant

preoperative acidosis had significant increased risk of death with RSCL, just as in the non-RSCL group.

Of the 162 non-RSCL emergent laparotomies, 27 (17 %) required unplanned re-explorations. Mortality in this unplanned take-back group was significantly higher than in the patients who did not require re-exploration (33.3 % vs 17.8 %; $p = 0.04$). Of the 33 deaths in the non-RSCL cohort, 27.3 % were patients necessitating unplanned re-explorations. Compared to the non-RSCL patients who did not undergo re-exploration, the unplanned take-back group had significantly higher rates of pre-operative severe sepsis / septic shock (44.4 % vs 11.9 %; $p < 0.0001$). Of all severe sepsis / septic shock patients in the non-RSCL group, 42.9 % (12) required re-exploration ($p < 0.0001$).

Discussion

The negative downstream consequences of inflammation are well established in acute care surgery. In the trauma patient population, severe physiologic derangements, particularly the lethal triad (hypothermia, acidosis, and coagulopathy), guide management decisions [22]. Research into these postinjury systemic inflammatory states has established the importance, for example, of the damage

Table 4 Logistic regression analyses predicting in-hospital mortality for non-RSCL patients

Variable[a]	Unadjusted model[a]		Adjusted multivariable model[b]	
	OR (95 % CI)	*p*-value[c]	OR (95 % CI)	*p*-value[c]
Preoperative inflammatory status:				
No inflammation	0.30 (0.12–0.71)	0.0060	1.00	-
Sepsis	0.71 (0.31–1.62)	0.4146	0.18 (0.02–1.95)	0.1583
Severe sepsis/septic shock	7.44 (3.04–18.17)	<0.0001	12.32 (1.19–127.33)	0.0350
Patient Characteristics:				
Male Gender	2.72 (1.14–6.47)	0.0240	23.98 (2.00–287.34)	0.0122
Race, White	1.25 (0.47–3.32)	0.6579	0.25 (0.01–5.64)	0.3857
Age (≥70)	4.13 (1.86–9.19)	0.0005	13.77 (1.30–145.70)	0.0293
No comorbidities	1.48 (0.69–3.18)	0.3201	1.00	-
1 comorbidity	0.001 (0.001–999.99)	0.9546	0.001 (0.001–999.99)	0.9132
2 comorbidities	1.07 (0.284.09)	0.9181	0.04 (0.01–4.13)	0.1746
≥3 comorbidities	1.21 (0.55–2.66)	0.6299	0.07 (0.01–0.57)	0.0139
Preoperative metrics:				
Acidosis (pH ≤ 7.25)	3.94 (1.51–10.30)	0.0052	11.08 (1.02–120.64)	0.0484
Lactate (≥3)	2.68 (1.06–6.82)	0.0378	0.62 (0.08–4.78)	0.6425
Coagulopathy (INR ≥ 1.7)	2.08 (0.62–6.97)	0.2333	2.11 (0.22–20.43)	0.5183
ASA score, 1 or 2	0.001 (0.001–999.99)	0.9672	1.00	-
ASA score, 3	0.21 (0.08–0.57)	0.0022	999 (0.001–999.99)	0.9574
ASA score, 4 or 5	10.10 (3.65–27.95)	<0.0001	999 (0.001–999.99)	0.9416

RSCL rapid source control laparotomy, *PRBC* packed red blood cells, *C* Celsius, *INR* international normalized ratio, *ASA* American Society of Anesthesiologists
[a]Unadjusted univariate analyses were used to test an independent variables's predictive ability on in-hospital mortality
[b]Model covariates for mortality were chosen by full selection
[c]*P*-value of <0.05 significant

Table 5 Logistic regression analyses predicting in-hospital mortality for RSCL patients

Variable[a]	Unadjusted model[a]		Adjusted multivariable model[b]	
	OR (95 % CI)	*p*-value[c]	OR (95 % CI)	*p*-value[c]
Preoperative inflammatory status:				
No inflammation	1.26 (0.32–5.01)	0.7397	1.00	-
Sepsis	0.44 (0.15–1.32)	0.1415	0.60 (0.07–5.39)	0.6446
Severe sepsis/septic shock	2.30 (0.68–7.80)	0.1811	3.29 (0.26–41.92)	0.3596
Patient Characteristics:				
Male Gender	0.96 (0.32–2.85)	0.9416	0.55 (0.07–4.28)	0.5708
Race, White	0.58 (0.12–2.88)	0.5022	0.26 (0.01–8.47)	0.4509
Age (≥70)	1.59 (0.51–4.92)	0.4230	5.19 (0.75–35.74)	0.0942
No comorbidities	1.20 (0.40–3.57)	0.7448	1.00	-
1 comorbidity	1.22 (0.07–20.55)	0.8915	999 (0.001–999.99)	0.9848
2 comorbidities	0.89 (0.18–4.45)	0.8900	0.58 (0.05–6.08)	0.6458
≥3 comorbidities	0.85 (0.28–2.58)	0.7739	0.06 (0.01–0.70)	0.0252
Preoperative metrics:				
Acidosis (pH ≤ 7.25)	1.92 (0.60–6.15)	0.2703	19.42 (1.74–216.65)	0.0159
Lactate (≥3)	0.79 (0.26–2.40)	0.6831	0.10 (0.01–0.93)	0.0431
Coagulopathy (INR ≥ 1.7)	1.53 (0.36–6.55)	0.5680	2.14 (0.27–16.83)	0.4682
ASA score, 1 or 2	-	-	1.00	-
ASA score, 3	0.14 (0.02–1.20)	0.0729	1.00	-
ASA score, 4 or 5	7.32 (0.83–64.43)	0.0729	26.45 (0.82–857.50)	0.0650

RSCL rapid source control laparotomy, *PRBC* packed red blood cells, *C* Celsius, *INR* international normalized ratio, *ASA* American Society of Anesthesiologists
[a]Unadjusted univariate analyses were used to test an independent variables's predictive ability on in-hospital mortality
[b]Model covariates for mortality were chosen by full selection
[c]*P*-value of <0.05 significant

control (DC) laparotomy for early definitive source control [1–6], and more recently the concept of DC resuscitation [23]. In critically ill patients, the substantial benefits of blunting the proinflammatory immune response has led to such key practices as early goal-directed therapy [24] and standardized treatment protocols for sepsis [25–27].

In EGS patients, upregulation of the systemic inflammatory response leads to a cascade of physiologic insults, and is a prime contributor to death, with mortality rates for severe sepsis / septic shock of over 40 % [14, 19]. However, unlike in trauma and critically ill patients, where physiologic derangements are aggressively acted on with specific corrective interventions, in EGS patients similar preoperative derangements are often recognized but may not be targeted with explicit restorative management techniques [28].

One solution to mitigating the negative downstream effects of physiologic insults seen preoperatively in EGS patients has been the application of DC techniques. Akin to the DC concept in trauma, it has been theorized that EGS patients needing operative intervention may benefit from an abbreviated laparotomy (i.e. rapid source control laparotomy; RSCL) with planned take-back. Such an operation is one of the first stages on a continuum of care that prioritizes the restoration of physiologic normality and homeostasis, and deemphasizes the importance of immediate organ repair and definitive anatomic reconstruction.

To guide the use of the staged RSCL in EGS patients, trauma's lethal triad has been applied as the standard criteria for operative decision-making. The data to support this, however, is limited [29]. Furthermore, "expert opinion" about the timing of nontraumatic surgical emergencies has been published to guide surgical interventions in EGS patients [30]. To date, no data or empirical evidence has specifically defined a unique set of criteria on which to base the use of RSCL techniques to improve the poor survival rates of physiologically decompensated EGS patients.

Our results represent such data, and suggest that the acute physiologic indicators which help guide operative decisions in trauma patients may not confer a similar survival advantage to decompensated EGS patients undergoing an emergent laparotomy. In the 53 patients who underwent a staged RSCL based on the lethal triad, adjusted multivariable regression analysis shows that when used alone, no component of the lethal triad independently improved survival (Table 3). Therefore, contrary to current practices, application of the lethal triad does not appear to improve survival rates in EGS patients, and may possibly lead to overuse of RSCL with higher mortality rates (Table 2).

These data also illustrate that the indications for performing a staged RSCL in EGS patients should be founded on a set of unique preoperative physiologic parameters, coupled with inherent patient traits, which collectively define an EGS patient as physiologically decompensated (Tables 4 & 5). Our results suggest a profile of a patient who may realize a survival benefit from a RSCL: a patient with preoperative severe sepsis / septic shock, with an elevated lactate (≥3); acidosis (pH ≤ 7.25); elderly (≥70); male gender; and multiple comorbidities (≥3).

Patients with severe sepsis / septic shock had equally high unadjusted mortality rates in both cohorts: 53.6 % in the non-RSCL group and 60.0 % in the RSCL group (Table 2). In the risk-adjusted analyses for the non-RSCL group, presence of severe sepsis / septic shock was independently related to higher mortality rates, with an adjusted odds ratio for death of 12.3 (Table 4). In contrast, in the RSCL group, severe sepsis / septic shock was not independently predictive of increased risk of death (Table 5).

Collectively, our study suggests that emergency operative patients with severe sepsis / septic shock may benefit from a staged, abbreviated laparotomy, and may have an increased risk of death with an unstaged operative approach. Furthermore, in the non-RSCL cohort, 44.4 % of all patients who required unplanned re-explorations had severe sepsis / septic shock preoperatively, compared to only 11.9 % in the patients who were successfully unstaged. These data also document that nearly 50 % of patients with severe sepsis/septic shock undergoing laparotomy with primary fascial closure will require re-exploration (known as an on-demand re-laparotomy).

Similar patterns exist in the data for males and the elderly; these inherent patient traits independently and significantly increased the risk of mortality in emergent non-RSCL, but were not significantly related to mortality in the RSCL cohort (Tables 4 & 5). As such, men and those over the age of 70 may have poorer outcomes when they undergo unstaged, non-RSCL at the time of initial operation. Another inherent patient trait, multiple comorbidities, was independently associated with improved survival for both the non-RSCL and RSCL groups (Tables 4 & 5). Taken together, these data indicated that the elderly (≥70), males, and patients with multiple comorbidities (≥3) may see lower odds of mortality with RSCL emergent operations.

Acidosis (pH ≤ 7.25) and elevations in lactate (≥3) often occur in concert with each other, but presence of one does not necessarily mean presence of the other. We therefore modeled these variables independently from one another, as there was not a significant interaction between these variables in our analyses. In the RSCL group, elevated lactate independently improved chances of survival in patients undergoing abbreviated laparotomies; lactate was not significantly predictive of survival benefit in the non-RSCL cohort. Patients with acidosis (pH ≤ 7.25), on the other hand, have a very poor prognosis across all emergent operations (Table 2). Acidosis was the one variable associated with poor outcomes in both the non-RSCL and RSCL groups (Tables 4 & 5). Because odds of mortality go up significantly and independently with acidosis, and because survival is 50 % in acidotic patients, we have included it as an indication for RSCL.

The data further confirm that certain emergency patients will not benefit from RSCL, and in fact could be harmed by undergoing abbreviated operations. Specifically, patients without physiologic evidence of preoperative inflammation, as defined by the SIRS criteria, should not be considered candidates for RSLC. This cohort can, in most scenarios, safely undergo a non-staged operation; this is akin to the principle of on-demand re-laparotomy [17].

This study has limitations. First, our conclusions are drawn from retrospective data, and are thus constrained by the limitations and biases therein, including selection bias. Second, the definition of an emergency patient is a construct of the study, as well as the individual assessments of the attending surgeon and anesthesiologist. Therefore, generalizing to all emergency surgical patients may not be valid, as definitions of "emergency patient" are not standardized [31]. Thirdly, the data are from one institution, which is a tertiary medical center and large academic hospital; this may not be representative of a national sample from which to make conclusions. Fourth, our conclusions are drawn from a small sample size of 215 patients; we therefore lack the necessary power to show potentially significant differences. And finally, there may be other peri-operative risk factors and physiologic variables not identified here which more accurately predict the need for RSCL in EGS patients.

Conclusions

In conclusion, when correctly applied, the staged RSCL may help to improve survival in decompensated EGS patients. The best candidates for staged RSCL are those patients with severe sepsis / septic shock, who are also male, over age 70 years old, with multiple comorbidities, and have an elevated lactate with acidosis. Use of the staged RSCL can also avoid unplanned re-explorations, which occurred in nearly 50 % patients with severe sepsis / septic shock who underwent primary fascial closure at the initial operation. Patients without evidence of preoperative inflammation may not benefit from staged

RSCL. These results further reinforce the concept that EGS patients represent a unique patient-population, and that operative decision-making in these patients should be guided by EGS-specific preoperative and intraoperative physiologic metrics and variables.

Abbreviations

ASA: American Society of Anesthesiologist Score; DC: Damage control; EGS: Emergency general surgery; ICU: Intensive Care Unit; NSQIP: National surgical quality improvement program; RSCL: Rapid source control laparotomy; SIRS: Systemic inflammatory response syndrome.

Competing interests

The authors declare that they have no competing interests.

Authors' contributions

Study conception and design: RDB, MCC. Acquisition of data: RDB, JRG, LPN, YS. Analysis and interpretation of data: RDB, ABP, JLS, JRG, LPN, YS, PRM, MCC. Drafting of manuscript: RDB, ABP, JLS, JRG, LPN, YS, PRM, MCC. Critical revision: RDB, ABP, JLS, JRG, LPN, YS, PRM, MCC. All authors read and approved the final manuscript.

Acknowledgements

None.

Author details

[1]Section of General Surgery, Trauma, and Surgical Critical Care, Department of Surgery, Yale School of Medicine, 330 Cedar Street, BB 310, New Haven, CT 06510, USA. [2]Department of Surgery, University of Pittsburgh School of Medicine, Pittsburgh, PA, USA. [3]Department of Surgery, University of North Carolina School of Medicine, Chapel Hill, NC, USA. [4]Department of Surgery, David Grant Medical Center, Travis Air Force Base, Fairfield, CA, USA. [5]Department of Surgery, Wake Forest University School of Medicine, Winston-Salem, NC, USA.

References

1. Lee JC, Peitzman AB. Damage-control laparotomy. Curr Opin Crit Care. 2006; 12:346–50.
2. Moore EE, Burch JM, Franciose RJ, Offner PJ, Biffl WL. Staged physiologic restoration and damage control surgery. World J Surg. 1998;22:1184–90. discussion 1190–1191.
3. Asensio JA, McDuffie L, Petrone P, Roldań G, Forno W, Gambaro E, et al. Reliable variables in the exsanguinated patient which indicate damage control and predict outcome. Am J Surg. 2001;182:743–51.
4. Rotondo MF, Schwab CW, McGonigal MD, Phillips 3rd GR, Fruchterman TM, Kauder DR, et al. "Damage control": an approach for improved survival in exsanguinating penetrating abdominal injury. J Trauma. 1993;35:375–82. discussion 382–383.
5. Johnson JW, Gracias VH, Schwab CW, Reilly PM, Kauder DR, Shapiro MB, et al. Evolution in damage control for exsanguinating penetrating abdominal injury. J Trauma. 2001;51:261–9. discussion 269–271.
6. Burch JM, Ortiz VB, Richardson RJ, Martin RR, Mattox KL, Jordan Jr GL. Abbreviated laparotomy and planned reoperation for critically injured patients. Ann Surg. 1992;215:476–83. discussion 483–484.
7. Rutherford EJ, Morris Jr JA, Reed GW, Hall KS. Base deficit stratifies mortality and determines therapy. J Trauma. 1992;33:417–23.
8. Dunham CM, Siegel JH, Weireter L, Fabian M, Goodarzi S, Guadalupi P, et al. Oxygen debt and metabolic acidemia as quantitative predictors of mortality and the severity of the ischemic insult in hemorrhagic shock. Crit Care Med. 1991;19:231–43.
9. Morris Jr JA, Eddy VA, Blinman TA, Rutherford EJ, Sharp KW. The staged celiotomy for trauma. Issues in unpacking and reconstruction. Ann Surg. 1993;217:576–84. discussion 584–586.
10. Baracco-Gandolfo V, Vidarte O, Baracco-Miller V, del Castillo M. Prolonged closed liver packing in severe hepatic trauma: experience with 36 patients. J Trauma. 1986;26:754–6.
11. Bender JS, Bailey CE, Saxe JM, Ledgerwood AM, Lucas CE. The technique of visceral packing: recommended management of difficult fascial closure in trauma patients. J Trauma. 1994;36:182–5.
12. Krige JE, Bornman PC, Terblanche J. Therapeutic perihepatic packing in complex liver trauma. Br J Surg. 1992;79:43–6.
13. Sharp KW, Locicero RJ. Abdominal packing for surgically uncontrollable hemorrhage. Ann Surg. 1992;215:467–74. discussion 474–475.
14. Becher RD, Hoth JJ, Miller PR, Meredith JW, Chang MC. Systemic inflammation worsens outcomes in emergency surgical patients. J Trauma Acute Care Surg. 2012;72:1140–9.
15. Ameican College of Surgeons (ACS) National Surgical Quality Improvement Program (NSQIP): Data Variables and Definitions from the "User Guide for the 2010 Participant Use Data File," accessed at: https://www.facs.org/~/media/files/quality%20programs/nsqip/ug10.ashx.
16. Levy MM, Fink MP, Marshall JC, Abraham E, Angus D, Cook D, et al. SCCM/ESICM/ACCP/ATS/SIS international sepsis definitions conference. Crit Care Med. 2001;2003(31):1250–6.
17. van Ruler O, Mahler CW, Boer KR, Reuland EA, Gooszen HG, Opmeer BC, et al. Comparison of on-demand vs planned relaparotomy strategy in patients with severe peritonitis: a randomized trial. JAMA. 2007;298:865–72.
18. Solomkin JS, Mazuski JE, Bradley JS, Rodvold KA, Goldstein EJC, Baron EJ, et al. Diagnosis and management of complicated intra-abdominal infection in adults and children: guidelines by the Surgical Infection Society and the Infectious Diseases Society of America. Surg Infect (Larchmt). 2010;11:79–109.
19. Becher RD, Hoth JJ, Miller PR, Mowery NT, Chang MC, Meredith JW. A critical assessment of outcomes in emergency versus nonemergency general surgery using the American College of Surgeons National Surgical Quality Improvement Program Database. Am Surg. 2011;77:951–9.
20. Schilling PL, Dimick JB, Birkmeyer JD. Prioritizing quality improvement in general surgery. J Am Coll Surg. 2008;207:698–704.
21. Ingraham AM, Cohen ME, Bilimoria KY, Raval MV, Ko CY, Nathens AB, et al. Comparison of 30-day outcomes after emergency general surgery procedures: potential for targeted improvement. Surgery. 2010;148:217–38.
22. Lenz A, Franklin GA, Cheadle WG. Systemic inflammation after trauma. Injury. 2007;38:1336–45.
23. Morrison CA, Carrick MM, Norman MA, Scott BG, Welsh FJ, Tsai P, et al. Hypotensive resuscitation strategy reduces transfusion requirements and severe postoperative coagulopathy in trauma patients with hemorrhagic shock: preliminary results of a randomized controlled trial. J Trauma. 2011; 70:652–63.
24. Rivers E, Nguyen B, Havstad S, Ressler J, Muzzin A, Knoblich B, et al. Early goal-directed therapy in the treatment of severe sepsis and septic shock. N Engl J Med. 2001;345:1368–77.
25. Shapiro NI, Howell MD, Talmor D, Lahey D, Ngo L, Buras J, et al. Implementation and outcomes of the Multiple Urgent Sepsis Therapies (MUST) protocol. Crit Care Med. 2006;34:1025–32.
26. Micek ST, Roubinian N, Heuring T, Bode M, Williams J, Harrison C, et al. Before-after study of a standardized hospital order set for the management of septic shock. Crit Care Med. 2006;34:2707–13.
27. ProCESS Investigators, Yealy DM, Kellum JA, Huang DT, Barnato AE, Weissfeld LA, et al. A randomized trial of protocol-based care for early septic shock. N Engl J Med. 2014;370:1683–93.
28. Moore LJ, Moore FA. Early diagnosis and evidence-based care of surgical sepsis. J Intensive Care Med. 2013;28:107–17.
29. Stawicki SP, Brooks A, Bilski T, Scaff D, Gupta R, Schwab CW, et al. The concept of damage control: extending the paradigm to emergency general surgery. Injury. 2008;39:93–101.
30. Kluger Y, Ben-Ishay O, Sartelli M, Ansaloni L, Abbas AE, Agresta F, et al. World society of emergency surgery study group initiative on Timing of Acute Care Surgery classification (TACS). World J Emerg Surg. 2013;8:17.
31. Becher RD, Meredith JW, Chang MC, Hoth JJ, Beard HR, Miller PR. Creation and implementation of an emergency general surgery registry modeled after the National Trauma Data Bank. J Am Coll Surg. 2012;214:156–63.

3

Benign cystic mesothelioma of the peritoneum

Hicham Elbouhaddouti*, Abdesslam Bouassria, Ouadii Mouaqit, El Bachir Benjelloun, Abdelmalek Ousadden, Khalid Mazaz and Khalid Ait Taleb

Abstract

Benign cystic mesothelioma of the peritoneum (BCM) is an uncommon lesion with some 130 cases reported since the first case described by Smith and Mennenmeyer in 1979. It is a rare intra abdominal tumor occurring predominantly in women of reproductive age. Due to the rarity of this tumor, similarity of patient presentation, and comparable features on imaging, the diagnosis of this pathology is difficult, and is based on histological findings. This tumor is known for local recurrence. It's agreed that surgery is the only effective treatment, but there are no evidence-based treatment strategies for BCM.

Introduction

Benign cystic mesothelioma of the peritoneum (BCM) is a rare intra abdominal tumor with a strong predilection for the peritoneum of pelvic organs. Symptoms are not specific, and the differential diagnosis is vast, including cystic lymphangioma, mucinous cystadenoma, cystic teratoma and pseudomyxoma retroperitonei. There are no evidence-based treatment strategies for BCM, and even if it is considered as a benign tumor, this tumor has a high local recurrence rate.

We report a new case of BCM, which appeared as a surgical emergency.

Case report

A 71 year-old woman presented to the emergency department complaining of history of abdominal pain since 2 days accompanied by diarrhea. Four months prior to presentation, she noticed an increase in abdominal girth. Moreover, she developed occasional abdominal discomfort, which slowly increased frequency. The patient also developed symptoms of constipation and severe reflux which were not improved by taking laxatives and a proton pump inhibitor. Our patient was hemodynamically stable with temperature at 37.9°C, and blood pressure was 130/80 mmHg. Abdominal examination was marked by diffuse abdominal distension, and tenderness. Computed tomography (CT) scanning showed a large spherical multi-loculated cystic mass in the abdomen which was not-communicating to any abdomen viscera, occupying nearly the entire abdominal cavity, displacing the hole bowel (Figure 1). Furthermore, on CT scan, there was a strong suspicion of central tumor necrosis (Figure 2). Therefore, our patient was taken to operating theatre. Laparotomy was done. Intraoperative examination showed a cystic mass extending from the pelvis inferiorly to the liver. There was a significant peritoneal thickening, and a peritoneal effusion, with many cystic lesions that makes dissection and resection very difficult. The mass and some of the free-floating cysts were carefully harvested and removed for histological examination. Benign cystic mesothelioma was revealed in the pathology report.

Our patient made an excellent recovery, and she was discharged home after 6 days. Our patient was seen in out patient clinic at 1 month and 3 months. She had no functional complaints and kept a slight abdominal distension.

This study was performed according to the declaration of Helsinki and approved by the Local Ethical Committee.

* Correspondence: h.elbouhaddouti@yahoo.fr
Department of Surgery, School of Medicine and Pharmacy of Fez, Sidi Mohammed Ben Abdallah University, University hospital HASSAN II, BP: 1893, Km2.200, Route de Sidi Hrazem FEZ 30000, Morocco

Discussion

Benign cystic mesothelioma of the peritoneum (BCM) was described first by Mennenmeyer and Smith [1].

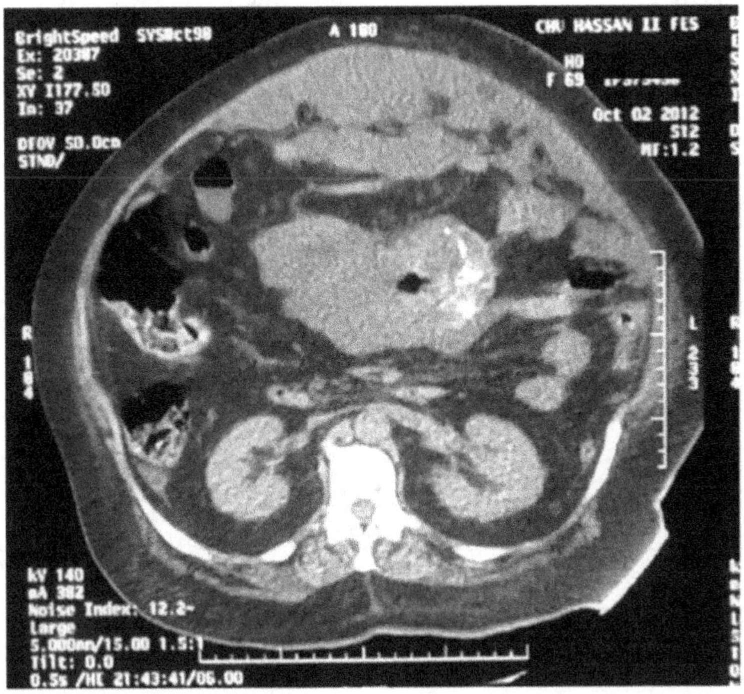

Figure 1 Large spherical multi-loculated cystic mass.

It's a rare pathological entity with about 130 cases reported in the literature [2,3] (Table 1). Several authors consider this tumor as benign [1,4], and it's prognosis is excellent [5]. There is only one reported death from BCM on the literature: Raafat and al. reported a case of a 14 years-old patient who had a subtotal resection of the abdominal mass, and died 12 years after refusing surgery for recurrence [6]. Indeed, BCM has a high local recurrence rate [7], and this recurrence rate is higher in women (40 – 50%) than in men (33%) [8]. The etiology remains unclear, but it is well known that many inciting factors may promote hyperplastic and neoplastic changes in mesothelial cells. The suggested provoking factors are

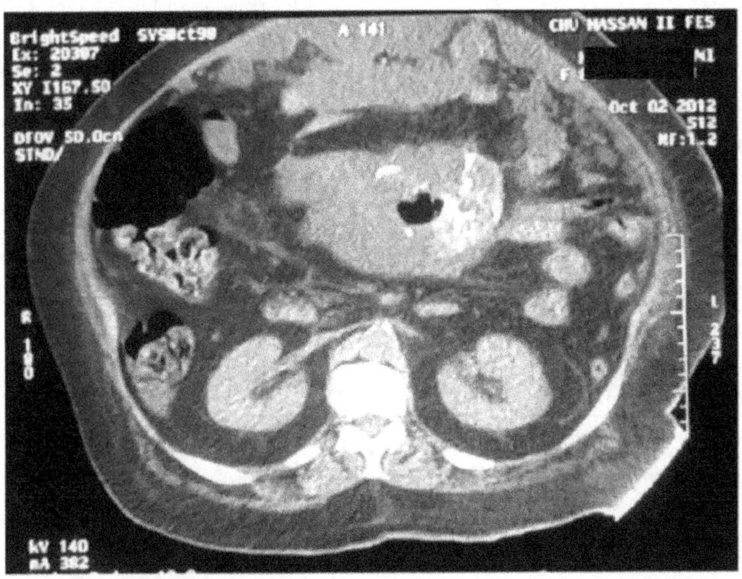

Figure 2 Suspicion of centro tumoral necrosis on CT scan.

Table 1 Review of the literature

Year	Authors	Number of cases
1982	Tasça and col. Benign peritoneal mesothelioma. Hystopathology in a case. Morphol Embryol; 28 (1): 47-9	1
1982	Katsube Y and col. Cystic mesothelioma of the peritoneum: a report of 5 cases and review of the literature. Cancer Oct 15; 50 (8)	5
1983	Schneider V and col. Benign cystic mesothelioma involving the female genital tract: report of four cases. Am J Obstet Gynecol; Feb 1; 145 (3)	4
1984	Philip G and col. Benign cystic mesothelioma. Case reports. British journal of Obstetrics and Gynaecology, Vol. 91, pp 932-938	2
1987	Pastormalo M and col. Benign cystic mesothelioma of the peritoneum. Minerva Ginecologia, Mar 39 (3)	1
1989	Betta PG and col. Benign cystic mesothelioma of the peritoneum. G Ital Oncol. Jan Mar; 9 (1)	1
1990	Hidvegi J and col. Benign cystic mesothelioma of the peritoneum. Orv Hetil. Feb 4; 131 (5)	1
1990	Chen YC and col. Benign cystic mesothelioma of the peritoneum: report of a case. J Formos Med Assoc. Jun; 89 (6)	1
1991	Hidvegi J and col. Peritoneal benign cystic mesothelioma. Pathol Res Pract. Jan; 187 (1)	1
1991	Pollack CV and col. Benign cystic mesothelioma presenting as acute abdominal pain in a young woman. J Emerg Med: 9 Suppl 1:21-5	1
1994	Kyzer S and col. Benign cystic mesothelioma of the peritoneum. Eur J Surg. May; 160 (5)	1
1995	Ricci F and col. Benign cystic mesothelioma in a male patient: surgical treatment by the laparoscopic route. Surg Laparosc endosc. Apr; 5 (2)	1
1995	Takenouchi Y and col. Report of a case of benign cystic mesothelioma. Am J Gastroenterol; Jul 90 (7)	1
1996	Tomasini P and col. Benign peritoneal multicystic mesothelioma. J Radiol; Jan 77 (1)	1
1996	Yaegachi N and col. Multilocular peritoneal inclusion cysts. J Obstet Gynaecol Res; Apr 22 (2)	1
1997	Cusatelli P and col. Benign cystic mesothelioma of the peritoneum: a case report. Eur J Gynaecol Oncol. 18 (2)	1
1997	Van Der Klooster and Col. Successful catheter drainage of recurrent benign multicystic mesothelioma of the peritoneum. Neth J Med, Jun; 50 (6)	1
1998	Abino JF and col. Peritoneal benign polycystic mesothelioma. Press Med, Apr 25; 27 (16)	1
1998	Letterie GS and col. The antiestrogen tamoxifen in the treatment of recurrent benign cystic mesothelioma. Gynecol Oncol, Jul; 70 (1)	1
1998	Kumar D and col. Benign cystic peritoneal mesothelioma in a man. Indian J Gastroenterol, Oct-Dec; 17 (4)	1
1999	Keiri-Vassilatou E and col. Benign cystic mesothelioma of the peritoneum an immunopathological study of three cases. Eur J Gyneacol Oncol. 20 (4)	3
1999	Jovovic M and col. Multicystic mesothelioma of the peritoneum. Vojnosanit Pregl. Mar-Apr; 56 (2)	1
1999	Park BJ and col. Treatment of primary peritoneal mesothelioma by continuous hyperthermic peritoneal perfusion (CHPP). Ann Surg Oncol, Sep;6(6):582-90.	18
2001	Petrou G and Col. Benign cystic mesothelioma in a 60 year old woman after cholecystectomy. ANZ J Surg, Oct; 71 (10)	1
2002	Hafner M and Col. Giant Benign cystic mesothelioma: a case report and review of the littérature. Eur J Gastroenterol Hepatol. 2002 Jan;14(1):77-80.	1
2002	Van ruth S and Col. Peritoneal Benign cystic mesothelioma: a case report and review of the literature. Eur J Surg Oncol. 2002 Mar;28(2):192-5	1
2002	Adolph AJ and col. Benign multicystic mesothelioma: a case report. J Obstet Gynaecol Can. 2002 Mar;24(3):246-7.	1
2002	Cavallaro A and col. Benign multicystic mesothelioma of the peritoneum: a case report. Chir Ital. 2002 Jul-Aug;54(4):569-72	1
2003	Shawn RN and col. Benign cystic mesothelioma of the peritoneum: a clinicopathologic study of 17 cases and immunohistochemical analysis of estrogen and progesterone receptor status. Hum Pathol. 2003 Apr;34(4):369-74.	17
2003	Bruni R and col. Benign cystic mesothelioma with multiple recurrences: a clinical case. Chir Ital. 2003 Sep-Oct;55(5):757-60	1
2004	Varma R and Col. Multicystic benign mesothelioma of the peritoneum presenting as postmenopausal bleeding and a solitary pelvic cyst--a case report. Gynecol Oncol. 2004 Jan;92(1):334-6.	1
2004	Baeyens P and col. Benign cystic peritoneal mesothelioma. JBR-BTR. 2004 May-Jun;87(3):114-5	1
2005	Szöllósi A and col. Benign cystic mesothelioma, a rare tumor of the peritoneum. Magy Seb. 2005 Feb;58(1):35-7	1
2005	Urbańczyk K and col. Mesothelial inclusion cysts (so-called benign cystic mesothelioma)–a clinicopathological analysis of six cases. Pol J Pathol. 2005;56(2):81-7.	6
2006	Svetlana M and col. Benign cystic mesothelioma of the peritoneum. Isr Med Assoc J. 2006 Jul;8(7):511-2	1
2006	Safioleas MC and col. Benign multicystic peritoneal mesothelioma: a case report and review of the literature. World J Gastroenterol. 2006 Sep 21;12(35):5739-42	New case: 1 Review: 130 cases
2007	Coskun A and col. Benign cystic mesothelioma presenting as a huge pelvic mass--a case report. Eur J Gynaecol Oncol. 2006;27(6):621-2	1
2007	Saad S and col. Benign peritoneal multicystic mesothelioma diagnosed and treated by laparoscopic surgery. J Laparoendosc Adv Surg Tech A. 2007 Oct;17(5):649-52	1
2008	Ashqar S and col. Benign mesothelioma of peritoneum presenting as a pelvic mass.J Coll Physicians Surg Pak. 2008 Nov;18(11):723-5	1
2008	Chammakhi-Jemli C and col. Benign cystic mesothelioma of the peritoneum. Tunis Med. 2008 Jun;86(6):626-8	1
2008	Stroescu and col. Recurrent benign cystic peritoneal mesothelioma. Chirurgia (Bucur). 2008 Nov-Dec;103(6):715-8	1
2009	Uzum N and col. Benign multicystic peritoneal mesothelioma.Turk J Gastroenterol. 2009 Jun;20(2):138-41	1

Table 1 Review of the literature *(Continued)*

2010	Limone A and col. Laparoscopic excision of a benign peritoneal cystic mesothelioma. Arch Gynecol Obstet. 2010 Mar;281(3):577-8	1
2010	Pitta X and col. Benign multicystic peritoneal mesothelioma: a case report. J Med Case Rep. 2010 Nov 29;4:385	1
2011	Akbayir O and col. Benign cystic mesothelioma: a case series with one case complicated by pregnancy. J Obstet Gynaecol Res. 2011 Aug;37(8):1126-31.	3
2012	Lari F and col. Benign multicystic peritoneal mesothelioma. A case report. Recenti Prog Med. 2012 Feb;103(2):66-8	1
2012	Stojsic Z and col. Benign cystic mesothelioma of the peritoneum in a male childJ Pediatr Surg. 2012 Oct;47(10):e45-9	1
2012	Khuri S and col. Benign cystic mesothelioma of the peritoneum: a rare case and review of the literature. Case Rep Oncol. 2012 Sep;5(3):667-70.	1
2013	Singh A and col. Multicystic peritoneal mesothelioma: not always a benign disease.Singapore Med J. 2013 Apr;54(4):e76-8	1

foreign fibres and dusts, inflammatory mediators, and mechanical injuries [9]. Proliferation and inward migration of peripheral mesothelial cells, proliferation and metaplasia of underlying connective tissue cells, and surface attachment and differentiation of free-floating mononuclear cells all have been postulated as the mechanism of mesothelial cell proliferation in pathological conditions [9]. This peritoneal lesion is characterized by the formation of multiple multilocular thin-walled cysts, which may form large intraabdominal masses [1]. The BCM affects women in 80% of cases, with an average age of 34 years [3]. The clinical presentation is unspecific: it is usually abdominal pain, increased abdominal girth and constipation. Physical examination revealed abdominal distension, abdominal tenderness or a palpable mass [10]. Imaging modalities that can be used include abdominal ultrasound (US), CT scan, or magnetic resonance imaging (MRI). They allow to visualize the lesion, but not to differentiate it from other cystic lesions of the peritoneum [11], especially lymphangiomas [9]. Laparoscopy remains the best diagnostic tool because it enables to perform biopsies and to establish the definitive diagnosis [12]. There are no evidence-based treatment strategies for BCM, but surgery, with complete enucleation of the cyst to prevent recurrence and possible malignant transformation remains the mainstay of treatment. However, some researchers advocate aggressive surgery followed by heated intraperitoneal chemotherapy (HIPEC) [12]. Indeed, for a long time, the treatment consist of full excision of the lesions (debulking surgery) [7]. Currently, some teams recommend aggressive surgery (extended peritonectomy) followed by HIPEC [3,13]. Two series are available on the results of extended peritonectomy followed by HIPEC. In the first one [13], 5 patients were asymptomatic, and 4 showed no recurrence with a follow up between 6 and 69 months. In the second series [14], 5 patients were asymptomatic, and 2 had got recurrence, with a follow up between 3 and 102 months.

Conclusion

Benign cystic mesothelioma of the peritoneum (BCM) is a rare tumor with a high local recurrence rate. It requires optimal care in a specialized center especially as there is no evidence-based treatment strategies.

Consent

Written informed consent was obtained from the patient for publication of this Case report and any accompanying images.

Competing interests

All authors declare that they have no competing interests.

Authors' contributions

EBH and AB participated in writing the case report and revising the draft, OM, EB, AO, KM and KAT participated in the follow up. All authors read and approved the final manuscript.

References

1. Mennemeyer R, Smith M: **Multicystic, peritoneal mesothelioma: a report with electron microscopy of a case mimicking intra-abdominal cystic hygroma (lymphangioma).** *Cancer* 1979, **44:**692–698.
2. Safioleas MC, Constantinos K, Michael S, Konstantinos G, Constantinos S, Alkiviadis K: **Benign multicystic peritoneal mesothelioma: a case report and review of the literature.** *World J Gastroenterol* 2006, **12**(35):5739–5742.
3. González-Moreno S, Yan H, Alcorn KW, Sugarbaker PH: **Malignant transformation of "benign" cystic mesothelioma of the peritoneum.** *J Surg Oncol* 2002, **79:**243–251.
4. Van Ruth S, Bronkhorst MWGA, Van Coeverden F, *et al*: **Peritoneal benign cystic mesothelioma: a case report and review of literature.** *Eur J Surg Oncol* 2002, **28:**192–195.
5. Bhandarkar DS, Smith VJ, Evans DA, Taylor TV: **Benign cystic peritoneal mesothelioma.** *J Clin Pathol* 1993, **46:**867–868.
6. Raafat F, Egan M: **Benign cystic mesothelioma of peritoneum. Immunohistochemical and Ultrastructural features in a child.** *Paediatr Pathol* 1988, **8:**321–9.
7. Schwartz AT, Peycru E, Tardat JP, Dufau J, Jarry F, Durand-Dastes: **Le mésothéliome kystique péritonéal: bénin ou malin ?** *J Chir* 2008, **145:**8.
8. Canty MD, Williams J, Volpe RJ, *et al*: **Benign cystic mesothelioma in a male.** *Am J Gastroenterol* 1990, **85:**311–15.
9. Pelosil G, Zannonil M, Caprioli F, Faccincani L, Battistoni MG, Balercia G, Bontempinil L: **Benign multicystic mesothelial proliferation of the peritoneum: Immunohistochemical and electron microscopical study of a case and review of the literature.** *Histol Histopath* 1991, **6:**575–583.
10. Vyas, *et al*: **Mesothelioma as a rapidly developing giant abdominal cyst.** *World J Surg Oncol* 2012, **10:**277.
11. Yang DM, Jung DH, Kim H, Kim JH, Hwang HY: **Retroperitoneal cystic masses: CT, clinical, and pathologic findings and literature review.** *Radio Graphics* 2004, **24:**1353–1365.

Impact of an acute care surgery service on timeliness of care and surgeon satisfaction at a Canadian academic hospital

Kerollos N Wanis, Allison M Hunter, Michael B Harington and Gary Groot*

Abstract

Introduction: In January 2012 an acute care surgery (ACS) model was introduced at St. Paul's Hospital, Saskatoon, Saskatchewan. The goal of implementing an ACS service was to improve the delivery of care for emergent, non-trauma surgical patients. We examined whether the ACS model improved wait time to surgery, decreased the proportion of surgeries performed after hours, and shortened post-surgical length of stay. We also assessed whether the surgeons working in an ACS system had higher on-call satisfaction than surgeons working in a non- ACS system.

Methods: A retrospective pre-post analysis was performed using data from the Discharge Abstract Database and the Organizing Medical Networked Information database. Surgeon satisfaction was evaluated using a questionnaire that was mailed to all general surgeons in Saskatoon.

Results: An ACS service significantly reduced wait time to surgery for patients with all acute general surgery diagnoses from 221 minutes to 192 minutes ($p = 0.015$; CI = 5.8-52.2). Post-surgery length of stay for patients operated on for acute appendicitis, or acute cholecystitis was not reduced. On average, patients with bowel obstruction had increased length of stay following ACS service implementation. Most surgeries in our study were performed between 16:00 hours and 08:00 hours but the introduction of an ACS significantly reduced the number of afterhours surgeries (60.0% vs. 72.6%) ($p < 0.0001$). Our survey had a response rate of 75%. Overall, surgeons on an ACS service had greater satisfaction with the organization of their call schedule than surgeons not on an ACS service.

Conclusion: Introduction of an ACS service in Saskatoon has decreased wait time to surgery and reduced the proportion of afterhours emergency surgeries, with no reduction in the length of post-surgery hospital stay. Satisfaction may be higher for surgeons in an ACS service.

Keywords: Acute care surgery, General surgery, Program evaluation, Surgeon satisfaction

Introduction

The acute care surgery (ACS) model is becoming the standard model for delivering emergency general surgery care in Canada [1]. Prior to implementation of this model, emergent surgical patients were attended to by the on-call surgeon who was simultaneously required to provide care for scheduled elective cases. Tight scheduling in elective practices made providing timely care increasingly challenging, and pushed care of emergent patients to the end of the day or during the night. This threatened patient care as well as undermined surgeon satisfaction.

ACS programs across Canada vary in their structure but share the goal of improving clinical outcomes for patients with general surgical emergencies. These programs require all general surgeons, regardless of subspecialty training, to participate in acute non-trauma surgical care for a fixed period of time (typically 7 days) while forgoing their subspecialty work [2]. Results from these services have been encouraging. Studies have demonstrated significantly reduced overall time spent by patients in the emergency department, shorter times to emergency consultation by the surgical team, reduced time to surgery, and reduced overall hospital length of stay [3-5]. In addition, a majority of surgeons feel that ACS has enabled

* Correspondence: garygroot@gmail.com
Department of Surgery, College of Medicine, University of Saskatchewan, 750 Spadina Cr. E, Saskatoon, SK S7K 3H3, Canada

a more manageable monthly call and a more predictable elective work schedule [6].

Australian ACS models, which are similar in structure to Canadian models, have similar results. They performed a greater proportion of operations during working hours, achieved a decreased length of hospital stay post-operatively, and had reduced complication rates for acute cholecystitis [7,8]. Furthermore, an American model with a similar structure found that ACS helped to reduce after-hours surgery and improved patient care [9]. The overall effect of an ACS system has resulted in improved time to surgery, increased the proportion of emergency procedures performed during daytime working hours, and reduced post-operative complications.

St. Paul's Hospital in the Saskatoon Health Region adopted an ACS model starting in January 2012. In this system, one surgeon dedicates an entire week to ACS while forgoing their elective practice. This surgeon is on-site during the day and takes home-call during the evenings. There are two 17:00–08:00 shifts during the week that are covered by a second surgeon.

This study compared data collected in a pre-ACS and post-ACS time frame to determine whether the introduction of an ACS service at St. Paul's Hospital reduced time to surgery for all emergent general surgery presentations. The post-surgery length of stay for patients presenting with acute appendicitis, acute cholecytitis, and bowel obstruction was also measured. In addition, this study evaluated surgeon satisfaction with the ACS system.

Methods

Data extracted from the Discharge Abstract Database (DAD) and the Organizing Medical Networked Information (OMNI) databases, were retrospectively examined. These data were compared from two time periods: January 1 2011 to December 31 2011 (Pre-ACS), and January 1 2012 to December 31 2012 (Post-ACS). In addition to collecting data from St. Paul's Hospital, we also collected data from Saskatoon's Royal University Hospital. The Royal University Hospital does not have an ACS service. The OMNI Data includes all emergent general surgery cases performed at both Saskatoon hospitals over a two year study period. From this data, we determined the average length of time patients waited, from when surgery was booked, to when surgery was initiated. In the OMNI data, there was a total of 419 patients from St. Paul's Hospital in the pre-ACS period and 468 in the post-ACS period. From Royal University hospital there was 446 cases in 2011 and 453 in 2012. DAD data consisted of time from surgery to time of discharge. In these data, only patients with a diagnosis of acute appendicitis, acute cholecystitis, or acute bowel obstruction were considered. In the DAD data, from St. Paul's Hospital, there was a total 286 patients in the pre-ACS period and 294 patients in the post-ACS period.

Surgeon satisfaction was determined using a series of questions relating to quality of work, teaching, and life while on-call. A questionnaire was emailed to all surgeons responsible for general surgery call in Saskatoon. The surgeons were asked to indicate their level of agreement (strongly agree, agree, neutral, disagree, strongly disagree) to nine statements. These statements were designed to assess work satisfaction and personal satisfaction with their respective call schedules. Twelve out of sixteen (75%), of the general surgeons taking call in our health region returned the survey. The levels of agreement, described above, were converted to number values out of five. The responses were anonymous and de-identified.

Statistical analysis was performed using IBM SPSS Statistics 20 for Windows. Comparison of means was performed using student t-test. Proportions were compared using Chi- squared test. A ρ value less than .05 was considered to represent statistical significance. Institutional ethics approval was obtained from the University of Saskatchewan Research Ethics Board.

Results

The OMNI database contained the wait time to surgery for 419 patients at St. Paul's Hospital in the pre-ACS-period, and 468 patients in the post-ACS period. The average wait time to surgery decreased from 221 minutes in the pre-ACS period to 192 minutes in the post-ACS period (ρ = 0.015; CI = 5.8-52.2) (Table 1). This was compared to the OMNI database data for Royal University hospital which did not implement an ACS service. At Royal University Hospital, there were 446 cases in 2011 and 453 in 2012. During this period, the average wait time to surgery decreased from 272 minutes to 250 minutes (ρ = 0.112) (Table 1).

Implementation of an ACS at St. Paul's Hospital had a significant effect on the proportion of surgeries performed after regular working hours (08:00 to 16:00). In the pre-ACS period, 304 of the 419 operations (72.6%) were performed afterhours (16:00 to 08:00). This proportion of cases decreased in the post-ACS period, as 281 of the 468 operations (60.0%) were performed after-hours. This difference was statistically significant with a ρ value less than 0.0001 (Table 2).

Table 1 Comparison of the average wait time to surgery for the two study periods

Hospital	Average wait time to surgery (minutes)		p-value
	Pre-ACS	Post-ACS	
St. Paul's Hospital	221	192	.015
Royal University Hospital	272	250	.112

Table 2 Comparison of the numbers of surgeries performed during-hours and after-hours

Time of surgery	Number of surgeries performed		p-value
	Pre-ACS	Post-ACS	
During hours (08:00–16:00 hours)	115	187	<0.0001
After hours (16:00–08:00 hours)	304	281	

Table 4 Comparison of the average post-operative length of stay for the two study periods

Diagnosis	Average length of stay (days)		p-value
	Pre-ACS	Post-ACS	
Appendicitis	1.78	1.69	.637
Cholecystitis	2.23	2.55	.392
Bowel obstruction	7.99	12.2	.010

At St. Paul's Hospital there were 286 patients in the pre-ACS period and 294 patients in the post-ACS period who had emergency surgery for either appendicitis, cholecystitis, or bowel obstruction. The demographic information for these patients is given in Table 3. The mean age of patients in the post ACS period was older (46.92 years, from 42.57 years) (ρ =0.001). There was no statistically significant difference in the ratio of male to female patients. As well, there was no statistically significant difference in the distribution of acute appendicitis, acute cholecystitic or bowel obstruction diagnoses. With respect to patients who underwent either appendectomy or cholecystectomy for acute cholecystitis, there was also no statistically significant difference in the post-surgery length of stay (Table 3). There was however, a statistically significant increase in post surgery length of stay for patients who were operated on for acute bowel obstruction (7.99 days pre-ACS and 12.2 days post-ACS; ρ = 0.010) (Table 4).

The surgeons at both St. Paul's Hospital and the Royal University Hospital were surveyed to identify their level of satisfaction with their call schedules. As shown in Table 5, the surgeons at St. Paul's Hospital who are working in the ACS system responded with higher average satisfaction to all of the questions in our survey.

Discussion

Emergency general surgery care is provided by two hospitals in Saskatoon: St. Paul's Hospital, and Royal University Hospital. In 2012, St. Paul's Hospital introduced an ACS service. The intention of creating this service in Saskatoon was to improve timeliness of care, with the added benefit of improving surgeon satisfaction. An improvement in timeliness of care would be identified as a reduction in the proportion of afterhours surgery, a decrease in wait time to surgery, and a reduction in post-surgery length of stay.

Table 3 Demographic characteristics for patients in the pre-ACS and post-ACS study groups

	Pre-ACS	Post-ACS	ρ value
Mean age	42.57	46.92	.001
Sex			.995
Male	140 (49.0%)	144 (49.0%)	
Female	146 (51.0%)	150 (51.0%)	
Diagnosis			.193
Appendicitis	142 (49.7%)	150 (51.0%)	
Cholecystitis	55 (19.2%)	70 (23.8%)	
Bowel obstruction	89 (31.1%)	74 (25.2%)	
Total	**286**	**294**	

In this study we had the advantage of being able to compare data for wait time to surgery between two hospitals: St. Paul's Hospital with the ACS service and Royal University Hospital without this service. After implementation of the ACS service we were expecting that there should be a reduction in the wait time to surgery for acute general surgery cases. We defined wait time to surgery as the time period from when surgery was deemed necessary and booked to when surgery was initiated. In the year following implementation of the ACS service, the wait time was shown to be decreased by an average of 29 minutes (Table 1). Every Monday through Friday, from 12:00 h – 17:00 h there is one dedicated operating theatre reserved for acute general surgical patients. Therefore, this statistically significant reduction is a reflection of the dedicated operating room time given to the ACS service. Wait time to surgery was compared to the non-ACS, Royal University Hospital data for this same period. It was noted that there was also a reduction in wait time to surgery; however, this reduction in wait time was not statistically significant. The statistically significant decrease in wait time to surgery at St. Paul's Hospital, but not at Royal University Hospital, is in keeping with what one would predict within an ACS system, and supports the findings of other Canadian studies [1].

Afterhours surgery is associated with increased morbidity and mortality [10-12]. One of the desired effects of an ACS service is to reduce afterhours surgery and to subsequently avoid complications. Our study supports previous findings [7] that with a dedicated ACS service, there are a greater proportion of emergency operations completed during normal work hours (Table 2).

Previous studies showed that within an ACS system there was a significant decrease in the post-operative length of hospital stay for patients who underwent surgery for appendicitis [11] or acute cholecystitis [8], but not for acute bowel obstruction [3]. Our data is not in keeping with these previous findings. As shown in Table 4, there was no statistically significant decrease in the length

Table 5 Satisfaction with call schedule for surgeons in an ACS service contrasted with those in a non-ACS service

Statements regarding satisfaction with organization of call schedule	ACS	No ACS
Elective practice and workload		
1. My current call schedule allows me to focus on my elective surgical practice when not on call	3.7	2.2
2. I find the number of calls I perform monthly to be manageable	4.3	2.3
3. I find the workload while on call to be manageable	3.8	3.3
4. I feel adequately equipped to deal with the cases I encounter while on call	4.3	4.0
Work environment		
5. While on call, I find that there is time during the day to teach residents and medical students	3.3	3.0
6. The call organization at my hospital provides for acceptable operating room accessibility	3.7	2.0
Personal satisfaction		
7. I feel adequately remunerated for my work while on call	2.5	2.0
8. I am satisfied with the variety of clinical cases seen while on call	4.0	2.8
9. I am satisfied with the amount of time I can spent with my family during my on call days	2.2	1.7

Legend: Average agreement with 9 statements, on a 5 point scale from strongly disagree to strongly agree, assessing surgeon satisfaction with call schedule. The average agreement of surgeons from St. Paul's hospital (ACS) are compared side-by-side with the average agreement of surgeons from Royal University hospital (No ACS).

of stay for patients who underwent an appendectomy, or cholecystectomy. This may be explained by the fact that the pre-ACS length of stay was already short, compared to these other studies [3,8,13]. An ACS service may have an impact on post-surgical length of stay, because of hypothesized reduction in complications, and more focused care of admitted acute care patients. Since our hospital already had a short length of stay for this subgroup of surgical patients, the effect of an ACS service may not have been great enough to decrease the length of stay further, given differences in patient factors. Note that Table 3 shows an increase of age of patients over this same time period, which may be associated with higher patient morbidity. With respect to the patients admitted with bowel obstruction, the post-operative length of stay actually increased (Table 4). We do not have enough data on the bowel obstruction cohort to know how long these patients were managed conservatively, with medical treatment, before going on to surgery. It is possible that, by extending hospital stay pre-operatively, these patients are at a higher risk for developing post-op complications and hospital acquired infections. By not knowing what factors were present in the post-operative recovery period, for this group of patients, one can only speculate on why post-operative length of stay was increased.

As well as assessing the clinical value of an ACS service on patient care, we were also interested in measuring the personal impact this service has with respect to surgeon satisfaction. In this study, our survey generated a 75% response rate from surgeons both at St. Paul's Hospital (ACS) and the Royal University Hospital (non-ACS). This response rate is similar to a prior study by Helewa, et al. [6] from which our survey was adapted. Overall, we found that the surgeons at St. Paul's Hospital, had higher average satisfaction with statements pertaining to the organization of their call schedule. The ACS surgeons still had low average satisfaction with the amount of time they can spend with family, and their remuneration while on call. However, this was still assessed to be of a higher level of satisfaction, compared to the non-ACS surgeons.

Introduction of an ACS service has not been without some drawbacks. One potential concern for ACS surgeons relates to the inherent unpredictability of working in this system. On any given day during the ACS week, the surgeon is not guaranteed to be booking surgical cases. This has economic consequences for surgeons who have less control over their income during the on-call week. Furthermore, our system includes only one dedicated operating room theater for emergency general surgery patients. Other services can book higher priority patients at the expense of general surgery cases. An obvious area of improvement, which is supported by the findings in our study, is the dedication of more than one operating room for acute general surgery patients. This will likely further improve time to surgery for patients. Overall, the satisfaction of surgeons in our service suggests that improvements in lifestyle and patient care outweigh potential concerns.

Limitations

Our study has a number of limitations. The patients in our post-ACS group had a significantly higher mean age than those in our pre-ACS group which may have influenced the length of stay, particularly for patients with bowel obstruction. As well, it was difficult to adequately comment on the increased length of stay for the bowel obstruction group without taking into consideration patient factors, such as pre-surgery admission time and other medical co-morbidities.

The survey which we mailed to all general surgeons in Saskatoon was not returned by 4 of the surgeons (25%). A deficiency in responses exposes our results to the possibility of non-response bias. Our conclusions, that surgeons in an ACS service are generally more satisfied than those with a traditional call schedule may be influenced by the fact that Royal University Hospital, our non-ACS centre is a trauma centre while St. Paul's Hospital is not. The surgeon who has to deal with trauma cases may respond differently to questions regarding workload and satisfaction while on call.

Conclusion

Introduction of an acute care surgery service at an academic Canadian center has resulted in decreased wait time to surgery for patients presenting with general surgical emergencies ($\rho = 0.015$; CI = 5.8-52.2 minutes). There was a statistically significant decrease in the proportion of afterhours surgeries following adoption of an acute care surgery service ($\rho < 0.0001$). Post-surgical length of stay for patients operated on for acute appendicitis, cholecyctitis, or bowel obstruction was not decreased. Surgeons operating in an acute care surgery system report high average agreement with statements regarding satisfaction with their call schedule.

Competing interests

The authors declare that they have no competing interests.

Authors' contributions

KW: study design, acquisition of data, data analysis and interpretation of data, drafting of the manuscript. AH: study design, acquisition of data, drafting of manuscript. MH: study concept, revision of manuscript. GG: supervised the study concept and design, revised the manuscript. All authors read and approved the final manuscript.

References

1. Hameed SM, Brenneman FD, Ball CG, Pagliarello J, Razek T, Parry N, Widder S, Minor S, Buczkowski A, MacPherson C, Johner A, Jenkin D, Wood L, McLoughlin K, Anderson I, Davey D, Zabolotny B, Seedia R, Bracken J, Nathens A, Ahmed N, Panton O, Warnock GL: **General surgery 2.0: the emergence of acute care surgery in Canada.** *Can J Surg* 2010, **53**(2):79–83.
2. Ball CG, Hameed SM, Brenneman FD: **Acute care surgery: a new strategy for the general surgery patients left behind.** *Can J Surg* 2010, **53**(2):84–85.
3. Faryniuk AM, Hochman DJ: **Effect of an acute care surgical service on the timeliness of care.** *Can J Surg* 2012, **56**(3):187–191.
4. Ball CS, MacLean AR, Dixon E, Quan ML, Nicholson L, Kirkpatrick AW, Sutherland FR: **Acute care surgery: the impact of an acute care surgery service on assessment, flow, and disposition in the emergency department.** *Am J Surg* 2012, **203**(5):578–583.
5. Qureshi A, Smith A, Wright F, Brenneman F, Rizoli S, Hsieh T, Tien HC: **The impact of an acute care emergency surgical service on timely surgical decision-making and emergency department overcrowding.** *J Am Coll Surg* 2011, **213**(2):284–293.
6. Helewa RM, Kholdebarin R, Hochman DJ: **Attending surgeon burnout and satisfaction with the establishment of a regional acute care surgical service.** *Can J surg* 2012, **55**(5):312–316.
7. von Conrady D, Hamza S, Weber D, Kalani K, Epari K, Wallace M, Fletcher D: **The acute surgical unit: improving emergency care.** *ANZ J Surg* 2010, **80**(12):933–936.
8. Lehane CW, Jootun RN, Bennett M, Wong S, Truskett P: **Does an acute care surgical model improve the management and outcome of acute cholecystitis?** *ANZ J Surg* 2010, **80**(6):438–442.
9. Garland AM, Riskin DJ, Brundage SI, Moritz F, Spain DA, Purtill MA, Sherck JP: **A county hospital surgical practice: a model for acute care surgery.** *Am J Surg* 2007, **194**(6):758–764.
10. Komen N, Dijk J, Lalmahomed Z, Klop K, Hop W, Kleinrensink GJ, Jeekel H, Ruud Schouten W, Lange JF: **After-hours colorectal surgery: a risk factor for anastomotic leakage.** *Int J Colorectal Dis* 2009, **24**(7):789–795.
11. Gray A: **United Kingdom national confidential enquiry into perioperative deaths.** *Minerva Anestesiol* 2000, **66**(5):288–292.
12. Lee A, Lum ME, O'Regan WJ, Hillman KM: **Early postoperative emergencies requiring an intensive care team intervention. The role of ASA physical status and after-hours surgery.** *Anaesthesia* 1998, **53**(6):529–535.
13. Earley AS, Pryor JP, Kim PK, Hedrick JH, Kurichi JE, Minoque AC, Sonnad SS, Reilly PM, Schwab CW: **Acute care surgery model improves outcomes in patients with appendicitis.** *Ann Surg* 2006, **244**(4):498–504.

Acute appendicitis in the elderly: risk factors for perforation

Abdelkarim H Omari[1*], Muhammad R Khammash[1], Ghazi R Qasaimeh[1], Ahmad K Shammari[1], Mohammad K Bani Yaseen[2] and Sahel K Hammori[3]

Abstract

Background: Acute appendicitis is the most common surgical emergency and becomes serious when it perforates. Perforation is more frequent in the elderly patients. The aim of this study was to identify the risk factors of perforation in elderly patients who presented with acute appendicitis.

Methodology: The medical records of 214 patients over the age of 60 years who had a pathologically confirmed diagnosis of acute appendicitis over a period of 10 years (2003-2013) were retrospectively reviewed. Patients were grouped into those with perforated and those with nonperforated appendicitis. Comparison was made between both groups in regard to demography, clinical presentation, and time delay to surgery, diagnosis, hospital stay and postoperative complications. Clinical assessment, Ultrasonography and Computerized tomography, in that order, were used for diagnosis. The incidence of perforation was also compared with a previous report from the same region 10 years earlier.

Results: During the study period, a total of 214 patients over the age of 60 years had acute appendicitis, 103 males and 111 females. Appendix was found perforated in 87 (41%) patients, 46 (53%) males and 41 (47%) females. Of all patients, 31% were diagnosed by clinical assessment alone, 40% needed US and 29% CT scan. Of all the risk factors studied, the patient's pre-hospital time delay was the most important risk factor for perforation. Perforation rate was not dependent on the presence of comorbid diseases or in-hospital time delay. Post operative complications occurred in 44 (21%) patients and they were three times more common in the perforated group, 33 (75%) patients in the perforated and 11 (25%) in the nonperforated group. There were 6 deaths (3%), 4 in the perforated and 2 in the nonperforated group.

Conclusion: Acute appendicitis in elderly patients is a serious disease that requires early diagnosis and treatment. Appendiceal Perforation increases both mortality and morbidity. All elderly patients presented to the hospital with abdominal pain should be admitted and investigated. The early use of CT scan can cut short the way to the appropriate treatment.

Keywords: Acute appendicitis, Perforated appendix, Acute appendicitis in the elderly, Age and appendicitis, Peritonitis

Introduction

Acute appendicitis is still the commonest abdominal surgical emergency with a lifetime incidence of 7%. Appendicitis is known to be the disease of the younger age groups with only 5-10% of cases occurring in the elderly population. However, the incidence of the disease in this age group seems to be rising due to recent increase in the life expectancy [1-11].

* Correspondence: akomari@just.edu.jo
[1]Department of General Surgery and Urology, King Abdullah University Hospital, Jordan University of Science and Technology, 22110 Irbid, Jordan
Full list of author information is available at the end of the article

As compared to younger age group, elderly patients have more underlying diseases and sluggish bodily physiological reactions resulting in a higher rate of morbidity and mortality [1,2].

Furthermore, the often atypical presentation and delay in seeking medical help have been associated with delay in diagnosis and treatment resulting in high morbidity and mortality rates [3,4]. The prognosis of uncomplicated appendicitis in both young and old age groups is nearly equal. However, perforation worsens the condition dramatically resulting in higher rates of morbidity and mortality [5-8].

In order to improve our clinical understanding of the factors leading to perforation and to reduce its incidence if possible, we reviewed the medical records of all our patients over the age of 60 years with a pathologically confirmed acute appendicitis over the past 10 years. We determined the rate of appendiceal perforation and factors associated with perforation including demographic data, delayed presentation to medical care, delayed diagnosis and treatment and the presence of co-morbid diseases. Also, we studied the presenting symptoms and physical findings, laboratory investigation, use of radiological evaluation, complications and postoperative hospital stay.

A comparison was made between perforated and non-perforated groups regarding those variables. In addition, we compared our result with another study that was done in this region 10 years back.

Methodology

The medical records of all patients (60 years and above) who underwent appendectomy at 3 major teaching hospitals in the north of Jordan from 1st January 2003 to the end of December 2012 were retrospectively reviewed. These three hospitals with a total of 1000 beds are affiliated to the Jordan University of Science and technology and draining an area of more than 1.5 million inhabitants. Data was collected through the computerized system of the King Abdulla University Hospital (KAUH) and manually from the patient's registry of Princess Basma and Prince Rashid hospitals.

We identified all patients who underwent appendectomy over the above mentioned study period. On a case by case basis and with the help of the histopathological and operative reports, we excluded all patients who had normal or incidental appendectomies in addition to those with incomplete medical records.

Chart review was done to collect information on patient's demographic data, initial clinical presentation and assessment, presence of co morbid diseases (diabetes mellitus, hypertension, cardiac, respiratory or renal diseases... etc), laboratory investigations, radiological studies with focus on Ultrasonography (US)and Computerized Tomography (CT) scan and whether the appendix was found perforated or not. Appendix was defined as perforated if it was described so in the operative notes and confirmed by the histopathological report.

At our three hospitals, patients with abdominal pain are usually seen first in the (ER) by the emergency physician and then by the surgeon on duty (if consulted) who admits or discharges the patient. Admitting diagnosis was based onhistory and clinical findings. These were defined as fever > 38°C, increased WBC > 10^9/L and right lower abdominal pain. The decision to use additional imaging studies as US or CT scan is usually taken by the surgeon, results of which are interpreted by a certified radiologist. Diagnosis of acute appendicitis was made on the appearance of its wall, surrounding inflammation and edema with or without the presence of intra abdominal free fluid. CT scan study was usually spared for those cases when the Clinical Assessment (CA) and (US) were inconclusive. Once the diagnosis of acute appendicitis was made, the patient was given a shot of intravenous broad spectrum antibiotic that covers aerobic and anaerobic organisms and prepared for surgery. Open appendectomy was done for all patients, through Mc Burney's or midline incisions. So far, neither the laparoscopic appendectomy nor the nonoperative management has been adopted for the treatment of acute appendicitis in the elderly patients at our hospitals.

The time interval from the onset of symptoms to the time of registration in the emergency room (ER) was coded in hours and defined as patient delay. The time from the (ER) visit to the operating room was defined as hospital delay and included time to diagnosis and time waiting for surgery.

Appendicitis was categorized into perforated (free or contained perforation, abscess formation) and nonperforated. A comparison between them was made in regard to demographic data, clinical presentation, investigations, patient's delay, hospital delay and post operative hospital stay and complications. Also a comparison of the incidence of perforated appendicitis was made between our present study and another work that was done 10 years back in this region.

Computer program, Statistical Package for the Social Sciences (SPSS 16) was used for statistical analysis. *P-Value* < 0.05 was considered statistically significant when comparing variables.

Ethical approval was granted from the institution review board (IRB) of Jordan University of Science and Technology and King Abdullah University Hospital.

Results

A total of 214 patients above the age of 60 years with histopathologically proven acute appendicitis during the period between January 2003 and December 2012 were analyzed retrospectively. There were 103 males and 111 females with a mean age of 64.4 ±2.7 years (range 60-95 years). A hundred and seventy seven (83%) patients were in their 60-69 years of age, 28 (13%) in the age group of 70-79, 8 (3%) patients in their 80-89 years and only one patient was 95 years old. Eighty seven (41%) patients proved to have perforated appendicitis, 46 (53%) males and 41 (47%) females (Table 1).

Of all patients, there were 92 (43%) who had concurrent chronic medical diseases; Hypertension 27 (13%), chronic cardiac diseases 26 (12%), diabetes mellitus 23 (11%), chronic obstructive airway disease 9 (4%), end stage renal disease 4 (2%) and malignant diseases in 3 (1%) patients. No significant statistical differences between the

Table 1 Patient's demographics, Co morbid diseases and post operative complications

Characteristics	Total population	Perforated	Non-perforated	Post. op complication
	100%	41%	59%	21%
Age	64.43 yr	65.23 yr	63.3 yr	64.3 yr
Sex				
Male	48	53	45)	61
Female	52	47	55	39
Co- morbidities	43	37	47	75
Diabetes	11	11	10	18
Hypertension	13	10	14	18
Cardiac diseases	12	9	16	18
Lung diseases	4	3	5	9
Renal diseases	2	2	2	7
Malignancies	1	2	1	5

risk of perforation and the presence of co morbid diseases were found (Table 1).

Regarding the time delay for treatment and as shown in Table 2, patients in the perforated group had a significantly longer Pre-hospital time delay than those in the nonperforated group (79.6 h and 47.3 h respectively) with <0.0001 *p*-value. At the same time, the table did not show a statistically significant difference between the two groups in regard to In-hospital delay (*p*-value 0.7923) (Table 2).

Regarding the clinical presentation, all patients were complaining of abdominal pain. However, the typical migratory pain that starts around the umbilicus and shifts later to the right lower abdomen was described only by 101 (47%) patients, 75 (59%) patients in the nonperforated and 26 (30%) in the perforated group. Anorexia was present in 74% of all patients but it could not differentiate perforated from nonperforated groups. Nausea and vomiting were present in 57% of the patients and were more significantly found in the non perforated group (Table 3).

Of all patients, 41% were febrile at presentation (>38°C). Fever was seen more in the perforated group of patients (51%-34%). Localized tenderness in the right lower abdomen was present in 84% of all patients with 91% in the nonperforated compared to 75% in the perforated group.

Table 2 Delay in surgical intervention and post operative mean hospital stay

Variable	Perforated	Non perforated	P-value
	n = (87)	*n* = (127)	
Mean delay in surgical treatment			
Pre hospital delay	79.6 ± 62.4 hr	47.3 ± 43.7 hr	< 0.0001*
Hospital delay	19.2 ± 10.3 hr	18.7 ± 15.5 hr	0.7923
Post op hosp stay	7.4 ± 6.3 days	4.2 ± 3.1 days	<0.0001*

*The result is significant.

Although rebound tenderness was found in 75% of patients, it did not differentiate between both groups (Table 3).

Increased WBC count > 10^9/L, was seen in 143 (63%) of all patients at presentation. In the perforated group, Sixty two (71%) patients had high WBC with 94% shift to the left compared to 72 (57%) patients with 61% shift to the left in the non perforated group (Table 3).

Clinical Assessment (CA), Ultrasonography (US) and Computerized Tomography (CT) scan were used in that order for diagnosis. Of all patients 31% were diagnosed by CA alone, US detected another 40% and the remaining 29% were diagnosed by CT scan (Table 4). Although we couldn't calculate the sensitivity and specificity of each diagnostic test as we studied the positive cases only, we found that there were no false positive results when CT scan was used.

Mc Burney's incision was used in 168 and lower midline incision in 46 patients.

Post operative complications were seen in 44 (21%) patients. Complications were three times more frequent in the perforated as compared to the nonperforated group of patients, 33 (75%) and 11 (25%) respectively (Table 1). Four patients developed wound dehiscence and other eight had intra abdominal sepsis and collections, all in the perforated group except one. Other 22 patients in both groups had wound infection but all, except one, responded to antimicrobial treatment, debridement and dressings. Other complication as renal failure, chest infection, and respiratory failure, cardiovascular accidents were noted in both groups.

There were 6 (3%) deaths in both groups, four in the perforated and two in the nonperforated group. In the perforated group, two patients developed multiple intra abdominal abscess collections and died due to uncontrollable sepsis. Of the other two, one was already on chemotherapy treatment for lymphoma and died due to

Table 3 Comparison between perforated and nonperforated groups in regard to clinical picture

Variables	Total	Perforated	Non perforated	P-value
	n =214 (100%)	*n* = 87 (41%)	*n*= 127 (59%)	
Migrating pain	101 (47)	26 (30)	75 (59)	<0.0001*
Anorexia	150 (70)	64 (74)	86 (68)	0.3588
Nausea & vomiting	122 (57)	37 (43)	85 (67)	0.0004*
Tender right lower abdomen	180 (84)	65 (75)	115 (91)	0.0018*
Rebound tenderness	160 (75)	70 (80)	90 (71)	0.1125
Fever > 38°C	87 (41)	44 (51)	43 (34)	0.0145*
WBC count	143 (63)	62 (71)	72 (57)	0.0304*
WBC shift to left	159 (74)	82(94)	77 (61)	<0.0001*

*The result is significant.

uncontrollable atypical pneumonia while the other had an advanced cardiovascular disease and died due to congestive heart failure. In the nonperforated group, one patient died due to uncontrolled intra abdominal sepsis and the other due to massive myocardial infarction. As expected, the hospital stay was longer for patients in the perforated group (7.4 ± 6.3 and 4.2 ±3.1 days in perforated and nonperforated groups respectively) (Table 2).

Discussion

Acute appendicitis continues to be the commonest cause of surgical abdominal emergency. It was often thought to be the disease of the young but as a result of recent increases in lifetime expectancy, the incidence of acute appendicitis also increased in the elderly [1-11].

The incidence of appendiceal perforation in acute appendicitis is estimated to be in the range of 20-30% which increases to 32-72% in patients above 60 years of age [3-9,12-14]. The reasons behind this high rate were postulated to be due to the late and atypical presentation, delay in diagnosis and surgical intervention, presence of comorbid diseases and to the age-specific physiological changes [1-8,13,15-18]. In our study, perforated appendicitis was found in 87 (41%) patients, a result that lies within the range reported by many other reports [3,4,7,8,13,14,18]. Also found in the study was the absence of sex predilection for perforation; 46 (53%) patients were males and 41 (47%) were females. Although 92 (43%) of all patients had co morbid diseases at presentation, the risk of perforation did not appear to depend upon their presence (Table 1). These results were in conformity to the finding of Storm-Dickerson *et al.* [4].

Table 4 Number and percentage of patients diagnosed with appendicitis

Variable	Total	Perforated	Nonperforated
	n =214 (100%)	*n* = 87 (41%)	*n* = 127 (59%)
Diagnostic tools:			
Clinical assessment	66 (31)	27 (31)	39 (31)
Ultrasonography	85 (40)	29 (33)	56 (44)
Computerized scan	63 (29)	31 (36)	32 (25)

Delay in presentation was found by many authors to be the reason behind the higher rate of perforation seen in the elderly population [2,3,6,7,13,15-17]. Our study showed that perforation rate correlated well with delayed presentation (pre-hospital delay) but did not correlate with the in-hospital delay.

The triad of right lower abdominal pain and tenderness, fever and leukocytosis is reported to be present in not more than 26% of patients above 60 years [4,19,20]. In this study, all patients presented to the hospital with abdominal pain. However, the classical migratory pain of appendicitis was present in only 47% of them. Localized tenderness in the right lower abdomen which is considered to be the most constant diagnostic physical sign for appendicitis was present in 84% of cases. Both features (migratory pain and localized tenderness) were seen more often in the nonperforated rather than in the perforated group (Table 3). This finding may be explained by the fact that patients with perforated appendix would show poor localization of pain as well as more generalized lower abdominal tenderness and guarding.

Our study showed that, fever (>38°C) was present in 41% of all patients and was much higher in the perforated group (Table 3), a result which is in agreement with the findings of other studies [4,6,21].

Also in the study, WBC was found elevated in 63% of all patients with 74% shifts to left. As expected, values were higher in the perforated group as 71% of them had high WBC with 94% shift to left (Table 3). Again, a result in agreement with many other studies [1,4,21].

There are many scoring systems that have been used in the diagnosis of acute appendicitis like Alvarado, Kharbanda and Lintula scores [22-24]. In general, these clinical scoring systems have better Likelihood ratios (LRs) than individual symptoms or signs alone. However, they don't have sufficient discriminatory or predictive ability to routinely be used alone to diagnose appendicitis. They have been used to determine the need for further radiologic studies or as a guide for dictating clinical management [25-27]. The policy of our hospitals has not adopted the use of any scoring system so far.

Advances in diagnostic skills and improvements in diagnostic facilities (CT) scan and (US) advocated improving the diagnosis in patients with suspected appendicitis [16,20,28]. US can often diagnose an inflamed appendix and detects free fluid in the pelvis but this simple method is influenced by the operator's experience, the body built and co-operation of the patient. The wider use of CT scan for patients with suspected appendicitis has been shown to improve the accuracy of the diagnosis and decrease the negative laparotomy rates [3,4,17]. Recent studies reported a high sensitivity of 91-99% in this age group [20]. Storm-Dickerson TL *et al.* reported that the incidence of perforation declined over the past 20 years from 72% to 51% in his patients due to the earlier use of CT scan [4]. In our patients, CT scan was only used in those with equivocal findings and in whom the diagnosis was not reached after repeated CA and US. We could not calculate the sensitivity and specificity of CA, US and CT scans in our patients because we studied the positive cases. However, we did not find any false positive result when the CT scan was used.

Elderly patients have a higher risk for both mortality and morbidity following appendectomy. It was estimated to be around 70% as compared to 1% in the general population [1,4,9-11].

In our study, the overall post operative complication rate was 21%, a figure which is a bit lower than 27-60% reported by others [6,20,29]. As expected, complications were three times more frequent in the perforated as compared to the nonperforated group. This finding is in consistency with several other studies that have shown that perforation per se was the most predictive factor for post operative morbidity in the elderly patients with acute appendicitis [1,7,14,20].

The mortality rate in elderly patients following perforated appendicitis was reported between 2.3%-10%. Death is often related to septic complications compounded by the patient's co morbidities [3,6,7,29,30].

In this study, there were 6 (3%) deaths in both groups, four in the perforated and two in the nonperforated group. Three patients died due to septic complications while the others due to respiratory and cardiovascular causes.

As compared to younger age groups, the length of the hospital stay is usually longer in the elderly patients. This is usually ascribed to the higher rate of complications, prolonged need of antibiotics, treatment of other comorbidities and difficulties in communication [6,16,31]. Our result of 7.4 and 4.2 days for perforated and nonperforated groups was found in agreement with these studies.

When comparing our result to a previous study that was done in the same region 10 years back [32], we found that the incidence of appendiceal perforation did not decrease over the past ten years in spite of improved health care programs and diagnostic facilities. We think that this failure was due to the underestimation of the seriousness of the abdominal pain in this age group by both the patients and the primary health care providers.

Other factors that may influence the patient outcomes were not specifically addressed in this analysis, but are relevant to medical decision making in cases of appendicitis.

Reports in the literature had appeared describing the advantages of laparoscopic surgery over the open technique in terms of decreasing post operative pain, time to recovery, wound complications and post operative hospital stay, while others found that referring an elderly patient with complicated appendicitis to laparoscopic surgery will increase the operative time, conversion rate and length of hospital stay [19,31,33]. In a recent study published in 2013, Wray CJ *et al.* concluded that, the question of whether or not appendectomy should be performed via an open or laparoscopic technique has been inherently difficult to answer because both approaches offer similar advantages, namely, a small incision, low incidence of complications, a short hospital stay, and rapid return to normal activity [25]. At our hospitals, the laparoscopic approach has been adopted for the treatment of appendicitis in the younger age groups but so far, not for the elderly patients.

Despite the fact that appendectomy has been regarded as the standard treatment for appendicitis for more than 100 years, several reports have appeared in the literature over the last few years describing nonoperative management of acute, uncomplicated appendicitis. This conservative treatment which consists of nil by mouth, intravenous fluids and broad spectrum antibiotics had proved effective with less pain but had high recurrence rate, a risk that should be compared with the complications after appendectomy [27,34-38]. However, Wray CJ *et al.* considered that the available evidence regarding this nonoperative management is provocative and that level 1 data to suggest this is an alternative treatment option are not universally accepted [25]. Although the main object of our study was not the management of acute appendicitis in elderly patients, but after reviewing the literature, we think that the non operative management of acute appendicitis in this age group should be comprehensively studied.

The result of this study should be read with limitations. First, it is a retrospective study and in order to highlight the risk factors leading to appendiceal perforation one would ideally collect clinical data before and not after perforation occurred. Second, the rate of perforation differs according to the patient's accessibility to medical health services.

Conclusion

Acute appendicitis should still be considered in the differential diagnosis of abdominal pain in the elderly patients. Delay in presentation to the hospital is associated with higher rates of perforation and post operative complications. All elderly patients presented with abdominal pain should be admitted and investigated. The early use of CT scan can cut short the way to the appropriate treatment.

Abbreviations

ER: Emergency room; CA: Clinical assessment; US: Ultrasonography; CT scan: Computed tomography scan.

Competing interests

The authors declare that they have no competing interests.

Authors' contributions

AO: participated in collecting data, design and coordination of the study, helped to draft the manuscript and reviewed the literature. MK: participated in planning, design and coordination of the study. AS: participated in collecting data, GQ: participated in literature review and coordination, MB: collected data from princess Basma teaching Hospital, SH: collected data from Prince Rashid Military Hospital. All authors read and approved the final manuscript.

Author details

[1]Department of General Surgery and Urology, King Abdullah University Hospital, Jordan University of Science and Technology, 22110 Irbid, Jordan. [2]Department of General Surgery, Princess Basma Teaching Hospital, 22110 Irbid, Jordan. [3]Department of General Surgery, Prince Rashid Military Teaching Hospital, 22110 Irbid, Jordan.

References

1. Horattas M, Guyton D, Diane W: **A reappraisal of appendicitis in theelderly.** *Am J Surg* 1990, **160**:291–293.
2. Smithy WB, Wexner SD, Daily TH: **The diagnosis and treatment of acute appendicitis in the aged.** *Dis Colon Rectum* 1986, **29**:170–173.
3. Franz MG, Norman J, Fabri PJ: **Increased morbidity of appendicitis with advancing age.** *Am Surg* 1995, **61**:40–44.
4. Storm-Dickerson TL, Horattas MC: **What we have learned over the past 20 years about appendicitis in the elderly?** *Am J Surg* 2003, **185**:198–201.
5. Lunca S, Bouras G, Romedea NS: **Acute appendicitis in the elderly patient: diagnostic problems, prognostic factors and out-comes.** *Rom J Gastroenterol* 2004, **13**:299–303.
6. Lee JF, Leow CK, Lau WY: **Appendicitis in the elderly.** *ANZ J Surg* 2000, **70**:593–596.
7. Sherlock DJ: **Acute appendicitis in the over-sixty age group.** *Br J Surg* 1985, **72**:245–246.
8. Lau WY, Fan ST, Yiu TF, Chu KW, Lee JM: **Acute appendicitis in the elderly.** *SurgGynecolObstet* 1985, **161**:157–160.
9. Yamini D, Vargas H, Bongard F, Klein S, Stamos MJ: **Perforated appendicitis: is ittruly a surgical urgency?** *Am Surg* 1998, **64**:970–975.
10. Hardin D: **Acute appendicitis: review and update.** *Am FamPhys* 1999, **60**:2027–2036.
11. Tehrani H, Petros JG, Kumar RR, Chu Q: **Markers of severe appendicitis.** *Am Surg* 1999, **65**:453–455.
12. Temple C, Huchcroft S, Temple W: **The natural history of appendicitisin adults, a prospective study.** *Ann Surg* 1995, **221**:279–282.
13. Ryden CI, Grunditz T, Janzon L: **Acute appendicitis in patients above and below 60 years of age.** *Acta ChirScand* 1983, **149**:165–170.
14. Paajanen H, Kettunen J, Kostiainen S: **Emergency appendictomies in patients over 80 years.** *Am Surg* 1994, **60**:950–953.
15. Watters JM, Blackslee JM, March RJ, Redmond ML: **The influence of age on the severity of peritonitis.** *Can J Surg* 1996, **39**:142–146.
16. Korner H, Sondenaa K, Soreide JA, Andersen E, Nysted A, Lende TH, Kiellevold KH: **Incidence of acute nonperforated and perforated appendicitis: age-specific and sex-specific analysis.** *World J Surg* 1997, **21**:313–317.
17. Eldar S, Nash E, Sabo E, Matter I, Kunin J, Mogilner JG, Abrahamson J: **Delay of surgery in acute appendicitis.** *Am J S* 1997, **173**:194–198.
18. Thorbjarnarson B, Loehr WJ: **Acute appendicitis in patients over the age of sixty.** *SurgGynecolObstet* 1967, **125**:1277–1280.
19. Paranjape C, Dalia S, Pan J, Horattas M: **Appendicitis in the elderly: a change in the laparoscopic era.** *SurgEndosc* 2007, **21**:777–781.
20. Pooler BD, Lawrence EM, Pickhardt PJ: **MDCT for suspected appendicitis in the elderly: diagnostic performance and patient outcome.** *Emerg Radio* 2012, **19**:27–33.
21. Sheu BF, Chiu TF, Chen JC, Tung MS, Chang MW, Young YR: **Risk factors associated with perforated appendicitis in elderly patients presenting with signs and symptoms of acute appendicitis.** *ANZ J Surg* 2007, **77**:662–666.
22. Alvarado A: **A practical score for the early diagnosis of acute appendicitis.** *Ann Emerg Med* 1986, **15**:557–564.
23. Kharabanda AB, Taylor GA, Fishman SJ, Bachur RG: **A clinical decision rule to identify children at low risk of appendicitis.** *Pediatrics* 2005, **116**:709–716.
24. Lintula H, Kokki H, Pulkkinen J, Kettunen R, Grohn O, Eskelinen M: **Diagnostic score in acute appendicitis. Validation of a diagnostic score (Lintula score) for adults with suspected appendicitis.** *Langenbecks Arch surg* 2010, **395**:495–500.
25. Wray CJ, Kao LS, Millas SG, Tsao K, Ko TC: **Acute appendicitis: controversies in diagnosis and management.** *CurrProblSurg* 2013, **50**:54–86.
26. Rezak A, Abbas HM, Ajemian MS, Dudrick SJ, Kwasnik EM: **Decreased use of computed tomography with a modified clinical scoring system in diagnosis of pediatric acute appendicitis.** *Arch Surg* 2011, **146**:64–67.
27. Farahnak M, Talaei-Khoei M, Gorouhi F, Jalali A: **The Alvarado score and antibiotics therapy as a corporate protocol versus conventional clinical management: randomized controlled pilot study of approach to acute appendicitis.** *Am J Emerg Med* 2007, **25**:850–852.
28. Ilves I, Paajanen HE, Herzig KH, Fagerstrom A, Miettinen PJ: **Changing incidence of acute appendicitis and nonspecific abdominal pain between 1987 and 2007 in Finland.** *World J Surg* 2011, **35**:731–738.
29. Freund HR, Rubinstein E: **Appendicitis in the aged: is it really different?** *Am Surg* 1984, **50**:573–576.
30. Blomqvist PG, Andersson RE, Granath F, Lambe MP, Ekbom AR: **Mortality after appendectomy in Sweden, 1987-1996.** *Ann Surg* 2001, **233**:455–460.
31. Kirstein B, Perry ZH, Mizrahi S, Lantsberg L: **Value of laparoscopic appendectomy in the elderly patient.** *World J Surg* 2009, **5**:918–922.
32. Qasaimeh GR, Khader Y, Matalqah I, Nimri S: **Acute appendicitis in north of Jordan- A 10 year survey.** *J Med J* 2004, **42**:149–154.
33. Hui TT, Major KM, Avital I, Hiatt JR, Margulies DR: **Outcome of elderly patients with appendicitis- effect of computed tomography and laparoscopy.** *Arch Surg* 2002, **137**:995–998.
34. Hansson J, Korner U, Khorram-Manesh A, Solberg A, Lundholm K: **Randomized clinical trial of antibiotic therapy versus appendicectomy as primary treatment of acute appendicitis in unselected patients.** *Br J Surg* 2009, **96**:473–481.
35. Malik AA, Bari SU: **Conservative management of acute appendicitis.** *J GastrointestSurg* 2009, **13**:966–970.
36. Styrud J, Eriksson S, Nilsson I, Ahlberg G, Haapaniemi S, Neovius G, Rex L, Badume I, Granstrom L: **Appendectomy versus antibiotic treatment in acute appendicitis. a prospective multicenter randomized controlled trial.** *World J Surg* 2006, **30**:1033–1037.
37. Papandria D, Goldstein SD, Rhee D, Salazar JH, Arlikar J, Gorgy A, Ogtega G, Zhang Y, Abdullah F: **Risk of perforation increases with delay in recognition and surgery for acute appendicitis.** *J Surg Res* 2013, **184**:723–729.
38. Liu K, Fogg L: **Use of antibiotics alone for treatment of uncomplicated acute appendicitis: a systemic review and meta-analysis.** *Surgery* 2011, **150**:673–683.

6

How to mend a broken heart: a major stab wound of the left ventricle

Mari-Liis Kaljusto* and Theis Tønnessen

Abstract

A 28-year-old male admitted with a stab wound under his left nipple, underwent emergency surgery because of confusion, a decreasing blood pressure and increasing tachycardia. A median sternotomy incision was made and after establishing cardiopulmonary bypass, a 7 cm wound in the left ventricle and a smaller wound in the left atrium were repaired. An injured segment of lung was resected and the left anterior descending and circumflex arteries were grafted after weaning from cardiopulmonary bypass was initially unsuccessful. Although the patient suffered a stroke, probably due to prehospital hypoperfusion, he eventually recovered without major sequelae. In addition to the case report we present a literature review of the last 15 years pertaining the management of penetrating cardiac injury.

Background

Onehundred and sixteen years ago Alex Cappelen repaired a penetrating injury of the left ventricle through a left anterior thoracotomy in Christiania (former name of Oslo), in one of the world`s least violent countries [1]. Cappelen`s operation is considered to be the first report of a cardiac surgical procedure. Today trauma centers all over the world perform complex cardiac repairs due to penetrating trauma but the mortality is still high [2-5].

We report the case of a young man who suffered a large stab wound (SW) in the left ventricle and left atrium in addition to a lung injury for approximately 2 h before undergoing reparative surgery. In addition we present a literature review of penetrating cardiac injuries from 1997 – 2012 (Table 1). As data source we used all available English-language articles from peer-reviewed journals in the Ovid MEDLINE and PubMed databases. The articles selected were relevant case reports, original articles and reviews focusing on the clinical presentation of penetrating cardiac injury, initial management, operative technique, complications and follow up.

* Correspondence: m.l.kaljusto@medisin.uio.no
Department of Cardiothoracic Surgery, Oslo University Hospital, Ullevål PB 4956 Nydalen and University of Oslo, Oslo, 0424, Norway

Case presentation

A 28-year-old male was admitted to the emergency department (ED) with a 5 cm stab wound (SW) under his left nipple. Pre-hospital treatment included insertion of a left chest drain due to dyspnoea, but this was clamped during transport because of massive hemorrhage. On admission, he was self-ventilating, with palpable carotid pulses, but without a measurable blood pressure. He was agitated and pale with a Glasgow coma score of 12 since he could open his eyes, localize pain and speak. The blood pressure ranged from 80/60 to 100/60 mmHg after starting intravenous fluid therapy and he had a tachycardia of 100–120 beats per minute. When the clamp was removed from the chest drain, 650 ml of blood was rapidly drained. The chest x-ray showed persisting hemothorax and atelectasis and an additional drain was inserted. The arterial saturation varied from 86% to 98% and blood gas analysis showed a haemoglobin of 12.6 g/l, pH 7.17, base excess -9 and lactate 5.5 mmol/l. Focused Assessment with Sonography in Trauma (FAST) revealed no blood in the pericardium and upper abdomen. The neck veins were not distended and so the patient received transfusion of 1500 ml of crystalloid fluid and 250 ml of red cells. The blood pressure decreased as soon as the intravenous therapy was reduced, the tachycardia did not resolve and the patient was therefore transferred to the operating room.

After intubation, the ECG showed ST elevation and a median sternotomy incision was rapidly performed. The

Table 1 Overview of the papers on penetrating cardiac injury from 1997 to 2012

Ref nr, author, year, journal and study origin. Study type	Patients/patient group/injury site	Outcomes/performed surgery	Key results	Comments
[2] Asensio et al. (1998), J Trauma, USA. Prospective evaluation	2-year prospective evaluation of 105 penetrating cardiac injuries	65% GSW (survival 16%), 35% SW (survival 65%). EDT in 76 pts with 10 survivors (16%)	Presence of cardiac tamponade and the anatomical site did not predict outcome, presence of sinus rythm when the pericardium was opened did	
[6] Baker et al. (1998), Arch Surg, USA. Retrospective study + review	106 pts with penetrating heart injury (1989–1995): 60 GSW, 46 SW, 55% overall survival.	6 patients on CPB (4 gunshots, 2 stabs, only 2 GSW survived)	Few survivors due to long time from injury to CPB. Those who were resuscitated >5 min prehospitally had a very poor outcome. SR at admission-good prognostic sign. CPB no good to reverse outbled situation/profound shock, but necessary to repair multichamber injuries/large injuries	
[7] Bar et al. (2009), Ind J Thorac Cardiovasc Surg, Israel. Retrospective study	14 pts with penetrating cardiac wound requiring operation (1999–2006) (9 SW, 2 GSW and 2 schrapnel injuries, 1 multipl trauma)	4 sternotomies, 10 anterolat thoracotomies (8 with sternum transsection). 5LV, 6RV, 3RA injuries - all single chamber injuries, no combined.	No CPB, 100% survival, all discharged	Mean interval from injury to surgery 37 min
[8] Barbosa et al. (2011), Interact Cardiovasc Thorac Surg, Argentina. Case report	18 yr male, SW in 4th ic space in the left midclavicular line	Left thoracotomy, suture of right ventricular wound at admittance	Developed pneumonia/lung edema postop, after 30 days AVR for penetrated aortic valve and closure of shunt (RV -> aorta)	
[9] Bowley et al. (2002), Ann Thorac Surg, South Africa. Case report	24 yr male, multiple stab wounds	No vital signs, PEA, at EDT: tamponade. 2 cm LV wound with LAD transsection, transsected PDA on the opposite side (RV)	Initially Foley catheter in the wound, mattress sutures, LAD ligation, PDA ligation. VF, hypotension: OPCAB with right gastroepiploic artery. Died of respiratory complications due to Brown-Sèquard lesion (another stab injury to the spinal cord)	
[10] Burack et al. (2007), Ann Thorac Surg, USA. Retrospective study	207 pts with mediastinal penetrating trauma 1997–2003, 72 (35%) unstable.	72 unstabel pts, 15% had cardiac injury with 18% survival when explored in ED and 71% when reached OR	With penetrating mediastinal trauma the mortality is 85% when moribund at arrival and 55% when unstable (overall data, not injury specific)	

Table 1 Overview of the papers on penetrating cardiac injury from 1997 to 2012 *(Continued)*

[11] Carr et al. (2011), J Trauma, USA. Retrospective study	2000-2009 penetrating cardiac injuries, both GSW and SW	28 SW with 17 survivors (61%), no information about anatomical site	Functional outcome (5yrs) after: if coronary arteries were not involved - good chance to normal cardiac function at follow up.	
[12] Chughtai et al. (2002), Can J Surg, Canada. Review + case report	Cases of 9 pts, 8 managed with CPB in trauma setting from 1992-1998	Only 2 pts of the presented had a sole cardiac injury (LV + coronary artery, RA + intrapericardial vena cava)	The patient with LV and coronary artey injury died (no CPB), the other patient survived without sequele	
[3] Clarke et al. (2011), J Thorac Cardiovasc Surg, South Africa. Retrospective study	All patients with penetrating cardiac injury requiring operation from 2006-2009	Of 1062 stab wounds, 104 were operated, 76 had cardiac injury, overall mortality 10%. Approx 50% median sternotomy, 50% left thoracotomy	When data put together with mortuary data: mortality of 30% for SW (in the mortuary cohort of 548 patients with SW, 38% had penetrating cardiac injury). Less than 25% with penetrating cardiac injury reach hospital alive, of these ca 90% survive.	Mostly SW, also mortuary data analyzed. The center has no availability for CPB.
[13] Claassen et al. (2007), J Trauma, USA. Case report	2 male pts : 21 yr and 27 yr	Pas 1: SW in 5th right ic space (axilla) (+ in abdomen), 400ml on chest tube + knife blade in thorax: laceration of right ventricular outflow tract (sutured) + lung resection	Pas 2: SW in left supraclav midline. Tamponade at FAST: pericardial drainage, thereafter stable. Sternotomy after transfer, laceration of the pulmonary outflow tract, sutured, further repaire of aortopulmonary shunt (thrill + TEE)	Think outside the box: SW outside the precordium
[14] Comoglio et al. (2010), Int J Emerg Med, Italy. Case report	75 yr male with chest pain and syncope, had been working with a nailgun	Stable, underwent CT where the nailgun nail was found imbedded in the left ventricular wall. Removed through median sternotomy, suture without CPB	The pt underwent formal coronary angiography to rule out underlying coronary disease	
[15] Desai et al. (2008), J Thorac Cardiovasc Surg, Canada. Brief communication	22 yr male, single SW in the left chest	Severe shock, loss of vital signs in the ED. EDT, ROSC after opening of pericardium. Tamponde + through-and-through laceration of the RV, stapled and transferred to OR	CPB, staples had occluded the PDA, the wound in close proximity. Staples removed, wound sutured. Intraoperative fluorescence coronary angiography showed widely patent PDA	
[16] Fedalen et al. (2001), J Trauma, USA. Case report	30 yr male, isolated SW to left anterior chest wall	Tension pneumothorax, hypotension, cardiac tamponade. Transfer to OR	Median sternotomy, proximal laceration of LAD with posterior wall of the vessel intact. OPCAB with SVG, intraluminal shunt. Laceration used as	

Table 1 Overview of the papers on penetrating cardiac injury from 1997 to 2012 *(Continued)*

			anastomotic site. Discharge at postop day 8
[17] Fulton et al. (1997), Ann Thorac Surg, South Africa. Case report	61 yr male, a single SW in right 2nd ic space parasternally. History of right-sided empyema 18 yrs ago treated by thoracotomy and decortication	Stable, enlargened mediastinum at chest X-ray. Arcography showed laceration to innominate artery, left common carotid artery and left subclavian artery. Distal cannulation, repair in deep hypothermic arrest	Uneventful postoperatively, discharge at day 10
[18] Hibino et al. (2003), Journal of Cardiac Surgery, Japan. Case report	39 yr male, SW anterior chest wall, suicide attempt.	Median sternotomy at OR. Injury of the right ventricular outflow tract, repair without CPB	2 yr after aorto-right ventricular fistula (dyspnea), repair with patch and AVR. The authors suggest long term follow-up to detect unindentified lesions
[19] Ito et al. (2009), Gen Thorac Cardiovasc Surg, Japan. Case report	51 yr male, SW in left 5th ic space with the ice pick still in place, suicidal attempt	Ice pick was moving synchronously with heart beat, echo showed tip in right ventricle, cardiac tamponade	CPB, mattress stich. Heart murmur day 12, 5mm ventricular septal defect detected. No surgery, follow up
[20] Jodati et al. (2011), Interact Cardiovasc Thorac Surg, Iran. Case report	24 yr construction worker, shortness of breath and palpitations, unaware of the pneumatic nailgun injury	Nail through RV outflow tract, interventricular septum, through the mitral valve at TEE and CT.	Median sternotomy, CPB. Entry point on RV, nail tip barely visible, not exit wound after LA was opened. Nail removed, anterior leaflet of mitral valve repaired. Discharge at postop day 5
[21] Kang et al. (2009), Injury, New Zealand/Canada. Review	Review about causes of penetrating cardiac injury, pathophysiology, sequelae, initial and operative management	Hihglighted key points for every section, outlining of prognostic factors	Few other conditions in medicine are as lethal; death occurs from cardiac tamponade or exsanguination; the greatest danger is missing the dgn; resuscitation is of limited value; immediate operative intervention is the only meaningful treatment
[22] Karin et al. (2001), Eur J Emerg Med, Israel. Case report and literature review	1. 29 yr male with single SW in left chest. 2. 35 yr male, stabbed in left lower thorax	1. Cardiac tamponade, ED thoracotomy: SW in the LV transsecting LAD (ligated, sutured). CPB with SVG in OR 2. Hemopneumothorax, respiratory distress, chest tubes. FAST: tamponade. Left thoracotmy at OR, distal LAD transsection, ligated.	Both had normal echocardiographies postoperatively and were discharged respectively 10th and 7th postop day

Table 1 Overview of the papers on penetrating cardiac injury from 1997 to 2012 *(Continued)*

[23] Kurimoto et al. (2007), Surgery today, Japan. Case report	57 yr male, SW in 5th ic space parasternally, suicide attempt	Arrest prehospitally, EDT at admission + pericardiotomy, further percutaneous CPB + repair at ED. 3 cm left ventricular wound near coronary artery	Postop encephalopathy, 3 yrs afterwards at rehabilitation home	
[24] Lau et al. (2008), Singapore Med J. Case report	31 yr male, 2 SW: in the left 4th ic space and in the right 2nd ic space	Pulseless with PEA, EDT, SW in the RV, internal cardiac massage to ROSC, transfer to the OR. Suture of the laceration	Discharged to further rehabilitation due to hypoxic encephalopathy	
[4] Molina et al. (2008), Interact Cardiovasc Thorac Surg, USA. Retrospective study	237 pts (2000–2006) with EDT for penetrating injury, of these 94 with penetrating cardiac injury	GSW 87%, SW 13%, overall survival 8% (5% for GSW, 33% for SW)	None of the patients who reached OR needed CPB. Predictors of survival: sinus rythm, signs of life at ED, SW vs GSW, transport by police, higher GCS	Mostly GSW -very poor outcome
[25] Moore et al. (2007), Am Surg, USA. Case report	16 yr male, multiple stab wounds	Tachycardia and hypotension, left hemothorax. FAST: pericardial and infraabdominal fluid. LAD injury (ligation), RV (suture).	OPCAB (SVG) due to evolving large anteroseptal MI. Abdominal packing. Discharge postop day 17.	
[26] Nwiloh et al. (2010), Ann Thorac Surg, USA/Nigeria. Case report	11 yr boy, arrow in the 4th ic space	Pt admitted 3 days after hunting with arrow in the midline. Attempted retracted at local hospital, referred to the visiting cardiothoracic team from USA. TTE: arrow through right ventricle, ventricular septal shunt	CPB, retraction of the arrow and suture of the RV. Shunt was insignificant, not repaired	
[27] O'Connor et al. (2009), J R Army Med Corps, USA. Review	History, demographics and outcome, repair techniques, special occasions etc.			Refer to iv adenosin infusion for temporary arrest to facilitate the repair
[28] Parra et al. (2010), J Thorac Cardiovasc Surg, USA. Case report	81 yr male struck by a stingray in his left chest	CT: left pneumothorax, foreign body through mediastinum. Left anterior thoracotomy at the OR, the barb was found imbedded in the heart, the entry was repaired and pt transferred to a cardiac center	At cardiac center: CPB, barb through both right and left ventricles. RA was accessed and the barb pulled out in an antegrade fashion. Ventricular septal and RV defects closed with pledgeted sutures. Discharge 60 days postop	Splenectomy due to hemorrhage postop day 1 (unidentified injury, the pt fell when attacked by the sting ray)
[29] Seamon et al. (2009), J Trauma, USA. Retrospective study	283 pts with cardiac or great vessel penetrating injury	88% GSW (survival 2,8%), 12% SW (survival 24,2%)	Predictors of survival in multivariate	Multiple GSW almost unsalvagable

Table 1 Overview of the papers on penetrating cardiac injury from 1997 to 2012 *(Continued)*

	requiring EDT (2000–2007)		analysis: GSW and GCS
[30] Sugiyama et al. (2011), Ann Thorac Surg, USA. Case report	20 yr male, SW in left chest (nipple level)	Cardiac arrest at ED, left anterior thoracotomy, suture of right ventricle	Postop instable, 7. day - 1,9 cm septal defect with left to right shunt (3,7-1), ARDS etc., shunt=VSD repaired 2 mnths afterwards
[5] Tang et al. (2011), Arch Surg, USA. Retrospective study	406 pts with penetrating cardiac injury from 2000-2010	74% SW, 26% GSW. Overall survival 27%.	Focusses on postdischarge complications, 17% had an abnormal echocardiogram at follow-up; all managed conservatively
[31] Tasdemir et al. (2011), Acta Cardiol, Turkey. Case report	19 yr male, SW left chest	Presented in shock, tamponade and complete bilat visual loss. SW of LV with LAD injury,	CPB, SV graft to LAD, visus gradually regained
[32] Toda et al. (2007), Interact Cardiovasc Thor Surg, Japan. Case report	50 yr male, 3 SW by 30 cm sashimi knife, (Neck, 4th ic space, right upper quadrant of abdomen), suicidal attempt	Hypotensive, FAST negative, CT showed pneumopericardium and left hemothorax	Median sternotomy, RV laceration, repair by pledgeted sutures. LV laceration near posterolateral branch of CX, without bleeding, covered with TachoComb.
[33] Topal et al. (2010), J Trauma, Turkey. Retrospective study	Penetrating cardiac injury (57 SW, 4 GSW), 2002-2009	53 left thoracotomies, 4 median sternotomies. 2 LAD injuries, ligated. Total mortality 15% (isolated RV –11%, isolated LV 31% (mixed SW and GSW).	95% injury in 1 chamber. Focusses on predictors of outcome: > mortality when uncouncious, BP<50, low Hct, Na, temp and PH. Patients pronounced "dead on arrival" were not assessed in this study.
[34] Topaloglu et al. (2006), Tex Heart Inst J, Turkey. Case report	19 yr male, SW with skrewdriver in 5th left ic space	Dyspnea and hypotension, 1500ml chest tube output. Left anterior thoracotomy at OR, RV wound repair.	1 week later a cardiac murmur occurred, transfer to a cardiac center, TTE: perforation of membranous septum and anterior leaflet of the mitral valve. Median sternotomy, CPB, LA access: pericardial patch repair of the leaflet, suture of the septal defect through RA. Discharged postop day 5.
[35] Topcuoglu et al. (2009), Thorac Cardiovasc Surg, Turkey. Case report	14 yr male, SW in right 6th icr paravertebrally, stable with knife in place	Right posterolat thoracotomy (knife in situ), at removal bleeding from atrio-inferiocaval junction	Repair on CPB, discharged on 7th postop day

Table 1 Overview of the papers on penetrating cardiac injury from 1997 to 2012 *(Continued)*

[36] Gwely et al. (2010), Thorac Cardiovasc Surg, Egypt. Retrospective study	73 pts operated for cardiac SW (1998–2008)	Unstable 35%, 20% cardiac arrest prior to EDT. Mortality 23%	Poor prognosis: cardiopulmonary resuscitation (mortality rate 68%), EDT (67%) and shock (50%) on admission	Dead on arrival excluded

AVR - aortic valve replacement, CABG - coronary artery bypass, CPB - cardiopulmonary bypass, CX - circumflex artery, ED - emergency department, EDT - emergency department thoracotomy, FAST - focused assessment with sonography in trauma, GCS - Glasgow coma scale, GSW - gunshot wound, LA - left atrium, LAD - left anterior descendent artery, LV - left ventricle, OPCAB - off pump coronary artery bypass, OR - operating room, PDA - posterior descendent artery, RA - right atrium, ROSC - return of spontaneous circulation, RV - right ventricle, SVG - saphenous vein graft, TEE - transesophaegeal echocardiography, VF – ventricular fibrillation.

pericardium was opened and although there was a clot ventral to the heart, there were no signs of cardiac tamponade. There was a 6 cm cut in the lateral pericardium corresponding to the stab wound in the chest and a 7 cm, almost transmural wound in the left ventricle, parallel to a major diagonal branch (Figure 1). The wound was not bleeding. A 5 cm stab wound in the left lung (Figure 2) was sutured and cardiopulmonary bypass (CPB) was established. The cardiac injury ended close to the origin of the left main stem and crossed the left atrium. The ventricular wound was repaired with single mattress sutures reinforced by strips of bovine pericardium (Figures 3, 4) without arresting the heart and without cross-clamping the aorta. The left atrium was sutured using 5/0 Prolene (Ethicon). Blood appeared in the tracheal tube and bronchoscopy revealed ongoing bleeding from the left lung which required resection of the lingula. Weaning from CPB was initially unsuccessful and we suspected that there had been injury to the left main stem either caused by the initial stab or by the hemostatic sutures. The left anterior descending artery was grafted using the internal mammary artery and a vein graft was anastomosed to the circumflex artery. The patient was thereafter successfully weaned from CPB.

Post-operatively, the patient had signs of a stroke and a CT scan revealed a cerebral infarction. One week after surgery he was transferred to the neurological intensive care unit. After three weeks he was awake and self-ventilating. He was moved to his local hospital and was discharged after 6 weeks with only a minor deficit affecting the left upper extremity.

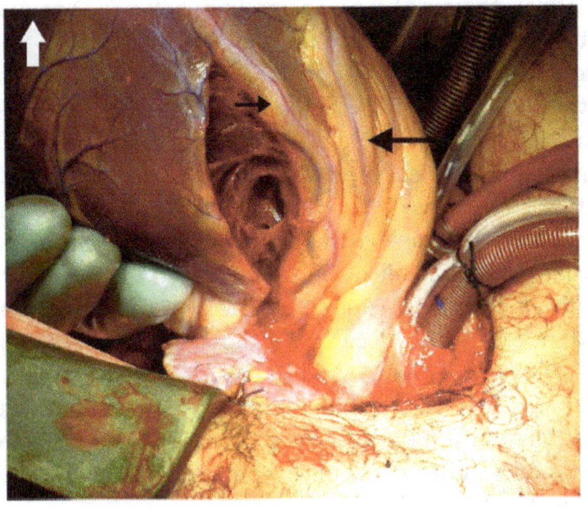

Figure 1 The left ventricular injury almost penetrating the left ventricular wall, notice the left anterior descending coronary artery (large black arrow) with the first diagonal branch (small black arrow). All the photos are taken from the anaesthesiologist point of view and the white arrow indicates the caudal direction.

Discussion

We report the case of a young male patient with a major cardiac stab wound combined with lung injury. Our patient was stabbed during a violent quarrel, thus being a typical stab victim, however, in Japan suicide attempts seem to be equally frequent [18,23]. In large series, gunshot wounds (GSW) are the predominant cause of cardiac penetrating trauma [2,4,6,29]. In Norway, this type of injury is obviously less common but still existing [37-39].

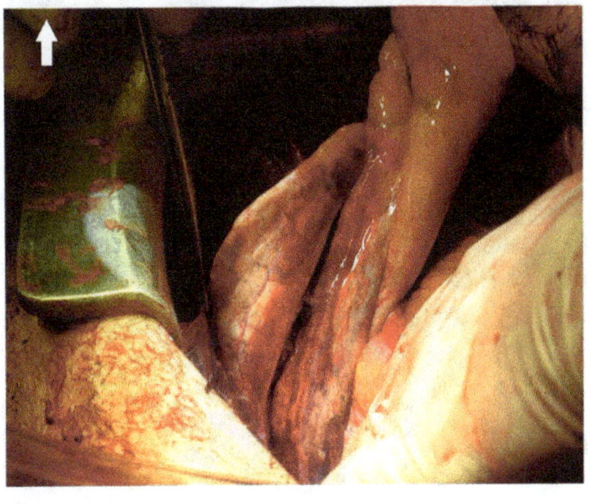

Figure 2 The injured left lung (upper lobe, lingula).

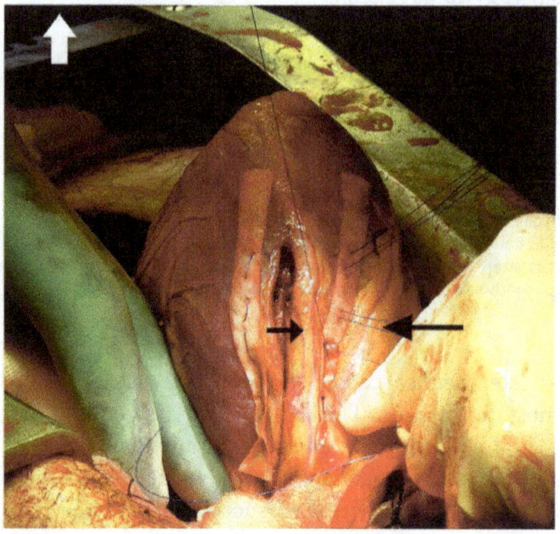

Figure 3 The wound repair with bovine pericardial strips.

Knife is the most common weapon for stab injuries, followed by other sharp items such as screwdrivers [34], ice picks [19], chopsticks, pneumatic nailgun nails [14,20,40] but also curiosities as barb from a sting ray [28]. Fractured ribs or sternum are also reported to cause cardiac penetration [41]. Pneumatic nails might be shot without the patient noticing and cause surprise when detected by CT scan or eccocardiography imbedded in the heart [14,20]. The iatrogenic penetrations of the heart due to different medical devices (pacemaker leads, intracoronary stents, Amplatzer devices) are not discussed in this paper.

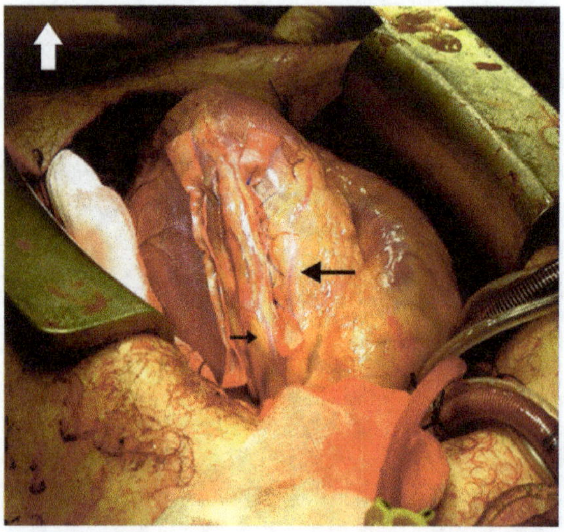

Figure 4 The completed repair of the left ventricular wound.

Penetrating cardiac wounds are mostly fatal either due to cardiac tamponade, exsanguination or coronary artery injury [1]. Clarke reports that of 1064 patients with stab wounds to the chest 104 were operated and 76 were found to have a cardiac injury [3]. The overall mortality was 10% giving an impression of low mortality in this particular group of cardiac injuries. However, when the data was put together with the mortuary report for the same time, the mortality for penetrating cardiac stab wounds was found to be 30%. Most of the studies are retrospective and the patient selection is determined by the survivors arriving at the hospital and ignorance of the mortuary data. Topal et al. report a mortality rate of 15% in 61 penetrating cardiac cases with predominantly stab wounds but state that "patients pronounced dead on arrival were not assessed in this study" [33]. The only known prospective study reports another reality with a mortality rate of 97% when multichamber penetrating injury is present [2]. Also Molina et al. reports high mortality (67%) in a cohort with mainly stab wounds throughout the last decennium [4].

Our patient maintained suboptimal circulation for approximately two hours before undergoing surgery. The time span taken into consideration, our patient was extremely lucky as the outcome is usually poor when the time from trauma to surgery increases [5,6]. An Israeli study of 14 patients reports 100% survival (9 SW, 2 GSW, 1 shrapnel injury and 1 multi trauma) with the mean time from injury to surgery of 37 min [7]. In addition to fast admission to surgery, this outstanding result may also be due to the fact that all patients had single chamber injuries and no coronary artery injury. According to Burack et al., patients with penetrating mediastinal trauma triage themselves between operative intervention or evaluation and observation as they present either stable or unstable on admission. In this retrospective study the authors present 207 patients of which 72 were unstable [10]. Of these 15% had cardiac injury with 18% survival when explored in the ED. The survival rate was 71% when patients with penetrating cardiac injury reached the operating room. All patients having cardiac injury in this study were unstable (authors criteria: traumatic cardiac arrest or near arrest and an emergency department thoracotomy (EDT); cardiac tamponade; ATLS grad III shock despite fluid resuscitation; chest tube output >1500 ml at insertion; chest tube output >500 ml in the initial hour; massive hemothorax after chest tube input). The study does not report the use of CPB.

In our patient, there was a large stab wound of the left ventricle running parallel to the diagonal artery as well as a stab wound in the left atrium. Regarding the location of penetrating cardiac injury, the right ventricle is the most common due to its ventral anatomical position, followed by the left ventricle, right atrium and left atrium [2,3,11]. The patients with a single right ventricle injury are mostly salvagable whereas those with multichamber injuries have a very high mortality [2,4,21]. The concomitant injury of the lung in our patient is not a rarity [3]. Our patient did not suffer from cardiac tamponade as there was a large opening to the left pleural cavity through the wound in the pericardium. This probably saved his life, although profound hypovolemia can conceal signs of cardiac tamponade leading to delayed diagnosis [36]. However, cardiac tamponade in the reviewed studies is not a prognostic factor regarding survival [2,33].

The role of CPB has been debated in trauma surgery, espescially when it comes to penetrating cardiac wounds [6,21]. Some series present large cohorts of penetrating cardiac injury without use of CPB [3-5]. In case of complex cardiac injuries with multichamber lacerations the advantages of a bloodless and still operating field is obvious [6,20,21]. The required heparinisation for CPB might be deleterious in a trauma patient. However, if the bleeding source or sources can be controlled, the risk of further profound haemmorhage is low. On the other hand, full heparisation might cause severe morbidity, and CPB might initiate consumptive coagulopathy and profound systemic inflammatory reaction [28]. Off pump cardiopulmonary bypass is an alternative when it comes to coronary artery lesions [16,22,25]. Establishing CPB in arrested patients or patients in deep haemorrhagic shock is not favourable for the outcome [6]. It could be debated whether or not the aorta should have been cross-clamped in our patient during repair of the left ventricular wall and coronary bypass surgery, but the ECG changes and the suspicion of pre-existing ischemia due to sustained pre-operative hypoperfusion, persuaded us to leave the aorta unclamped in this particular case.

Peroperative fluorescent angiography is a reliable tool to identify suspect coronary artery involvement peroperatively either caused by the injury itself or the surgical procedure [15], unfortunately this technique was not available at our OR. Cardiac stabbings might lead to initially unidentified additional injuries which become apparent first several weeks to years later [8,18]. One study with a large series of patients report that these injuries seldom need surgical treatment [5]. There is consensus that echocardiographic assessment should be provided during the hospital stay [5,11].

On admission to the ED, our patient was given a high Glasgow coma score (GCS), yet post-operatively was found to have had a cerebral injury. Unfortunately, the patient was foreign, and despite speaking, nobody could assess his verbal response adequately. Furthermore, he received an intravenous injection of Ketalar a few minutes after admission, following which he needed assisted manual ventilation and was no longer able to communicate. The initial GCS was later reconsidered and probably the patient suffered from major hypoxia in the pre-hospital phase. Nevertheless the patients with lower GCS have poor outcome, Asensio still reports a high mortality rate (27%) for patients with Glasgow Coma Scale >8 [2]. However, in an emergency room thoracotomy material GCS was found to be a predictor of survival, despite none of the patients had a score >7 [29]. In our patient, it is possible that CPB might have caused cerebral injury by embolization or by giving an insufficient cerebral perfusion pressure. With pre-existing cerebral damage, the standard perfusion pressure during CPB in our patient (mean arterial pressure 50–60mmHg) might not have been high enough to meet the needs of the brain already damaged by hypoperfusion.

Patients with a simple penetrating cardiac injury might be successfully managed without a cardiac surgeon present [2,3]. However, repair of a severe wound of the left ventricle and the complications that can arise will require the surgical skills of a cardiac surgeon, as demonstrated in the present study and the likelihood of survival will be considerably increased by the immediate availability of a cardiac surgical service. The cases where initial tamponade was managed at a lower trauma care center with further transfer for definite surgery, witness of general surgeon`s competence of the initial management of these patients [13,28]. In our level I trauma center, a cardiothoracic surgeon in the trauma team has been practiced for decades and we believe provides optimal management of patients with penetrating cardiac trauma.

Conclusions

We present a complicated case of a young male patient with a chest stab wound who served the trauma team both diagnostic and treatment challenges. We provide the reader a review of literature of the last 15 years publications on penetrating cardiac injury, focusing on stab wounds. Our patient suffered a stroke which origin could be multigenetic, prehospital hypoperfusion, air emboli due to major lung injury and/or insufficient perfusion pressure or microemboli during the cardiopulmonary bypass. The patient in our study survived with minor sequelae due to coordinated work of the trauma team in charge. In conclusion, if the patient with a penetrating stab wound in the heart is not obviously dead on arrival, an attempt for cardiac repair should be done with or without CPB.

Competing interests

The authors declare that they have no competing interests.

Authors' contribution

Both authors were operating surgeons regarding the presented patient case. TT provided the idea of the article. M-L K drafted the initial manuscript while both authors worked on improvement and refining of the final manuscript. Both authors read and approved the final manuscript.

References

1. Asensio JA, Petrone P, Pereira B, Pena D, Prichayudh S, Tsunoyama T, *et al*: **Penetrating cardiac injuries: a historic perspective and fascinating trip through time.** *J Am Coll Surg* 2009, **208:**462–472.
2. Asensio JA, Berne JD, Demetriades D, Chan L, Murray J, Falabella A, *et al*: **One hundred five penetrating cardiac injuries: a 2-year prospective evaluation.** *J Trauma* 1998, **44:**1073–1082.
3. Clarke DL, Quazi MA, Reddy K, Thomson SR: **Emergency operation for penetrating thoracic trauma in a metropolitan surgical service in South Africa.** *J Thorac Cardiovasc Surg* 2011, **142:**563–568.
4. Molina EJ, Gaughan JP, Kulp H, McClurken JB, Goldberg AJ, Seamon MJ: **Outcomes after emergency department thoracotomy for penetrating cardiac injuries: a new perspective.** *Interact Cardiovasc Thorac Surg* 2008, **7:**845–848.
5. Tang AL, Inaba K, Branco BC, Oliver M, Bukur M, Salim A, *et al*: **Postdischarge complications after penetrating cardiac injury: a survivable injury with a high postdischarge complication rate.** *Arch Surg* 2011, **146:**1061–1066.
6. Baker JM, Battistella FD, Kraut E, Owings JT, Follette DM: **Use of cardiopulmonary bypass to salvage patients with multiple-chamber heart wounds.** *Arch Surg* 1998, **133:**855–860.
7. Bar I, Papiashvili M, Jeroukhimov I, Muhanna AY, Alzaanin AA: **Strategies in the management of penetrating cardiac trauma based on 14 surviving patients from a strife-ridden area.** *Ind J Thorac Cardiovasc Surg* 2009, **25:**23–26.
8. Barbosa FM, Quiroga JM, Otero AE, Girela GA: **Aortic valve regurgitation with aorto-right ventricular fistula following penetrating cardiac injury.** *Interact Cardiovasc Thorac Surg* 2011, **13:**653–654.
9. Bowley DM, Saeed M, Somwe D, Boffard KD, Naidoo K, Davis SC: **Off-pump cardiac revascularization after a complex stab wound.** *Ann Thorac Surg* 2002, **74:**2192–2193.
10. Burack JH, Kandil E, Sawas A, O'Neill PA, Sclafani SJ, Lowery RC, *et al*: **Triage and outcome of patients with mediastinal penetrating trauma.** *Ann Thorac Surg* 2007, **83:**377–382.
11. Carr JA, Buterakos R, Bowling WM, Janson L, Kralovich KA, Copeland C, *et al*: **Long-term functional and echocardiographic assessment after penetrating cardiac injury: 5-year follow-up results.** *J Trauma* 2011, **70:**701–704.
12. Chughtai TS, Gilardino MS, Fleiszer DM, Evans DC, Brown RA, Mulder DS: **An expanding role for cardiopulmonary bypass in trauma.** *Can J Surg* 2002, **45:**95–103.
13. Claassen CW, O'connor JV, Gens D, Sikorski R, Scalea TM: **Penetrating cardiac injury: think outside the box.** *J Trauma* 2010, **68:**E71–E73.
14. Comoglio C, Sansone F, Boffini M, Ribezzo M, Rinaldi M: **Nail gun penetrating injury of the heart mimicking an acute coronary syndrome.** *Int J Emerg Med* 2010, **3:**135–137.
15. Desai ND, Moussa F, Singh SK, Chu P, Fremes SE: **Intraoperative fluorescence angiography to determine the extent of injury after penetrating cardiac trauma.** *J Thorac Cardiovasc Surg* 2008, **136:**218–219.
16. Fedalen PA, Bard MR, Piacentino V III, Fisher CA, McCarthy JR, Schina MJ Jr, *et al*: **Intraluminal shunt placement and off-pump coronary revascularization for coronary artery stab wound.** *J Trauma* 2001, **50:**133–135.
17. Fulton JO, Brink JG: **Complex thoracic vascular injury repair using deep hypothermia and circulatory arrest.** *Ann Thorac Surg* 1997, **63:**557–559.
18. Hibino N, Tsuchiya K, Sasaki H, Matsumoto H, Nakajima M, Naito Y: **Delayed presentation of injury to the sinus of valsalva with aortic regurgitation resulting from penetrating cardiac wounds.** *J Card Surg* 2003, **18:**236–239.
19. Ito H, Saito S, Miyahara K, Takemura H, Sawaki S, Matsuura A: **Traumatic ventricular septal defect following a stab wound to the chest.** *Gen Thorac Cardiovasc Surg* 2009, **57:**148–150.
20. Jodati A, Safaei N, Toufan M, Kazemi B: **A unique nail gun injury to the heart with a delayed presentation.** *Interact Cardiovasc Thorac Surg* 2011, **13:**363–365.
21. Kang N, Hsee L, Rizoli S, Alison P: **Penetrating cardiac injury: overcoming the limits set by Nature.** *Injury* 2009, **40:**919–927.
22. Karin E, Greenberg R, Avital S, Aladgem D, Kluger Y: **The management of stab wounds to the heart with laceration of the left anterior descending coronary artery.** *Eur J Emerg Med* 2001, **8:**321–323.
23. Kurimoto Y, Kano H, Yama N, Nara S, Hase M, Asai Y: **Out-of-hospital cardiopulmonary arrest due to penetrating cardiac injury treated by percutaneous cardiopulmonary support in the emergency room: report of a case.** *Surg Today* 2007, **37:**240–242.
24. Lau CK, Chin HF, Ong FH, Eng KH: **Emergency department thoracotomy for pericardiac tamponade.** *Singapore Med J* 2008, **49:**e382–e384.
25. Moore FO, Berne JD, Turner WF, Villarreal DH, McGovern T, Rowe SA, *et al*: **Off-pump coronary artery bypass is an alternative to conventional cardiopulmonary bypass when repair of traumatic coronary artery injuries is indicated.** *Am Surg* 2007, **73:**296–298.
26. Nwiloh J, Edaigbini S, Danbauchi S, Aminu MB, Oyati A: **Arrow injury to the heart.** *Ann Thorac Surg* 2010, **90:**287–289.
27. O'Connor J, Ditillo M, Scalea T: **Penetrating cardiac injury.** *J R Army Med Corps* 2009, **155:**185–190.
28. Parra MW, Costantini EN, Rodas EB, Gonzalez PJ, Salamen OJ, Catino JD, *et al*: **Surviving a transfixing cardiac injury caused by a stingray barb.** *J Thorac Cardiovasc Surg* 2010, **139:**e115–e116.
29. Seamon MJ, Shiroff AM, Franco M, Stawicki SP, Molina EJ, Gaughan JP, *et al*: **Emergency department thoracotomy for penetrating injuries of the heart and great vessels: an appraisal of 283 consecutive cases from two urban trauma centers.** *J Trauma* 2009, **67:**1250–1257.
30. Sugiyama G, Lau C, Tak V, Lee DC, Burack J: **Traumatic ventricular septal defect.** *Ann Thorac Surg* 2011, **91:**908–910.
31. Tasdemir K, Everekliogl C, Kaya MG: **Transient cortical blindness and successful recovery after coronary bypass surgery.** *Acta Cardiol* 2011, **66:**661–664.
32. Toda K, Yoshitatsu M, Izutani H, Ihara K: **Surgical management of penetrating cardiac injuries using a fibrin glue sheet.** *Interact Cardiovasc Thorac Surg* 2007, **6:**577–578.
33. Topal AE, Celik Y, Eren MN: **Predictors of outcome in penetrating cardiac injuries.** *J Trauma* 2010, **69:**574–578.
34. Topaloglu S, Aras D, Cagli K, Ergun K, Deveci B, Demir AD, *et al*: **Penetrating trauma to the mitral valve and ventricular septum.** *Tex Heart Inst J* 2006, **33:**392–395.
35. Topcuoglu MS, Poyrazoglu HH, Yaliniz H: **A unusual case of right lung and right atrio-inferiocaval injury caused by stabbing.** *Thorac Cardiovasc Surg* 2009, **57:**248–249.
36. Gwely NN, Mowafy A, Khalaf S, Amer S, Hamza U, El-Saeed M: **Management of stab wounds of the heart: analysis of 73 cases in 10 years.** *Thorac Cardiovasc Surg* 2010, **58:**210–214.
37. Hougen HP, Rogde S, Poulsen K: **Homicide by firearms in two Scandinavian capitals.** *Am J Forensic Med Pathol* 2000, **21:**281–286.
38. Pahle AS, Pedersen BL, Skaga NO, Pillgram-Larsen J: **Emergency thoracotomy saves lives in a Scandinavian hospital setting.** *J Trauma* 2010, **68:**599–603.
39. Braathen B, Bøen A, Thorsen T, Tønnessen T: **Gunshot through the left ventricle.** *Resuscitation* 2009, **80:**615–616.
40. Carr CS, Alkhafaji S, Alkhulaifi A, Carr CS, Alkhafaji S, Alkhulaifi AM: **Penetrating cardiac nail gun injury.** *BMJ Case Rep* 2009, **2009:**bcr2006040121.
41. Grieve P: **Cardiac perforation secondary to a fractured rib sustained in a ram attack in New Zealand: a review of ovine fatalities and an important lesson regarding the severely injured chest.** *N Z Med J* 2006, **119:**U2315.

7

Efficacy of extra-peritoneal pelvic packing in hemodynamically unstable pelvic fractures, a Propensity Score Analysis

Osvaldo Chiara[1,3*], Emanuele di Fratta[1], Anna Mariani[1], Bertuzzi Michaela[2], Lucia Prestini[2], Fabrizio Sammartano[1] and Stefania Cimbanassi[1]

Abstract

Background: An option for emergency control of pelvic hemorrhage is Extra-peritoneal Pelvic Packing (EPP), which addresses the retroperitoneal source of exsanguination in pelvic fractures. The aim of this study was to demonstrate the efficacy of early EPP in reducing mortality due to hemorrhage from pelvic fractures, and to evaluate the impact of packing on transfusion requirements within the first 24 h and ICU length of stay (ICU-LOS).

All data pertaining trauma patients admitted from October 2002 and December 2103 with hemodynamic instability and pelvic fractures were selected from the Hospital Trauma Registry. Patients with severe brain injury and bleeding from extra-pelvic sources were excluded. Patient population was divided into two groups: EPP group, including patients admitted from 2009 to 2013, with EPP as part of the treatment algorithm, and NO-EPP group, from 2002 to 2008, without EPP as atherapeutic option. Descriptive statistical analysis was performed on allpatients. Twenty-five patients of each group with similar features were matched using Propensity Score Analysis (PSA).

Results: Six hundred eighty out of 4659 major trauma (14.6 %) presented a pelvic fracture. In 78 hemodynamically unstable patients (30 in EPP group,48 in NO-EPP group) the major source of bleeding was the pelvis. Among patients selected by PSA early mortality was significantly reduced in EPP group (20 vs 52 %, $p = .03$) compared to NO-EPP, notwithstanding similar hemodynamic impairment. No difference was observed in transfusion requirements and ICU-LOS.

Conclusions: The EPP is a safe and quick procedure, able to improve hemodynamic stabilization and to reduce acute mortality due to hemorrhage in patients with pelvic fracture, in combination with optimized transfusion protocol. EPP may be useful as a bridge for time-consuming procedures, such as angio-embolization.

Keywords: Pelvic fracture, Hemodynamic instability, Extra-peritoneal pelvic packing, Propensity score analysis

Background

Hemodynamically unstable pelvic fractures still represents a diagnostic and therapeutic challenge for trauma surgeons. Pelvic ring disruption is always a marker of high energy impact mechanism, often associated with life-threatening injuries in other body districts. Despite the multidisciplinary approach mortality remains as high as 40 %, with one third of patients dying because of an uncontrolled hemorrhage [1, 2]. Bleeding in pelvic fractures originates in 85 % of cases from cancellous bone and low-pressure veins, and in the remaining 15 % from arteries [3]. Arterial bleeding may be predominant in patients with persistent hemodynamic instability after mechanical stabilization [4]. Data on pelvic injury treatments suggest that the use of angio-embolization has a success rate between 80 and 100 % in arterial bleeding control. However, this procedure is less effective when used to stop venous and bone bleeding [3]. Additionally, angio-embolization requires a lengthy set up, specialized equipment and personnel, that may not be

* Correspondence: ochiara@yahoo.com
[1]SC Trauma Team, Niguarda Trauma Center, Ospedale Niguarda Ca' Granda Milano, Milano, Italy
[3]Trauma Team Ospedale Niguarda, Piazza Ospedale Maggiore 3, Milano 20162, Italy
Full list of author information is available at the end of the article

promptly available in all hospitals. In this situation, it is not advised to transfer hemodynamically unstable patients to interventional radiology suites or to higher level facilities [5].

Extra-peritoneal Pelvic Packing (EPP) is a quick and effective procedure for the emergency control of pelvic hemorrhage that directly addresses the bleeding coming from the retroperitoneal space in severe pelvic injuries. This technique was first described in Germany in 1994 [6] and subsequently adopted by several European groups [7, 8]. In the United States, EPP was originally adopted by the Denver group and when used in association with pelvic stabilization, it showed a reduction of the mortality rate and need for transfusions and angiography [9].

The EPP is an easy and fast procedure, feasible in emergency room [7, 10]. A recent Italian Consensus Conference [8] assigned a pivotal role to EPP in the acute management of hemorrhagic shock consequent to unstable pelvic fractures, but the treatment strategy and effects on the survival still remain controversial.

The purpose of this study was to demonstrate the efficacy of early EPP in reducing the mortality due to hemorrhagic shock from pelvic fractures. The Propensity Score Analysis [11] was used to adjust the baseline characteristics and severity of different patient groups. The impact of pelvic packing on transfusion requirements within the first 24 h and ICU length of stay (ICU-LOS) were the secondary end points.

Methods

Patients selection

All patients in this study received a standardized protocol and were selected from the hospital Trauma Registry. Hemodynamic instability was defined as a persistent systolic blood pressure (SBP) of < 90 mmHg during initial resuscitation despite pelvic binder and ≥ 2000 ml of intravenous crystalloids and transfusion of ≥ 2 units of packed red blood cells (PRBCs). All demographic data, Injury Severity Score (ISS), Organ Injury Scale (OIS), Abbreviated Injury Scale (AIS), mechanism of injury, emergency room time, physiologic indices, lactates and base excess (BE) on admission, units of blood transfused, length of ICU-LOS, concomitant injuries, were taken into account. The pattern of pelvic fracture was classified according to Tile (A,B,C) [12] and Young & Burgess class (antero-posterior compression, APC, lateral compression, LC, vertical shear, VS, combined mechanism, CM) [13]. Coagulation status was checked with standards exams (INR, PTT, Platelets count), while TEG/ROTEM [14, 15] was available since 2006.

Patients with pelvic fracture consecutively admitted to our level 1 Trauma Centre from October 2002 to December 2013 were selected from the hospital Trauma Registry and only those with persistent hemodynamic instability were considered for this study. The aim was to investigate the best treatment option to address bleeding exclusively or mostly caused by pelvic fracture, thus the following two categories were excluded: (a) patients with concomitant extra-pelvic bleeding requiring damage control surgery for hemorrhage and non-operated deceased patients where autopsy demonstrated a significant (about 1 L or more) extra-pelvic source of bleeding, (b) patients affected by brain injury AIS ≥ 4, deceased and non.

Protocol of treatment

Pelvic injury patients were initially treated in our Trauma Centre by a hospital trauma team composed of a general surgeon, anesthesiologist, radiologist, radiology technician and two nurses. An orthopedic surgeon was always notified of the admission of a patient with a pelvic fracture and called to perform stabilization in emergency room and further surgical orthopedic procedures. Trauma team doctors were present in house 24 h and angio-embolization (AE) was ready available during working hours or within 60 min during weekends and nights. Hemodynamically unstable patients were transfused two 0 negative packed red blood cells followed by cross-matched packed red blood cells—fresh frozen plasma—platelets (PRBCs:FFP:PLT) at 1:1:1 ratio. Since 2008, crystalloid infusion was reduced and colloids avoided (both pre-hospital and in-hospital settings), cryoprecipitates were administered (1U/10 kg, after 20 PRBC U, or if fibrinogen < 2gr/L. This transfusion protocol did not change throughout the study period and the PRBC:FFP ratio was affected only by the overall number of PRBC (as the former were two 0 negative PRBC without FFP). Tranexamic acid (TXA) was routinely administered in class III- IV of shock only since 2011, with a loading dose of 1 gr, over 10 min, then infusion of 1 g over 8 h [16]. The source of bleeding was diagnosed with an antero-posterior chest and pelvis X-ray and Extended Focused Abdominal Sonography for Trauma (E-FAST). A total body contrast-enhanced CT-scan (CeCT) was carried out only after hemodynamic stabilization.

Before 2009 the treatment protocol of hemodynamically unstable patients with pelvic fracture consisted of: (a) temporary circumferential compression using a pelvic orthotic binder (T-POD, Bio Cybernetics International, La Verne, CA) at the level of the greater trochanters, (b) laparotomy in the operating room (OR) if E-FAST positive, (c) external fixation in the OR with the help of fluoroscopy, placed at the anterior inferior iliac spine, (d) AE if persistent instability or positive CeCT for arterial bleeding.

After 2009 early EPP was included in the treatment options: patients with pelvic fracture and persistent hypotension despite pelvic binder and two 0-negative

PRBCs would receive immediate EPP before laparotomy (if needed), followed by external fixation and AE when indicated by the presence of persistent hemodynamic instability or positive CeCT (Fig. 1).

The adopted surgical technique for EPP consisted in a vertical or supra-pubic skin incision, midline fascial cut, followed by placing 2–3 pads on each side of the bladder neck below the pelvic brim, suture of fascia and skin incision [6]. The EPP was performed directly in the emergency department (ED) inside the shock room if the patient was agonic or too unstable to be transported to the OR. The EPP was removed within 48 h in all patients.

Subjects whose hemodynamic status was stabilized by pelvic binding and 2 PRBCs transfusion underwent CeCT and AE if requested by a detectable arterial bleeding. These patients were not included in the present study.

Statistical analysis

In this study, patients were divided in 2 groups: (a) EPP group, including patients admitted from 2009 to 2013, with EPP as a part of the treatment algorithm, (b) NO-EPP group, including patients admitted from 2002 to 2008, without EPP among the therapeutic options.

The two groups were initially compared using descriptive statistics, considering the following values: time spent in the emergency room, lactate and BE levels, age, ISS, mechanism of trauma, pelvic fracture pattern, concomitant extra-pelvic injuries, mortality with early deaths (within 24 h) and late deaths (after 24 h), transfusion of PRBCs and ICU-LOS. All patients were followed until discharge or death.

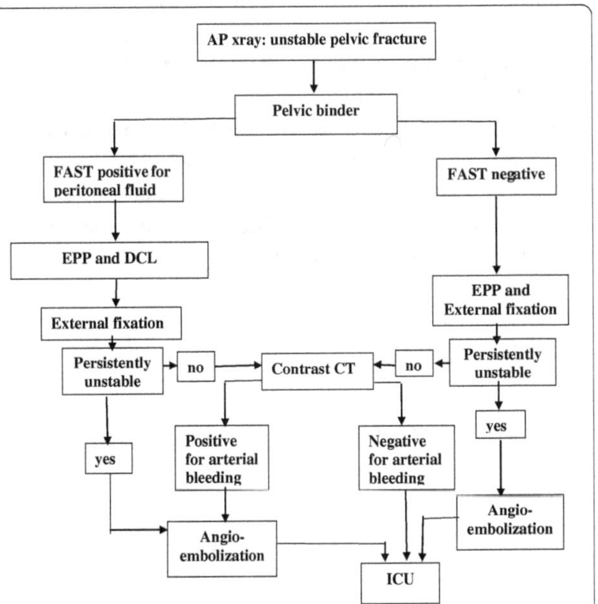

Fig. 1 Treatment algorithm of patients with pelvic fracture and hemodynamic instability since 2009 at Niguarda Trauma Centre

The Propensity Score Analysis was used to adjust the differences in the baseline characteristics and severity of condition at admission between the two groups. The Propensity Score was estimated modeling for potential confounders: age, ISS, pattern of pelvic fracture and non bleeding extra-pelvic injuries. With regard to exclusion criteria, only head injuries AIS 3 or less, pneumothorax, lung contusion, rupture of thoracic aorta with mediastinal hemorrhage confined, abdominal parenchymal injuries treated with non-operative management, hollow viscus injuries and fractures of the extremities were taken into consideration. A one-to-one matched analysis using nearest-neighbor matching was performed based on the estimated Propensity Score of each patient. A match occurred when one patient in the EPP group had an estimated score within 0.1 standard deviation (SD) of another in the NO-EPP group. Hence, the second study period was considered concluded when the number of EPP group was enough for the one-to-one matching with the patients selected in the NO-EPP group.

Continuous variables were compared using t-test and categorical variables with Fisher's exact test. A p value of < 0.05 was considered statistically significant.

Results

From October 2002 to December 2013, 4659 major trauma were admitted at the Niguarda Trauma Center: 680 (14.6 %) patients showed pelvic ring fractures and 111 (16.3 %) of them were hemodynamic unstable. Thirty-three patients (6 in EPP and 27 in NO-EPP group) were excluded from the study as follows: 12 for severe traumatic brain injury AIS > 3 and 21 for extra-pelvic sources of significant bleeding. In these cases pelvic fracture was considered only partially affecting hemodynamic status and the causes of instability were identified as multifactorial. Of the remaining 78 patients, 30 were in EPP group and 48 in NO-EPP. Males were 17 (57 %) in EPP and 35 (73 %) in NO-EPP group.

All patients sustained a blunt trauma (Table 1) and common causes of pelvic fractures were falls from height, pedestrian struck and motorcycle crash. The average time inside the emergency room from the admission to the conclusion of the emergency procedures

Table 1 Mechanisms of injury in the two groups

Mechanism	EPP *n* (%)	NO-EPP *n* (%)
Car	2 (6.6)	5 (10.4)
Motorcycle	7 (23.3)	10 (20.8)
Bicycle	2 (6.6)	8 (16.6)
Pedestrian	9 (30)	10 (20.8)
Fall	10 (33.3)	13 (27.1)

was 22 ± 8 min. in EPP and 19 ± 10 min. in NO-EPP (p ns). The age and ISS were not significantly different between groups (Table 2). Tile B1 fractures (Young & Burgess APCI/II), Tile B2 (LC I/II) and B3 (LC III) were more frequent in NO-EPP group while an increased number of Tile C fractures (Young & Burgess APCIII or VS or CM) was observed in EPP group. Extra pelvic injuries were similar between groups, in fact more than 70 % of patients were affected by injuries in other body regions. The overall mortality was higher in NO-EPP group, but not statistically significant.

Only 25 patients in each group resulted eligible according to the propensity Score matching. Table 3 shows the patients who were selected. Baseline characteristics were well balanced with homogeneity of potential confounders and Propensity Scores were all within 0.1 SD in the two groups. In Table 4 matched patients are compared. The BE and lactate were not different in the two groups, indicating a similar degree of hemodynamic impairment, but the admission INR was significantly lower in the EPP group. It was possible to evaluate the type of bleeding in 19 of NO-EPP and 22 of EPP patients. A prevalence of arterial bleeding was demonstrated in both groups, particularly in EPP patients. Overall mortality was significantly decreased in EPP group. Time distribution of deaths between packed and non-packed patients was different: EPP patients showed fewer early deaths and two late deaths due to organ failure while NO-EPP patients died exclusively within 24 h. In the EPP group the systolic blood pressure increased immediately after packing from 64.1 ± 15.3 to 105.5 ± 16.5 ($p < .0001$) and heart rate decreased from 119.9 ± 23.8 to 99.23 ± 20.5 ($p < .002$). In deceased patients, the elapsed time from admission to death was significantly longer in patients who received pelvic packing. Thus, the EPP group showed a decreased rate of acute deaths due to hemorrhage by more than 50 %. Moreover, patients in the NO-EPP group underwent less AE procedures than EPP patients because of the increased rate of acute mortality: eight (32 %) NO-EPP patients died before angiography and five (20 %) died despite of embolization. Conversely, in EPP patients only 3 (12 %) did not survive until angiography and 4 (16 %) died after interventional radiology. No complications related to EPP were observed.

There were no differences of PRBC requirement within the first 24 h after admission: packed and non-packed patients were both substantially transfused, with a mean of 14 and 13 units respectively. The PRBC:FFP ratio was 1.16 ± 0.8 in survived and 1.28 ± 0.09 (p ns) in non-survived patients. All the patients in this study were admitted to ICU and ICU LOS was not different among the two groups.

Discussion

Despite the advances in the acute management of hemodynamic unstable pelvic fractures, the mortality rate of the affected patients is still higher than 40 % [6], with exsanguination being the main cause of acute deaths and multi-organ failure of late deaths. We hypothesized that early EPP is a "bridging treatment" in pelvic fractures with severe hemodynamic instability, useful to stabilize the source of bleeding thus increasing the safety of diagnostic and hemostatic procedures, such as ceCT-scan, angio-embolization, DCL and external fixation. Moreover, EPP may be indicated as a life-saving procedure in peripheral hospitals, before transferring the patient to higher level facilities. In our Trauma Centre patients with unstable pelvic fractures are splinted with the pelvic binder, adapted to the fracture type after initial AP x-Ray. The pelvic binder is further closed in Tile B1 (Young & Burgess APC I-II) and optimized with a posterior compression in Tile C (Young & Burgess APC III/VS/CM) fractures. The EPP is immediately performed by a trauma surgeon in the emergency room in hemodynamically unstable non-responder patients after pelvic binder and transfusion of two 0-negative PRBCs. The T-POD is left in place during EPP to avoid the displacement of pelvic fragments [17, 18]. The highly significant hemodynamic effect of EPP is demonstrated in our clinical series by the significant increase in systolic blood pressure after the maneuver.

Table 2 General characteristics of group 1 and 2 patients selected from Trauma Registry

	EPP Group ($n = 30$)	NO-EPP Group ($n = 48$)	p
Age (years)	55.3 ± 21.8	48.5 ± 20.8	0.1393
ISS	44.93 ± 10.06	40.57 ± 15.53	0.142
Tile Young & Burgess			0.076
A APCI-LCI	1 (2 %)	5 (10 %)	
B APCI-II, LCI-III	9 (29 %)	24 (50 %)	
C APCIII,VS,CM	20 (69 %)	19 (40 %)	
Extra-pelvic injuries	23 (77 %)	33 (70 %)	0.626
Mortality	10 (33 %)	21 (49 %)	0.092

Table 3 Potential confounders in patients matched with Propensity Score Analysis and calculated Propensity Scores

EPP GROUP						NO-EPP GROUP					
ID	Age	ISS	Tile/Y&B	Extra-pelvic injuries yes/no	Propensity Score	ID	Age	ISS	Tile/YB	Extra-pelvic injuries yes/no	Propensity Score
P.D.	19	50	C1/APCIII	yes	0.27	P.M.	15	68	C3/CM	Yes	0.27
C.G.	46	50	C2/VS	yes	0.52	B.E.	62	59	C3/CM	Yes	0.48
T.A.	77	41	B3/LCIII	yes	0.44	P.A.	85	50	B3/LCIII	No	0.39
A.J.	20	43	C2/VS	yes	0.44	F.S.	35	41	C2/VS	No	0.41
P.G.	60	48	C1/APCIII	yes	0.51	P.M.	38	45	C2/VS	yes	0.52
E.A.	85	38	B2/LCI	yes	0.55	B.M	46	38	C2/VS	No	0.50
P.A.	79	41	B2/LCI	yes	0.35	I.C.	52	25	B2/LCI	No	0.36
A.L.	59	45	C1/APCIII	yes	0.40	M.P.	41	25	B3/LCIII	No	0.40
V.M.	55	38	C1/APCIII	yes	0.59	F.G.	63	25	B3/LCIII	yes	0.66
S.G.	76	43	B2/LCII	yes	0.31	C.P.	42	50	B3/LCIII	yes	0.29
C.A.	63	34	C1/VS	yes	0.54	Z.F.	35	32	C2/VS	No	0.50
C.E.	84	38	B3/LCIII	yes	0.51	A.F.	36	32	C2/VS	yes	0.51
L.P.	72	50	B2/LCII	yes	0.35	F.A.	80	43	B2/LCI	No	0.34
I.A.	27	57	C1/VS	yes	0.16	L.P.	30	59	C1/APCIII	yes	0.15
P.L.	69	38	B2/LCII	yes	0.32	T.D.	38	34	B2/LCII	yes	0.33
M.P.	77	25	C2/VS	no	0.79	C.I.	65	26	C3/CM	No	0.80
B.A.	52	34	C2/VS	no	0.58	G.P.	60	59	C2/CM	yes	0.50
N.B.	69	25	B2/LCI	No	0.46	C.A.	29	59	C3/CM	yes	0.43
P.L.	70	38	C2/VS	yes	0.76	A.G	81	26	C2/VS	No	0.80
G.G.	53	25	C1/APCIII	no	0.58	G.R.	62	19	B2/LCI	No	0.48
M.L.	34	43	C2/VS	yes	0.52	M.G	79	29	B2/LCI	No	0.47
A.A.	82	38	C2/CM	yes	0.36	B.G.	83	75	C1/APCIII	yes	0.36
P.M.	80	29	C3/CM	no	0.84	C.M	88	41	C2/VS	yes	0.81
C.M.	55	25	B2/LCII	no	0.38	R.D.	40	57	C3/CM	yes	0.37
G.J.	24	41	C2/VS	yes	0.48	G.Z.	36	45	C1/APCIII	yes	0.40

Table 4 Comparisons of the two groups matched with Propensity Score Analysis. Continuous data are expressed as mean values ± SD

	EPP Group (25 pts)	NO-EPP Group (25 pts)	*p*
Base Excess (mEq/L)	−4.33 ± 3.78	−4.88 ± 3.38	0.29
Lactate (mmol/L)	5.18 ± 2.55	5.80 ± 3.38	0.23
INR	1.91 ± 090	1.46 ± 0.33	0.03
Arterial bleeding	22 (88 %)	19 (76 %)	-
Number of total deaths	7 (28 %)	13 (52 %)	0.01
Deaths >24 h	2 (8 %)	0	-
Deaths < 24 h	5 (20 %)	13 (52 %)	0.03
Hours from admission to death	122.8 ± 63.11	7.38 ± 10.43	0.003
n. of angio-embolizations	21 (84 %)	14 (56 %)	0.05
n. of PRBCs < 24 h	13.00 ± 11.00	14.10 ± 11.00	0.71
ICU-LOS (days)	19.80 ± 12.60	18.70 ± 11.00	0.73

The Italian Consensus Conference on the management of hemodynamically unstable pelvic trauma held in April 2013 gives a key role to EPP in the treatment of these patients [8]. Osborn et al. [19] in a retrospective analysis of pelvic trauma patients treated with either early angiography or direct retroperitoneal packing demonstrated that EPP significantly reduces transfusion requirements over 24 h post-intervention with no early deaths. In a review of two decades literature Papakostidis and Giannoudis [20] concluded that there is not a clear superiority of EPP over angio-embolization on patient outcome and both procedures could play a complementary role to each other. The review by Suzuki et al. [21] proposed EPP as first intervention in hemodynamically unstable patients, whereas angiography could be the first choice in stabilized patients. Tai et al. [22] in a retrospective study suggested that early EPP with subsequent angiography if needed was associated with a non-significant decrease in mortality in respect to an early angiography (from 69.2 to 36.3 %). External fixation plus EPP has been indicated by Burlew et al. [23] as optimal for life-threatening hemorrhage from unstable pelvic fracture. EPP is a level III recommendation in the guidelines from Eastern Association for the Surgery of Trauma [24], with the need of future comparative studies to define the best strategy. In a recent paper, Marzi et al. [25], suggested that angiographic embolization could be used as the first line treatment in hemodynamically stable patients with arterial blush at ceCT, while pelvic packing and mechanical stabilization are immediately carried out in hemodynamically unstable patients.

The concept of pelvic packing was originally described by Pohlmann et al. [6] in Hannover, then modified by Ertel et al. [7] in Zurich and extensively applied by Moore et al. [26] in Denver. It is a quick and easy procedure with a short learning curve and a minimal blood loss. For instance, in our series, the time required to carry out EPP was 15 min (range 8–20). It can be performed either in emergency and operating room and is especially suited for austere settings where angiography is unavailable or unable to be done expeditiously. A survey done in Wales [27], showed that only 18 % of hospitals had a formal interventional radiology service available 24 h a day, while 58 % of general surgeons and 34 % of orthopedic surgeons were able to perform EPP.

In this retrospective observational study we considered the 78 patients with hemodynamic instability and pelvic fractures admitted at the Trauma Centre of Niguarda Hospital in Milan from October 2002 to December 2013. The EPP was introduced in our hospital protocol since 2009 in addition to other techniques of hemostatic emergency procedures, such as external fixation and angio-embolization. As a randomized study was not possible for ethical and practical reasons, we used the Propensity Score Analysis to reduce potential confounders related to outcome. Propensity Score Analysis was first described by Rosembaum and Rubin in 1983 [28] and has been used increasingly in medical research [11]. The Propensity Score represents the probability (between 0 and 100 per cent) of receiving treatment A rather than B for patients in a non-randomized trial. It is based on observed baseline characteristics (potential confounder factors) and summarizes all measured confounders in a single score. Hence, Propensity Score Analysis attempts to reconstruct a situation similar to randomization.

In the present study all patients with extra-pelvic sources of bleeding and severe traumatic brain injury were excluded to avoid interference on hemodynamic status from factors other than pelvic hemorrhage. The two groups were then compared for general characteristics, such as mechanism of trauma, age, pattern of fracture, ISS, associated extra-pelvic injuries. Finally the Propensity Analysis matched 25 EPP with 25 NO-EPP patients and this "quasi-randomization" [29] pointed out the effects of early EPP in the emergency treatment of unstable pelvic fracture patients. It was evident that, given a similar hemodynamic impairment at admission, in EPP group acute deaths within the 24 h following treatment were markedly reduced, notwithstanding a higher rate of arterial bleeding.

The refinement of the transfusion protocols and expertise of the trauma team undoubtedly increased survival in the second period of the study. EPP group had a lower INR value at admission, probably due to the improved pre-hospital care (shorter time, less fluids, no colloids) in the second phase of the study. In all patients in both groups massive transfusion protocol was performed accordingly to the European guidelines [30]. The 1:1:1 ratio was always started in the emergency room after two 0 negative units since the beginning of the study. Only after 2009, in the second period of the study, TXA and cryoprecipitates were used and thromboelastometry was extensively applied for further decision making. However, EPP seemed to be very effective, as demonstrated by immediate hemodynamic improvement with increase in systolic blood pressure after packing. Most likely, the early bleeding control by EPP combined with the improved transfusion protocol contributed to the decrease of early deaths. The EPP appears to be effective in the immediate recovery of hemodynamic parameters and may be life-saving in very sick patients. The refinements of transfusion protocol can be considered of fundamental importance to recover and preserve the coagulation activity with the prevention of further bleeding in the long term.

The external fixation was always performed by orthopedic surgeons in the OR after EPP, at the end of laparotomy, if needed, and before angiography because closed bone reduction could reduce the need for embolization or, inversely, could produce new bleeding points [23]. An angiography was always performed if the patient was hemodynamically unstable after EPP and pelvic fixation. In the case of hemodynamic stabilization, even if partial, we preferred to obtain a ceCT and angiography only when ongoing arterial bleeding was detected.

Our data show that EPP did not reduce the number of transfusions needed, probably due to the different acute mortality between groups. The higher early mortality and the shorter time from admission to death in NO-EPP compared to EPP group (respectively 7.38 ± 10.43 and 122.8 ± 63.11 h) allowed less time in NO-EPP patients to receive units of blood notwithstanding a supposed higher transfusion requirement. The higher survival rate in the acute phase in EPP patients increased the risk of late multiple organ failure: two patients of this group died respectively after 43 and 53 days from injury while NO-EPP patients did not show any late mortality. This observation explains also why EPP did not reduce the mean ICU-LOS in this group.

This study presents several weaknesses. First, it is a retrospective analysis of data retrieved from a Trauma Registry. However, all patients have been prospectively included in the Registry and received two types of standardized treatments, which were compared.

Second, an inherent bias may be due to the introduction of a new technique, which can lead to a more efficient practice of this regimen.

Third, the long study period and changes in transfusion protocol represent a bias in the evaluation of EPP efficacy. However EPP is highly effective on systolic blood pressure and has an unquestionable role in this clinical series on early hemodynamic stabilization, before the effects of hemostatic resuscitation.

Finally, although the study included a small population, the patients were highly representative of the optimal treatment of pelvic hemorrhage. By using the Propensity Score Analysis we were able to match for principal confounder factors, obtaining a statistical significant result.

Conclusions

Our data suggest that EPP is a safe and quick procedure, that can be easily performed in different hospital settings.

It can significantly decrease the mortality from hemorrhagic shock in pelvis fractures when used in combination with other emergency room and damage control resuscitation strategies.

In view of its immediate hemodynamic effect, EPP should be considered particularly in highly hypotensive patients, not responding to pelvic binder and initial resuscitation.

Increased awareness and training in techniques of emergency hemodynamic stabilization, such as pelvic binder compression, external fixation and EPP, will greatly improve the standard of treatment and care of patients affected by complex pelvic fractures.

Abbreviations

AE, angio-embolization; AIS, Abbreviated injury scale; APC, anterior posterior compression; CM, combined mechanical; CT, computed tomography; DCL, damage control laparotomy; EPP, extra peritoneal pelvic packing; FAST, focused abdominal sonography for trauma; FFP, fresh frozen plasma; ICU-LOS, intensive care unit-lenght of stay; ISS, Injury severity score; LC, lateral compression; OIS, Organ injury scale; PLT, platelets; PRBC, packed red blod cell; PSA, Propensity Score Analysis; TXA, tranexamic acid; VS, vertical shear.

Authors' contributions

OC and SC: design and drafting of manuscript. EdF, AM, FS: data retrieval and elaboration. MB and LP: statistical analysis. All authors read and approved the final manuscript.

Competing interests

The authors declare that they have no competing interests.

Author details

[1]SC Trauma Team, Niguarda Trauma Center, Ospedale Niguarda Ca' Granda Milano, Milano, Italy. [2]SC Quality Assessment Service, Ospedale Niguarda Ca' Granda Milano, Milano, Italy. [3]Trauma Team Ospedale Niguarda, Piazza Ospedale Maggiore 3, Milano 20162, Italy.

References

1. White CE, Hsu JR, Holcomb JB. Hemodynamically unstable pelvic fracture. Injury. 2009;40:1023–30.
2. Stein DM, O'Toole R, Scalea TM. Multidisciplinary approach for patients with pelvic fractures and hemodynamic instability. Scand J Surg. 2007;96:272–80.
3. Stahel PF, Mauffrey C, Smith WD, McKean J, Hao J, Burlew CC, et al. External fixation for acute pelvic ring injuries: Decision making and technical options. J Trauma Acute Care Surg. 2013;75(5):882–7.
4. Lustemberg T, Wutzler S, Stormann P, Laurer H, Marzi I. The role of angio-embolization in the acute treatment concept of severe pelvic injuries. Injury. 2015;46S4:S33–8.
5. Costantini TW, Bosarge PL, Fortlage D, Bansal V, Coimbra R. Arterial embolization for pelvic fractures after blunt trauma: are we all talk? Am J Surg. 2010;200:752–58.
6. Pohlmann T, Gansslen A, Bosch U, Tscherne H. The technique of packing for control of hemorrhage in complex pelvis frac- tures. Tech Orthop. 1995;9: 267–70.
7. Ertel W, Keel M, Eid K, Platz A, Trentz O. Control of severe hemorrhage using C-clamp and pelvic packing in multiply injured patients with pelvic ring disruption. J Orthop Trauma. 2001;15:468–74.
8. Magnone S, Coccolini F, Manfredi R, Piazzalunga D, Agazzi R, Arici C, Barozzi M, Bellanova G, Belluati A, Berlot G, et al. Management of hemodynamically unstable pelvic trauma: results of the first Italian consensus conference. World J Emerg Surg. 2014;9:18–26. doi:10.1186/1749-7922-9-18.
9. Cothren CC, Osborn PM, Moore EE, Morgan SJ, Johnson JL, Smith WR. Preperitoneal packing for hemodynamically unstable pelvic fractures: a paradigm shift. J Trauma. 2007;62:834–42.
10. Ron G, Epstein D, Ben-Galim P, Klein Y, Kaban A, Sagiv S. Extra-peritoneal pressure packing without external pelvic fixation: A life-saving standing-alone surgical treatment. J Emerg Trauma Shock. 2015;8(4):181–7.
11. Adamina M, Guller U, Weber WP, Oertli D. Propensity scores and the surgeon. British J Surg. 2006;93:389–94.

12. Tile M. Acute pelvic fracture I: causation and classification. J Am Acad Orthop Surg. 1996;4:143–6.
13. Young JWR, Burgess AR, Brumback RJ, et al. Pelvic fractures: value of plain radiography in early assessment and management. Radiology. 1986;160:445.
14. Kashuk JL, Moore EE, Sawyer M, Le T, Johnson J, Biffl WL, et al. Postinjury coagulopathy management. Ann Surg. 2010;251:604–14.
15. Mauffrey C, Cuellar III DO, Pieracci F, Hak DJ, Hammerberg EM, Stahel PF, et al. Strategies for the management of haemorrhage following pelvic fractures and associated trauma-induced coagulopathy. Bone Joint J. 2014; 96-B:1143–54.
16. CRASH-2 collaborators, Roberts I, Shakur H, Afolabi A, et al. The importance of early treatment with tranexamic acid in bleeding trauma patients: an exploratory analysis of the CRSAH-2 randomized controlled trial. Lancet. 2011;377:1096–101.
17. Prasarn ML, Horodyski M, Conrad B, Rubery PT, DuBose D, Small J, et al. Comparison of external fixation versus the trauma pelvic orthotic device on unstable pelvic injury: a cadaveric study of stability. J Trauma Acute Care Surg. 2012;72:1671–5.
18. Knops SP, Schep NWL, Spoore CW, VanRiel MPJM, Spanjesberg WR, Kleinrensink GJ, et al. Comparison of three different pelvic circumferential compression devices: a biomechanical cadaver study. J Bone Joint Surg Am. 2011;93:230–40.
19. Osborn PM, Smith WR, Moore EE, Cothren CC, Morgan SJ, Williams AE, Stahel PF. Direct retroperitoneal pelvic packing versus pelvic angiography. A comparison of two management protocols for hemodynamically unstable pelvic fractures. Injury. 2009;40:54–60.
20. Papakostidis C, Giannoudis PV. Pelvic ring injuries with hemodynamic instability: efficacy of pelvic packing, a systematic review. Injury. 2009;40:S53–61.
21. Suzuki T, Smith WR, Moore EE. Pelvic packing or angiography: competitive or complementary? Injury. 2009;40:343–53.
22. Tai DK, Li WH, Lee KY, Cheng M, Lee KB, Tang LF, Lai AK, Ho HF, Cheung MT. Retroperitoneal pelvic packing in the management of hemodynamically unstable pelvic fractures: a level I trauma center experience. J Trauma. 2011; 71:E79–86.
23. Burlew CC, Moore EE, Smith WR, Johnson JL, Biffl WL, Barnett CC, Stahel PF. Preperitoneal pelvic packing/external fixation with secondary angioembolization: optimal care for life-threatening hemorrhage from unstable pelvic fractures. J Am Coll Surg. 2011;212:628–35.
24. Cullinane DC, Shiller HJ, Zielinski MD, Bilaniuk JW, Collier BR, Como J, Holevar M, Sabater EA, Sems SA, Vassy WM, et al. Easter Association for the Surgery of Trauma practice management guidelines for hemorrhage in pelvic fracture-update and systematic review. J Trauma. 2011;71:329–38.
25. Marzi I, Lustenberger T. Management of bleeding pelvic fractures. Scand J Surg. 2014;103:104–11.
26. Jang JY, Shim H, Jung PY, Kim S, Bae KS. Preperitoneal pelvic packing in patients with hemodynamic instability due to severe pelvic fracture:early experience in a Korean trauma center. Scand J Trauma Resusc Emerg Med. 2016;24:3–7.
27. Metcalfe AJ, Davies K, Ramesh B, O'Kelly A, Rajagopal R. Hemorrhage control in pelvic fractures. A survey of surgical capabilities. Injury. 2011;42:1008–11.
28. Rosenbaum PR, Rubin DB. The central role of propensity score in observational studies for causal effects. Biometrics. 1983;70:41–55.
29. Braitman LE, Rosenbaum PR. Rare outcomes, common treatments: analytic strategies using propensity scores. Ann Intern Med. 2002;137:693–5.
30. Spahn DR, Cerny V, Coats TJ, Duranteau J, Fernandez-Mondejar E, et al. Management of bleeding following major trauma. A European guideline. Crit Care. 2007;11:R17. doi:10.1186/cc5686.

Thoracoscopic removal of dental prosthesis impacted in the upper thoracic esophagus

Luigi Bonavina*, Alberto Aiolfi, Stefano Siboni and Emanuele Rausa

Abstract

Dental appliances are the most common cause of accidental foreign body esophageal impaction, especially in the elderly population with decreased oral sensory perception. A 47-year-old man with history of oligophrenia and recurrent epileptic seizures was referred to our hospital following dislocation and ingestion of his upper dental prosthesis. Endoscopic removal and clipping of an esophageal tear had been unsuccessfully attempted. A chest CT scan confirmed entrapment of the dental prosthesis in the upper thoracic esophagus, the presence of pneumomediastinum, and the close proximity of one of the metal clasps of the prosthesis to the left subclavian artery. A video-assisted right thoracoscopy in the left lateral decubitus position was performed and the foreign body was successfully removed. The patient was then allowed to wear the retrieved prosthesis after dentistry consultation and repair of the wire clasps by a dental technician. At the 6-month follow-up visit the patient was doing very well without any trouble in swallowing.

Keywords: Esophagus, Esophageal perforation, Dental prosthesis, Thoracoscopy

Introduction

Accidental ingestion of foreign bodies is frequent in adult individuals with mental retardation or psychiatric disorders. Most of the little ingested foreign bodies pass the gastrointestinal tract without consequences. However, 10-20% of the patients may require endoscopic removal, and 1% or less may require surgery due to entrapment of the foreign body in the cervical (57%), thoracic (26%), or distal (17%) esophagus [1]. Dental appliances are the most common cause of accidental foreign body esophageal impaction, especially in the elderly population with decreased oral sensory perception [2]. The large size, sharp edges, and metal clasps of dental prostheses make endoscopic removal unsafe and carry a high risk of perforation in such circumstances. We present a case of successful thoracoscopic removal of dental prosthesis impacted in the upper thoracic esophagus.

Case report

A 47-year-old man with history of oligophrenia and recurrent epileptic seizures was referred to our hospital 3 days after dislocation and ingestion of his upper dental prosthesis. Before patient's referral, multiple flexible endoscopic attempts had been unsuccessfully performed, the last one leading to an intramural perforation partially repaired with endoclips. The patient's main complaints were dysphagia, odynophagia, and hypersalivation. He was afebrile, with normal leucocyte count, and slight elevation of C-reactive protein. Broad-spectrum antibiotic therapy (piperacillin + tazobactam) was started upon hospital admission. The physical examination did not reveal subcutaneous emphysema. A gastrografin swallow study showed extravasation of contrast at the level of the upper thoracic esophagus; a chest CT scan confirmed the presence of pneumomediastinum and the close proximity of one of the metal clasps of the prosthesis to the left subclavian artery (Figure 1A-B).

A video-assisted right thoracoscopy in the left lateral decubitus position was performed to remove the foreign body. Three ports were used: 10 mm optical port in the 6th intercostal space, 10 mm port in the 5th intercostal space, and 5 mm port in the 4th intercostal space, and. The exploration of the right chest showed a bulging of the upper mediastinal compartment above the confluence of the azygos vein into the superior vena cava (Figure 1C). There was no pleural contamination. After incision of the

* Correspondence: luigi.bonavina@unimi.it
Department of Biomedical Sciences for Health, Division of General Surgery, University of Milano Medical School, IRCCS Policlinico San Donato, Via Morandi 30, 20097, San Donato Milanese, (Milano), Italy

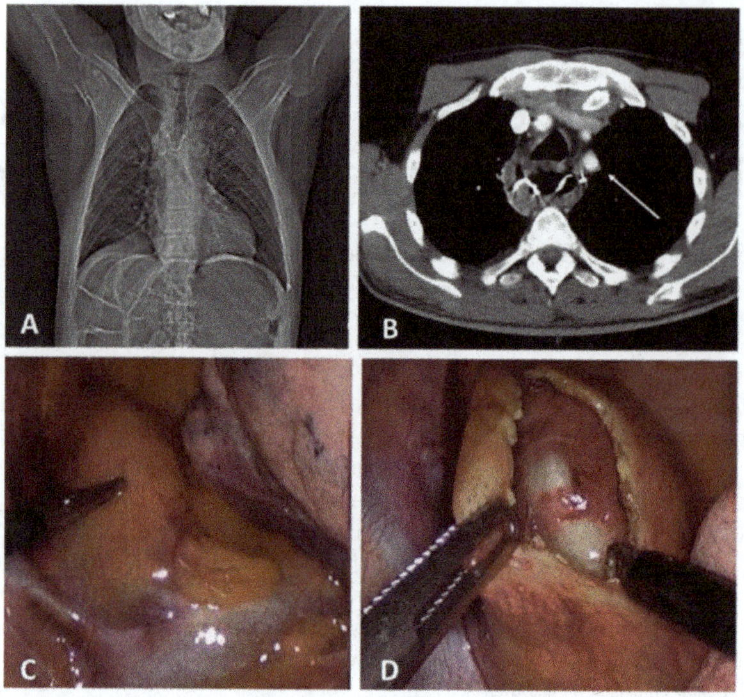

Figure 1 Appearance of the dental prosthesis at CT scan (A-B), and thoracoscopic exposure of the upper thoracic esophagus (C-D).

thickened mediastinal pleura (Figure 1 D), transillumination with a standard endoscope confirmed the site of impaction and the previous perforation. The esophagus was opened longitudinally for approximately 4 cm and the prosthesis (five dental elements with three metal clasps) was removed under direct endoscopic and thoracoscopic view using an endograsper (Figure 2A-B), and enveloped in a plastic bag. The edges of the esophagomyotomy appeared vital. The esophageal wound was closed with a double-layer running suture of Polydioxanone 3–0 including the mucosa and the muscle layers, and tested for air-leakage (Figure 2C-D). The mediastinal pleura was then approximated with a running suture. The plastic bag containing the dental prosthesis was removed from the anterior trocar site by slightly enlarging the incision. The postoperative course was uneventful. A gastrographin swallow study performed on postoperative day 3 showed a regular esophageal transit and the absence of leaks. The patient was then allowed to wear the retrieved prosthesis after repair of the wire clasps by a dental technician and dentistry consultation. He was discharged well from the hospital on postoperative day 8 on a free diet. At the 6-month follow-up visit the patient was doing very well without any complaint in swallowing.

Discussion

The frequency of removable dental prostheses among adults varies between 13 and 29% in Europe, with 3-13% of edentulous subjects wearing complete dentures in both jaws; interestingly, there is a trend towards an increasing use of removable partial dentures [3]. It is therefore reasonable to estimate that, with the growth of the denture-wearing population, the incidence of impacted dentures in the esophagus may increase in the future. Impacted dental prostheses in the esophagus can result in life-threatening conditions such as mediastinitis, pleural empyema, and aortoesophageal fistula [4]. The risk of severe complications is higher in patients with a delayed diagnosis and treatment, since long-standing impaction can lead to mucosal ulceration, transmural inflammation, esophageal perforation, and sepsis.

The diagnosis of denture impaction in the esophagus may be challenging in patients with mental disorders who may be unable to give a reliable medical history. Since dentures are made of acrylic resin, which is radiolucent, the patient work-up should routinely include a chest X-ray, a gastrografin swallow study, a computed tomography, and an upper endoscopy. These investigations are essential to define the anatomical site of impaction and the size, shape, and number of wire clasps of the prosthesis.

Attempts at endoscopic removal of the dental prosthesis may cause intramural perforation or a full-thickness tear due to the possible entrapment of the wire hooks in the esophageal wall. Esophagotomy through a right thoracotomy remains the safest therapeutic approach when the impaction occurs in the upper thoracic esophagus. Video-assisted thoracoscopy, either in the left lateral or prone decubitus position, allows a safe and minimally invasive

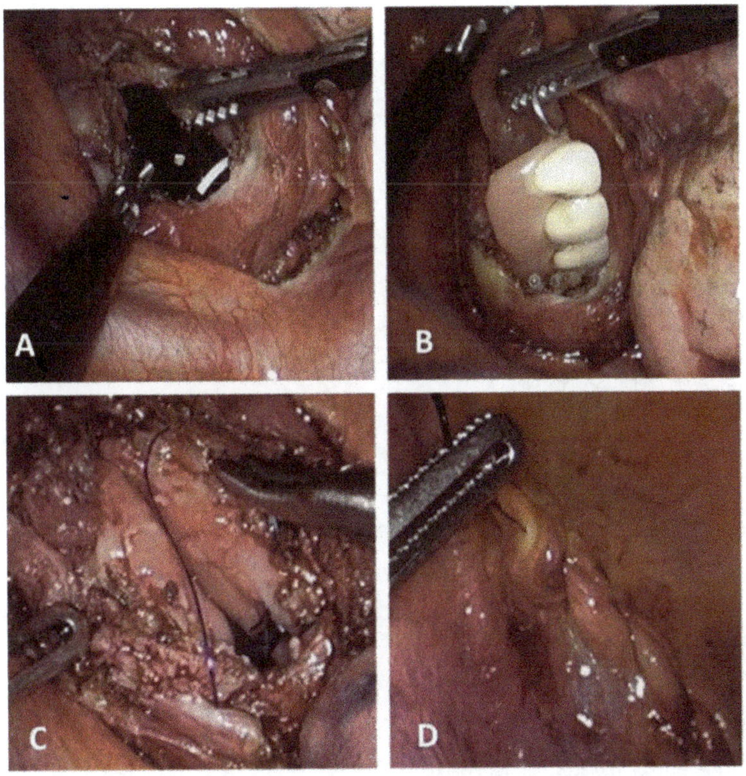

Figure 2 **Esophagotomy (A), removal of the dental prosthesis (B), and suture of the esophageal wall and mediastinal pleura (C-D).**

retrieval of the dental prosthesis followed by primary esophageal suture when there is no major pleural contamination and the edges of the esophagomyotomy appear vital. In the literature, a few cases of thoracoscopic removal of ingested foreign bodies have been reported; three of the 6 patients required an esophagotomy due to an impacted denture (Table 1). In our patient, thoracoscopic removal was successfully performed after previous failed endoscopic procedures complicated by intramural perforation. Exposure of the upper thoracic esophagus was possible without the need to divide the arch of the azygos vein.

Based on our experience and the available literature we conclude that thoracoscopic esophagotomy represents a safe and effective treatment for patients with impacted dentures in the esophagus. Multiple attempts at flexible and rigid esophagoscopy should definitely be abandoned in such patients, especially when a dental prosthesis has passed the cricophageal sphincter. Education and close follow-up of patients wearing removable dental prostheses is critical to prevent accidental impaction in the esophagus and the dangerous sequelae of esophageal perforation.

Table 1 Thoracoscopic management of ingested esophageal foreign bodies in adults: literature review

Author	Year	Description	Surgical approach	Operative decubitus	Treatment	Outcome
Davies B. [5]	2004	China cup fragment migrated in the mediastinum, with abscess	Right-side thoracoscopy (3-port access)	NS	Foreign body removal and abscess drainage	Good
Palanivelu C. [6]	2008	Impacted denture	Right-side thoracoscopy (3-port access)	Prone	Esophagotomy, foreign body removal and suture	Good
Rückbeil O. [7]	2009	Metallic needle migrated in the mediastinum	Right-side thoracoscopy (3- port access)	Left lateral	Foreign body removal	Good
Dalvi AN [8]	2010	Impacted denture	Right-side thoracoscopy (4-port access)	Left lateral	Esophagotomy, foreign body removal and suture	Good
Fujino K. [9]	2012	Fish bone migrated to lung	Right-side thoracoscopy (NS)	NS	Foreign body removal	Good
Present case	2013	Impacted denture	Right-side thoracoscopy (3-port access)	Left lateral	Esophagotomy, foreign body removal and suture	Good

(NS: non specified).

Competing interests

The authors declare that they have no competing interests.

Authors' contributions

LB designed and wrote the manuscript, AA, SS, and ER contributed to data collection and manuscript drafting. All authors read and approved the final manuscript.

References

1. Athanassiadi K, Gerazounis M, Metaxas E, Kalantzi N: **Management of esophageal foreign bodies: a retrospective review of 400 cases.** *Eur J Cardiothorac Surg* 2002, **21**:653–6.
2. Nwaorgu OG, Onakoya PA, Sogebi OA, Kokong DD, Dosumu OO: **Esophageal impacted dentures.** *J Natl Med Assoc* 2004, **96**:1350–53.
3. Zitzmann NU, Hagmann E, Weiger R: **What is the prevalence of various types of prosthetic dental restorations in Europe?** *Clin Oral Implants Res* 2007, **18**(Suppl 3):20–33.
4. Von Rahden BHA, Feith M, Dittler HJ, Stein HJ: **Cervical esophageal perforation with severe mediastinitis due to an impacted dental prosthesis.** *Dis Esoph* 2002, **15**:340–344.
5. Davies B, Black E, Vaughan R: **Thoracoscopic drainage of and foreign body removal from a posterior mediastinal abscess.** *Eur J Cardiothorac Surg* 2004, **25**(5):897–8.
6. Palanivelu C, Rangarajan M, Parthasarathi R, Senthilnathan P: **Thoracoscopic retrieval of a "smiling" foreign body from the proximal esophagus.** *Surg Laparosc Endosc Percutan Tech* 2008, **18**:325–328.
7. Ruckbeil O, Burghardt J, Gellert K: **Thoracoscopic removal of a transesophageal ingested mediastinal foreign body.** *Interact Cardiovasc Thorac Surg* 2009, **9**(3):556–7.
8. Dalvi AN, Thapar VK, Jagtap S, Barve DJ, *et al*: **Thoracoscopic removal of impacted denture: report of a case with review of literature.** *J Minim Access Surg* 2010, **6**(4):119–21.
9. Fujino K, Mori T, Yoshimoto K, Ikeda K, *et al*: **Esophageal fish bone migrating to the lung: report of a case.** *Kyobu Geka* 2012, **65**(10):5–922.

9

WSES Jerusalem guidelines for diagnosis and treatment of acute appendicitis

Salomone Di Saverio[1*], Arianna Birindelli[2], Micheal D. Kelly[3], Fausto Catena[4], Dieter G. Weber[5], Massimo Sartelli[6], Michael Sugrue[7], Mark De Moya[8], Carlos Augusto Gomes[9], Aneel Bhangu[10], Ferdinando Agresta[11], Ernest E. Moore[12], Kjetil Soreide[13], Ewen Griffiths[14], Steve De Castro[15], Jeffry Kashuk[16], Yoram Kluger[17], Ari Leppaniemi[18], Luca Ansaloni[19], Manne Andersson[20], Federico Coccolini[19], Raul Coimbra[21], Kurinchi S. Gurusamy[22], Fabio Cesare Campanile[23], Walter Biffl[24], Osvaldo Chiara[25], Fred Moore[26], Andrew B. Peitzman[27], Gustavo P. Fraga[28], David Costa[29], Ronald V. Maier[30], Sandro Rizoli[31], Zsolt J Balogh[32], Cino Bendinelli[32], Roberto Cirocchi[33], Valeria Tonini[2], Alice Piccinini[34], Gregorio Tugnoli[34], Elio Jovine[35], Roberto Persiani[36], Antonio Biondi[37], Thomas Scalea[38], Philip Stahel[12], Rao Ivatury[39], George Velmahos[40] and Roland Andersson[20]

Abstract

Acute appendicitis (AA) is among the most common cause of acute abdominal pain. Diagnosis of AA is challenging; a variable combination of clinical signs and symptoms has been used together with laboratory findings in several scoring systems proposed for suggesting the probability of AA and the possible subsequent management pathway. The role of imaging in the diagnosis of AA is still debated, with variable use of US, CT and MRI in different settings worldwide. Up to date, comprehensive clinical guidelines for diagnosis and management of AA have never been issued. In July 2015, during the 3rd World Congress of the WSES, held in Jerusalem (Israel), a panel of experts including an Organizational Committee and Scientific Committee and Scientific Secretariat, participated to a Consensus Conference where eight panelists presented a number of statements developed for each of the eight main questions about diagnosis and management of AA. The statements were then voted, eventually modified and finally approved by the participants to The Consensus Conference and lately by the board of co-authors. The current paper is reporting the definitive Guidelines Statements on each of the following topics: 1) Diagnostic efficiency of clinical scoring systems, 2) Role of Imaging, 3) Non-operative treatment for uncomplicated appendicitis, 4) Timing of appendectomy and in-hospital delay, 5) Surgical treatment 6) Scoring systems for intra-operative grading of appendicitis and their clinical usefulness 7) Non-surgical treatment for complicated appendicitis: abscess or phlegmon 8) Pre-operative and post-operative antibiotics.

Keywords: Acute Appendicitis, Guidelines, Consensus Conference, Alvarado Score, Appendicitis diagnosis score, Non-operative management, Antibiotics, Complicated appendicitis, Appendectomy, Laparoscopic appendectomy, Phlegmon, Appendiceal abscess

* Correspondence: salo75@inwind.it; salomone.disaverio@gmail.com
[1]Emergency and Trauma Surgery – Maggiore Hospital, AUSL, Bologna, Italy
Full list of author information is available at the end of the article

Background

Acute appendicitis (AA) is a common cause of acute abdominal pain, which can progress to perforation and peritonitis, associated with morbidity and mortality. The lifetime risk of appendicitis is 8.6 % for males and 6.7 % for females; however, the risk of undergoing appendectomy is much lower for males than for females (12 vs. 23 %) and it occurs most often between the ages of 10 and 30, with a male:female ratio of approximately 1.4:1 [1]. Despite numerous studies on AA, many unresolved issues remain, including aetiology and treatment. The diagnosis of AA is a constellation of history, physical examination coupled with laboratory investigations, supplemented by selective focused imaging. These can be used in combination in scoring systems. Various clinical scoring systems have been proposed in order to predict AA with certainty, but none has been widely accepted. The role of diagnostic imaging (ultrasound (US), computed tomography (CT) or magnetic resonance imaging (MRI)) is another major controversy.

The surgical treatment of AA has undergone a paradigm shift from open appendectomy to laparoscopic appendectomy, both in adults and now also in paediatric cases. Over the last decade non-operative treatment with antibiotics has been proposed as an alternative to surgery in uncomplicated cases [2], while the non-surgical treatment played an important role in the management of complicated appendicitis with phlegmon or abscess [3]. Another major issue in management still open to debate is the timing of appendectomy and the safety of in-hospital delay. Moreover, there are debated recommendations on the type of surgical treatment and the post-operative management including antibiotic therapy.

For these reasons the World Society of Emergency Surgery (WSES) decided to convene a Consensus Conference (CC) to study the topic and define its guidelines regarding diagnosis and treatment of AA.

Material and methods: organizational model

On August 2013 the Organizational Board of the 2nd World Congress of the World Society of Emergency Surgery (WSES) endorsed its president to organize the Consensus Conference (CC) on AA in order to develop WSES Guidelines on this topic. The WSES President appointed four members to a Scientific Secretariat, eight members to an Organizational Committee and eight members to a Scientific Committee, choosing them from the expert affiliates of the Society. Eight key questions on the diagnosis and treatment of AA were developed in order to guide analysis of the literature and subsequent discussion of the topic (Table 1). Under the supervision of the Scientific Secretariat, a bibliographic search related to these questions was performed through April 2015 without time or language restriction. The key words used for the electronic search are listed in Table 1. Additionally a manual literature search was performed by each of the members of the working groups involved in the analysis of the above-mentioned eight questions. Prior to the Consensus Conference, a number of statements were developed for each of the main questions, along with the Level of Evidence (LoE) and the Grade of Recommendation (GoR) for each statement. The 2011 Oxford Classification was used to grade the LoE and GoR. Provisional statements and their supporting evidence were then submitted for review to all the participating members of the Consensus Conference and to the WSES board members by email before the Conference. Modifications were performed when necessary based on feedback.

The Consensus Conference on AA was held in Jerusalem, Israel, on July 6th, 2015 during the 3rd World Congress of the WSES. During the first part of this CC, a member of each group (S. Di Saverio, M.D. Kelly, D. Weber, F. Catena, M. Sugrue, M. Sartelli, M. De Moya, C.A. Gomes) presented each of the statements along with LoE, GoR, and the literature supporting each statement. Each statement was then voted upon by the audience in terms of "agree" or "disagree" using an electronic voting system. The percentage of agreement was recorded immediately; in case of greater than 30 % disagreement, the statement was modified after discussion. Furthermore, comments for each statement were collected in all cases. Before the second part of the Consensus Conference, the president and representatives from the Organizational Committee, Scientific Committee and Scientific Secretariat modified the statements according to the findings of the first session of the CC. The revised statements were then presented again to the audience. During the Consensus Conference, a comprehensive algorithm for the treatment of AA was developed based on the results of the first session of the CC and voted upon for definitive approval (Fig. 1). The final statements, along with their LoE and GoR, are available in Appendix. All statements are reported in the following Results section, subdivided by each of the eight questions, with the relative discussion and supportive evidence.

Results

Diagnostic efficiency of clinical scoring systems

Diagnostic efficiency of clinical scoring systems and their role in the management of patients with suspected appendicitis - can they be used as basis for a structured management?(Speaker in Jerusalem CC Dr. D. G. Weber)

Multiple diagnostic scoring systems have been developed with the aim to provide clinical probabilities that a patient has acute appendicitis. These scores typically incorporate clinical features of the history and physical examination, and laboratory parameters. Most popular

Table 1 Key questions and key words used to develop the Consensus Conference on Acute Appendicitis (AA)

Key questions	Key words
1. Diagnostic efficiency of clinical scoring systems *Diagnostic efficiency of clinical scoring systems and their role in the management of patients with suspected appendicitis - can they be used as basis for a structured management?*	Derivation OR clinical OR predict OR decision AND rule OR algorithm OR tool OR model OR score OR indicator OR validation OR criteria AND appendicitis
2. Role of imaging *Routine vs selective imaging? CT or US or both? In what order?*	Diagnosis OR imaging AND selective OR routine AND ultrasound OR computed AND tomography OR US OR CT OR MRI AND adult OR child OR pregnant AND appendicitis
3. Non-operative treatment for uncomplicated appendicitis. *What is the natural history of appendicitis? Can appendicitis resolve without treatment? How common is it?*	Uncomplicated AND appendicitis AND pathogenesis OR antibiotics OR nonoperative OR conservative OR spontaneous AND resolution or self-limiting AND treatment OR management
4. Timing of appendectomy and in-hospital delay *Does in-hospital delay increasethe rate of complication or perforation? Is it safe to delay appendectomy? Timing of appendectomy*	Appendectomy AND delay OR perforation OR complication OR indicator OR criteria AND appendicitis
5. Surgical treatment *-open or laparoscopic?* *-lavage or aspiration of pus?* *-drains?* *-ligation or invagination of the stump?* *-primary or secondary closure of the wound?*	Surgery OR operative OR laparoscopy OR open OR treatment OR management AND elder OR comorbidities OR obese OR child OR pregnant AND complicated OR perforated OR abscess AND lavage OR aspiration OR suction OR drain OR mesoappendix OR sealing OR monopolar OR bipolar OR staple OR endoloop OR stump OR invagination OR ligation AND appendicitis
6. Scoring systems for intra-operative grading of appendicitis and their clinical usefulness *What are the histopathological criteria for appendicitis of clinical importance? Minor inflammatory changes, early appendicitis, catarrhal appendicitis. The criteria used will have an influence on the proportion of negative appendectomy, and also on evaluation of diagnostic performance.*	intra-operative AND grade OR score OR indicator OR criteria AND histopathology OR macroscopic AND diagnosis OR surgeon AND experience AND appendicitis
7. Non-surgical treatment of complicated appendicitis: abscess or phlegmone *Role of percutaneous drainage and Interval Appendectomy or immediate surgery.*	Abscess OR phlegmon AND drain OR percutaneous OR interval AND appendectomy AND conservative OR nonsurgical AND treatment OR management AND complicated AND appendicitis
8. Preoperative and Postoperative Antibiotics *Should Preoperative antibiotics prophylaxis be given? What antibiotics? When should postoperative antibiotics be given? What antibiotics? Duration?*	Antibiotic OR antimicrobial OR infection OR prophylaxis OR therapy OR treatment AND appendectomy OR surgery AND time OR day OR range OR duration AND complicated OR uncomplicated AND intravenous OR oral AND appendicitis

and validated examples include the Alvarado score (also known as the MANTRELS score) [4], the Paediatric Appendicitis Score (PAS) [5], the Appendicitis Inflammatory Response (AIR) Score [6], the Raja Isteri Pengiran Anak Saleha Appendicitis (RIPASA) score [7] and, most recently, the Adult Appendicitis Score (AAS) [8]. A comparison among these clinical scores is reported in Table 2. Alvarado and AIR scores are currently the most often used scores in the clinical settings. The primary data from which these scores have been derived are largely from retrospective and prospective cross-sectional studies, and represent either level 2 or 3 evidence.

More recently, attempts have been made to incorporate imaging findings into diagnostic scoring systems. Atema et al.[9] described a scoring system that successfully distinguished complicated from uncomplicated acute appendicitis, reporting a negative predictive value of 94.7 % (in correctly identifying patients with uncomplicated disease). A diagnostic scoring system that incorporates imaging to the primary clinical diagnosis of acute appendicitis has not yet been developed [10].

The Alvarado score is the most extensively studied score (though this statement is biased by time; the Alvarado score has been around much longer than some of the newer scores, e.g. the AAS). Its validity has been summarised in a recent meta-analysis [11] including 5960 patients in 29 studies. According to Ohle et al., the score's performance is dependent on the cut-off value: a

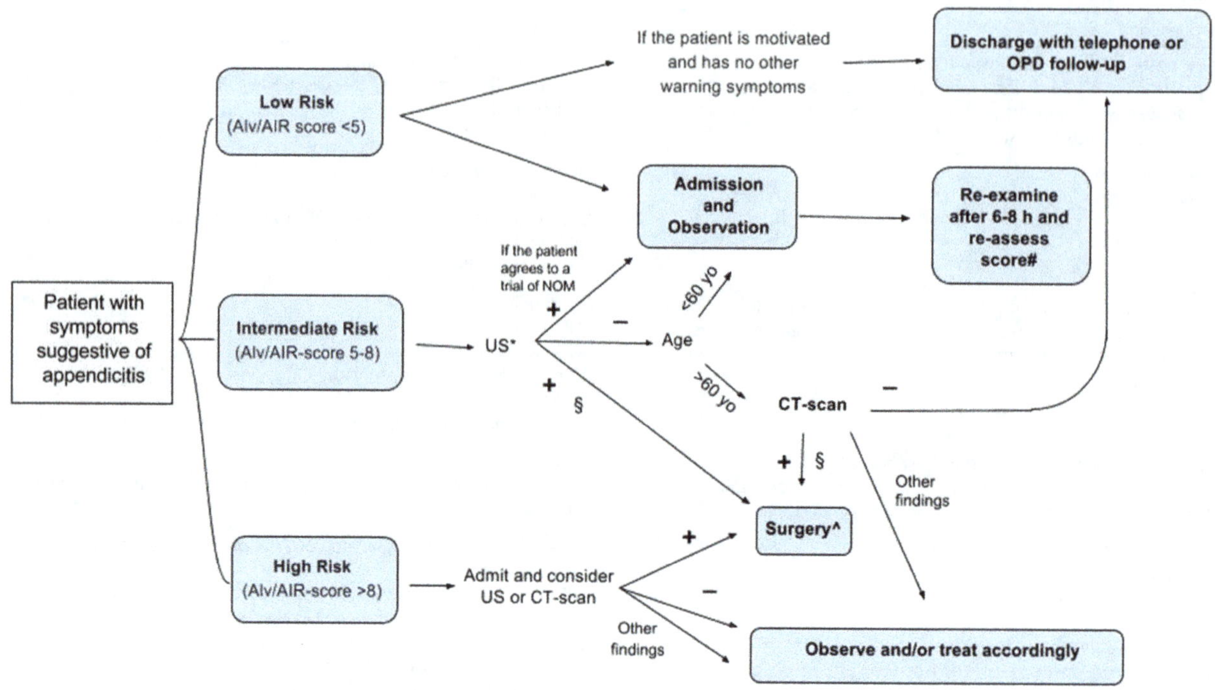

** If possible US Standard reporting templates for ultrasound and US 3 step sequential positioning; consider routine use of CT scan upon setting (e.g. USA) for Intermediate risk group; consider further imaging (US or CT) by carefully weighing risks/benefits of radiation exposure in low risk group*

 # If no improvements after observation and re-assessment, consider CT scan

§ Consider NOM + antibiotics in patients with severe comorbidities and high anesthesiological risk

^ Surgery is meant as Acute Appendectomy. In case of finding of abscess or phlegmon on US/CT, consider percutaneous drainage if interventional radiology is available.

Fig. 1 Practical WSES algorithm for diagnosis and treatment of patients with suspected acute appendicitis

clinical cut-off score of less than five can be applied to 'rule out' appendicitis with a sensitivity of 99 % (95 % CI 97 – 99 %) and a specificity of 43 % (36 – 51 %), while a cut-off score of less than seven results in a sensitivity of 82 % (76 – 86 %) and a specificity of 81 % (76–85 %), suggesting it is not sufficiently accurate to rule in or rule out surgery. Individual validation studies occasionally reported lower sensitivity, questioning the ability of the Alvarado score to reliably exclude appendicitis with a cut-off score of less than five [12, 13]. However, these concerns are not supported by the pooled meta-analysis of those data [11].

The Appendicitis Inflammatory Response (AIR) score has been proposed in 2008 by Andersson [6] and is based on eight variables, including C-reactive protein (CRP). The AIR score showed a significant better discriminating capacity when compared with the Alvarado score, with a ROC area of 0.97 vs. 0.92 for advanced appendicitis ($p = 0.0027$) and 0.93 vs. 0.88 for all appendicitis ($p = 0.0007$). According to the score, two cut-off points were identified to obtain three diagnostic test zones: a score <4 (low probability) has a high sensitivity (0.96) for appendicitis and can be used to rule out appendicitis; a score between five and eight identifies the intermediate probability patients, that require observation and eventual further investigations; a score >8 (high probability) has a high specificity (0.99) for appendicitis and can be used to rule in appendicitis. The AIR score has been also externally validated (ROC AIR 0.96 vs. Alvarado 0.82 $p < 0.001$) [14], especially in the high-risk patients, where a higher specificity and positive predictive value than the Alvarado score (97 vs. 76 % $p < 0.05$ and 88 vs. 65 % $p < 0.05$, respectively) has been reported [15]. The AIR score has demonstrated to be useful in guiding decision-making to reduce admissions, optimize utility of diagnostic imaging and prevent negative explorations [16].

Diagnostic scoring systems may perform differently in adult and paediatric patients. In fact, at a practical level, several of the predictor variables may be difficult to apply (e.g. asking an infant to describe migratory pain). The definition of a paediatric patient was not standardised among the studies, or clearly defined in the meta-analysis. Another systematic review compared the Alvarado score with the Paediatric Appendicitis Score, favouring the former [17].

Table 2 Comparison of the most popular and validated clinical scores for the diagnosis of AA

	Alvarado score[a]	AIR score[b]	PAS score[c]	RIPASA score[d]	AAS score[e]
Vomiting		1			
Nausea or vomiting	1		1	1	
Anorexia	1		1	1	
Pain in RIF[f]	2	1		0.5	2
Migration of pain to the RIF[f]	1		1	0.5	2
Rovsing's sign				2	
RIF[g] tenderness			2	1	
Women >50 years or men (any age)					3
Women <50 years					1
Rebound tenderness or muscular defense/guarding	1			1 + 2	
Light		1			2
Medium		2			4
Strong		3			4
Body temperature					
> 37.5 °C	1		1		
> 38.5 °C		1			
> 37– <39 °C				1	
WBC (white blood cell) count					
> 10.0 × 10⁹/l	2		1	1	
10.0–14.9 × 10⁹/l		1			
≥ 15.0 × 10⁹/l		2			
≥ .2 and <10.9 × 10⁹/l					1
≥ 10.9 and <14.0 × 10⁹/l					2
≥ 14.0 × 10⁹/l					3
Leukocytosis shift	1				
Polymorphonuclear leukocytes					
70–84 %		1			
≥ 75 %			1		
≥ 85 %		2			
≥ 62 % and < 75 %					2
≥ 75 % and < 83 %					3
≥ 83 %					4
CRP (C-reactive protein) concentration					
10–49 mg/l		1			
≥ 50 mg/l		2			
Symptoms <24 h and CRP (C-reactive protein) concentration					
≥ 4 and <11 mg/l					2
≥ 11 and <25 mg/l					3
≥ 25 and <83 mg/l					5
≥ 83 mg/l					1
Symptoms >24 h and CRP (C-reactive protein) concentration					
≥ 12 and <53 mg/l					2
≥ 53 and <152 mg/l					2
≥ 152 mg/l					1

Table 2 Comparison of the most popular and validated clinical scores for the diagnosis of AA *(Continued)*

Coughing/hopping/percussion pain			2		
Gender					
Male				1	
Female				0.5	
Age					
< 40 years				1	
≥ 40 years				0.5	
Duration of symptoms					
< 48 h				1	
> 48 h				0.5	
Negative urinalysis				1	
Total score	10	12	10	16.5	23

[a]Alvarado score: sum 0–4 = not likely appendicitis, sum 5–6 = equivocal, sum 7–8 = probably appendicitis, sum 9–10 = highly likely appendicitis
[b]Acute appendicitis response score (AIR): sum 0–4 = low probability, sum 5–8 = indeterminate group, sum 9–12 = high probability [161]
[c]Pediatric appendicitis score (PAS): ≥6 = appendicitis, ≤5 = observe
[d]Raja Isteri Pengiran Anak Saleha Appendicitis (RIPASA) score
[e]Adult Appendicitis Score (AAS): low risk (0–10 points), intermediate risk (11–15 points), high risk (≥16 points)
[f]*right iliac fossa*

The various derivation and validation studies investigating the different diagnostic scoring systems are troubled by various methodological weaknesses. Firstly, there is often inadequate definition of predictor variables, absence of reproducibility testing of predictor variables [18], lack of blinding and insufficient power [19]. Secondly, with regards to the participants, these studies often only include patients who an appendectomy was subsequently performed and for this reason potentially under-report false negatives. Such studies are questionable as the score is meant to be used on patients with suspicion of appendicitis, before all other diagnostic workup or selection. Thirdly, there is great variability in the study populations' level of appendicitis (ranging between approximately 10 – 80 %); studies with a high rate of disease should demonstrate a higher specificity in their diagnostic scoring system. Regrettably, due to these multiple factors, there is a great deal of heterogeneity among the diagnostic studies used to derive and validate the diagnostic scoring systems described. This heterogeneity, differences in treatment systems, and the fundamental demographic differences in treatment cohorts confound the direct applicability of these clinical studies in other practices.

No data are available to evaluate the ability of the published diagnostic scoring systems to improve clinical outcomes (e.g. length of hospital stay, perforation rate, negative appendectomy rate).

No cost analysis of diagnostic scoring system for the clinical diagnosis of acute appendicitis was identified.

The sensitivity and specificity of the diagnostic scoring systems are inversely related. At the expense of specificity, scoring systems may be given sufficiently sensitive cut-off scores to exclude disease (e.g. Alvarado score < 5). However, none of the current diagnostic scoring systems can reach enough specificity to identify with absolute certainty which patients warrant an appendectomy.

Statement 1.1 The Alvarado score (with cut-off score < 5) is sufficiently sensitive to exclude acute appendicitis. [EL 1, GoR A].

Statement 1.2 The Alvarado score is not sufficiently specific in diagnosing acute appendicitis [EL 1, GoR A].

Statement 1.3 An ideal (high sensitivity and specificity), clinically applicable, diagnostic scoring system/ clinical rule remains outstanding. This remains an area for future research. [EL 1, GoR B]

What is the value of clinical and laboratory findings in patients with suspected appendicitis?

The decision to do additional imaging of a patient with suspected appendicitis is based mainly on the complaints of the patient combined with findings at physical examination. The clinical presentation is, however, seldom typical and diagnostic errors are common. A thorough clinical examination is often stressed as an essential part of diagnosis, with laboratory examinations as an adjunct to the gathered clinical information. The review by Andersson [20] shows that each element of the history and of clinical and laboratory examinations is of weak discriminatory and predictive capacity. However, clinical diagnosis is a synthesis of information obtained from all these sources, and a high discriminatory and predictive power can be achieved by an accurate understanding of the relative importance of variables in combination.

When the values of two or more inflammatory variables found in laboratory are normal, appendicitis is unlikely. Conversely, appendicitis is very likely when the values of two or more inflammatory variables are increased [21]. Laboratory tests of the inflammatory response and the clinical descriptors of peritoneal irritation and migration of pain are the strongest discriminators and should be included in the diagnostic assessment of patients with suspected appendicitis.

Role of imaging

What is the optimum pathway for imaging in patients with suspected acute appendicitis? Routine vs. selective imaging? CT or US or both? In what order?(Speaker in Jerusalem CC Dr. M. Sugrue)

Diagnosis of AA is made by clinical history and physical examination the typical symptoms and laboratory signs may be absent in 20–33 % of patients and, when they are present, can be similar to other conditions, especially in early stage [22, 23] and the diagnosis can be particularly difficult in children, elderly patients, pregnant and childbearing age women.

Although several previous studies have shown discriminant factors in the differential diagnosis of AA and pelvic inflammatory disease (PID) in childbearing age women [24–29], imaging techniques such as US, CT or MRI may be required to reduce the negative appendectomy rate, with a low level of evidence currently available [30, 31]. Occasionally there is a role for diagnostic laparoscopy particularly in younger female patients [32].

In patients older than age 50 years diverticulosis is extremely common in the USA and Europe (about 8.5 % of the population) [33]. Right-sided diverticula occur more often in younger patients than do left-sided diverticula and because patients are young and present with right lower quadrant pain, they are often thought to suffer from acute appendicitis; it is difficult to differentiate solitary caecal diverticulitis from acute appendicitis. More than 70 % of patients with caecal diverticulitis were operated on with a preoperative diagnosis of acute appendicitis. In addition, selective focused imaging can be used for increasing the positive appendectomy rate imaging with aim to aid in diagnosing alternative diseases, who may not need surgery (e.g. omental infarction, solitary caecal diverticulum and torsion of appendix epilplocae). Nevertheless, delay in diagnosis later than 24 h increases risk of perforation, [34].

When recommending the choice of the imaging strategy, the patients' age and the potential radiation exposure are important. Although a careful balance of risk-benefit ratio is needed, particularly in young patients and women of childbearing age, routine use of CT scan has been demonstrated to be associated with lower negative appendectomy rates [35]. Furthermore, there is increasing evidence that spontaneous resolution of AA is common and that imaging can lead to increased detection of benign forms of the condition [36].

In view of the increased use of CT in children and concerns regarding radiation based imaging, the National Cancer Institute and the American Paediatric Surgical Association recommend use of non-radiation based imaging such as US where possible [37]. Currently, over 50 % of children undergoing appendectomy in North America have radiation based imaging [38]. This rate is too high [39] and a tailored approach based on risk is sensible, especially in children. Universal imaging of patients with CT, apart from consuming resources, is not without health risks. It has been estimated that the benefit of universal imaging in avoiding 12 unnecessary appendectomies could result in one additional cancer death [40].

In pregnant women with suspected appendicitis a positive US requires no further confirmatory test. However, in case of appendix non-visualization on US, MRI is the recommended imaging exam, since it yields a high diagnostic rate and accuracy [41–43].

In settings having availability of such resource, MRI can also be considered for pediatric appendicitis imaging being a non-radiative imaging modality potentially valuable in the setting of negative ultrasound.

Imaging is key in optimizing outcomes in appendicitis, not only as an aid in early diagnosis, but potentially reducing negative appendectomy rates. Combining appropriate imaging with history, physical examination and laboratory tests are crucial to this [8, 19, 44–49]. With use of novel scoring systems combining clinical and imaging features, 95 % of the patients deemed to have uncomplicated appendicitis were correctly identified as such [9]. Soreide in a recent PubMed search under the term appendicitis found over 20,000 articles, but few randomized trials, especially in imaging, have been undertaken with resultant variable level of evidence [50]. Wide variation in rates of imaging as low as a CT rate of 12 % in the UK, to 95 % in the US suggests a need for practice guidelines [51]. Only 25 % of Australian patients undergo imaging [52].

The surgeon has the responsibility of managing each case in the best way considering three possibilities: hospital discharge, admission for observation, surgical treatment. Estimating pre-image likelihood of appendicitis is important in tailoring management: low-risk patients could be discharged with appropriate safety netting, whereas high-risk patients are likely to require early senior review with a focus on timely surgical intervention rather than diagnostic imaging [16]. Using scoring systems to guide imaging can be helpful [49, 53].

Low risk patients being admitted to hospital and considered for surgery could have appendicitis ruled in or out by abdominal CT. A negative CT would generally allow the discharge of the patient with appropriate short outpatient-department follow-up [16].

Intermediate-risk classification identifies patients likely to benefit from observation and systematic diagnostic imaging. In the intermediate risk group an abdominal ultrasound would be the first line in imaging. A positive ultrasound would lead to appendectomy and a negative test to either CT or further clinical observation. A conditional CT strategy, where CT is performed after a negative US, will reduce number of CTs by 50 % and will correctly identify as many patients with appendicitis as an immediate CT strategy. However, conditional CT imaging results in more false positives [9, 54]. Overall sensitivity and specificity of US and CT is 58–76, 95 and 99, 84 % respectively [9, 55]. Performing serial US may improve accuracy and reduce the number of CT performed [56].

High-risk scoring patients may not require imaging in certain settings, nonetheless US or CT before surgery is routinely performed in western countries in such patients [16].

Standard reporting templates for ultrasound may enhance accuracy [40]. To optimize sensitivity and specificity three step sequential positioning or graded compression bedside may be beneficial [55], as opposed to radiology department. US lacks Level 1/2 evidence to support its use [57], The routine use of IV contrast to enhance the accuracy of CT is not clear [58], nor is the role of dose reduction techniques.

Findings suggestive of appendicitis include a thickened wall, a non-compressible lumen, diameter greater than 6 mm, absence of gas in the lumen, appendicoliths, hyperechogenic periappendicular fat, fluid collection consistent with an abscess, local dilation and hypoperistalsis, free fluid and lymphadenopathy [40]. The most sensitive sign seems to be a non-compressible appendix that exceeds 6 mm in diameter (up to 98 % sensitive), although some centres use 7 mm to improve their specificity [59]. As described earlier, ultrasound is inferior to CT in sensitivity and its negative predictive value for appendicitis and may not be as useful for excluding appendicitis [60]. This is particularly true if the appendix was never visualized. False negatives are also more likely in patients with a ruptured appendix. The potential adverse effect of high BMI on US accuracy is surprisingly not clear [61].

MRI is comparable to US with conditional use of CT in identifying perforated appendicitis. However, both strategies incorrectly classify up to half of all patients with perforated appendicitis as having simple appendicitis [62]. Scoring systems will enhance the ability to categorize whether appendicitis is simple or complex, showing that imaging is not a replacement for clinical examination. Finally, imaging may be undertaken by non-radiologists outside the radiology departments with variable results [63].

USA vs. EU perspective on appendicitis diagnosis

AA is rarely diagnosed by history/physical examination in the United States (USA). Unfortunately most of these patients in the USA are seen by emergency physicians and tests are ordered before the surgeon is called. In adults, it is rare to not obtain a CT scan unless a thin male (also rare in the USA). In children, an ultrasound is nearly always done. In the USA, logistics and legal concerns unfortunately impact our decision-making.

Despite the EU and the USA having similar access to health care, health technology and standards, they are very different healthcare systems with some inherent differences in the management strategies for appendicitis. One aspect that highlights this is the pre-operative imaging strategy for diagnosis. In the EU, only around 12.9 % of patients undergo pre-operative CT imaging [51]; which is typically reserved for elderly patients who might have cancer, atypical or delayed presentations or those who have suspected appendicular masses or abscesses. Young males with typical histories and examination findings would go straight to theatre without any imaging. Females would get an abdominal and pelvic ultrasound and laparoscopy if uncertainty exists. Perhaps as a consequence of this strategy, the rate of negative appendectomy in the UK is around 20 % [64]; this is in contrast to the USA. For instance, analysis of 3540 appendectomies form the Surgical Care and Outcomes Assessment Programme (SCOAP) in Washington State demonstrates that 86 % of patients underwent pre-operative imaging, 91 % of whom underwent CT [65]. In addition, in the UK, appendectomy is widely regarded as a training operation that most registrars would perform independently. From 2867 appendectomies in the recent UK audit, 87 % were performed by residents, and 72 % were performed unsupervised [66]. Laparoscopic appendectomy is performed, especially in high volume units, during the daytime and when a consultant is present in theatre, but overall 33.7 % of cases are performed as open procedures [51].

Statement 2.1 In patients with suspected appendicitis a tailored individualised approach is recommended, depending on disease probability, sex and age of the patient (EL 2 GoR B) Statement 2.2 Imaging should be linked to Risk Stratification such as AIR or Alvarado score. (EL2, GoR B)

Statement 2.3 Low risk patients being admitted to hospital and not clinically improving or reassessed score could have appendicitis rule-in or out by abdominal CT. (EL 2, GoR B)

Statement 2.4 Intermediate-risk classification identifies patients likely to benefit from observation and systematic diagnostic imaging. (EL 2, GoR B)

Statement 2.5 High-risk patients (younger than 60 years-old) may not require pre-operative imaging. (EL 2, GoR B)

Statement 2.6 US Standard reporting templates for-ultrasound and US three step sequential positioning-may enhance over accuracy. (EL 3, GoR B)

Statement 2.7 MRI is recommended in pregnant patients with suspected appendicitis, if this resource is available. (EL 2, GoR B)

Non-operative treatment for uncomplicated appendicitis

What is the natural history of appendicitis? Can appendicitis resolve without treatment? How common is it?(Speaker in Jerusalem CC Dr. F. Catena)

The analysis of the epidemiologic and clinical studies that elucidate the natural history of appendicitis performed by Andersson in 2007 showed that not all patients with uncomplicated appendicitis will progress to perforation and that spontaneous resolution may be a common event [36]. Also the recent review published in The Lancet investigated the natural history of appendicitis and distinguished between normal appendix, uncomplicated appendicitis and complicated appendicitis, according to their macroscopic and microscopic appearance and clinical relevance. Actually, if this is related to the natural history of appendicitis or not is still unknown, but according to the authors these may be two distinct forms of appendicitis: the first one is a mild simple appendicitis that responds to antibiotics or could be even self-limiting, whereas the other often seems to perforate before the patient reaches the hospital. Although the mortality rate is low, postoperative complications are common in case of complicated disease [67].

In order to elucidate the role of non-operative treatment of uncomplicated appendicitis, in 2012 Varadhan et al. performed a meta-analysis including four randomized controlled trials with a total of 900 patients (470 antibiotic treatment, 430 appendectomy): the antibiotic treatment was associated with a 63 % success rate at 1 year and a lower complication rate with a relative risk reduction of 31 % if compared with appendectomy (RR 0.69, I2 = 0 %, $P = 0.004$). Moreover, this risk reduction was found to be more relevant (39 %, RR 0.61, I2 = 0 %, $P = 0.02$), if the studies with crossover of patients between the antibiotic and surgical treatment were excluded. The analysis did not find significant differences for treatment efficacy, length of stay or risk of developing complicated appendicitis [2].

The observational NOTA (Non Operative Treatment for Acute Appendicitis) study treated 159 patients with suspected appendicitis with antibiotics [mean AIR (Appendicitis Inflammatory Response) score = 4.9 and mean Alvarado score = 6.2 (range 3–9) [68]] with a 2-year follow-up. The mean length of stay of those patients was 0.4 days and mean sick leave period was 5.8 days. The short-term (7 days) failure rate was 11.9 %. Of 22 patients with a long-term recurrence (13.8 %), 14 were successfully treated nonoperatively [69].

Recently, the RCT by Svensson et al. included 50 paediatric patients (24 antibiotic treatment, 26 appendectomy) with 92 % of success rate in the non-operative group. However, an 8 % short-term failure (two patients, one complicated appendicitis and one mesenteric lymphadenitis) and 38 % long-term (12 months) failure were reported in the non-operative group (one acute appendicitis, six patients with recurrent abdominal pain but no histopathological evidence of appendicitis and one for parental wish) [70].

The APPAC (Antibiotic Therapy vs Appendectomy for Treatment of Uncomplicated Acute Appendicitis) trial, published in JAMA in 2015, enrolled 350 patients with uncomplicated appendicitis confirmed by CT-scanning (257 antibiotic therapy, 273 appendectomy). The 1-year recurrence rate and appendectomy in the antibiotic group was reported as 27 %. The intention-to-treat analysis yielded a difference in treatment efficacy between groups of −27.0 %(95%CI, −31.6 % to ∞) ($P = .89$). The authors concluded that the antibiotic treatment did not meet the pre-specified criterion for non-inferiority compared with appendectomy [71].

In the recent review published in the New Engl J Med by Flum it is stated that appendectomy should be considered the first-line therapy in uncomplicated appendicitis and recommended to the patient. In the patients with equivocal clinical picture, or equivocal imaging, or in those who have strong preferences for avoiding an operation or with major comorbid medical problems it is reasonable to treat with antibiotics first [72].

However, an interesting still not well-studied topic is the role of spontaneous resolution of uncomplicated appendicitis. In fact, the effect of the antibiotic treatment could be biased due to spontaneous healing as a result of the expectant management [47].

Statement 3.1: Antibiotic therapy can be successful in selected patients with uncomplicated appendicitis who wish to avoid surgery and accept the risk up to 38 % recurrence. (EL 1, GoR A)

Statement 3.2: Current evidence supports initial intravenous antibiotics with subsequent conversion to oral antibiotics. (EL2, GoR B)

Statement 3.3: In patients with normal investigations and symptoms unlikely to be appendicitis but which do not settle:

- Cross-sectional imaging is recommended before surgery
  - Laparoscopy is the surgical approach of choice
  - There is inadequate evidence to recommend a routine approach at present (EL2 GoR)

Timing of appendectomy and in-hospital delay

Does in-hospital delay increase the rate of complication or perforation? Is it safe to delay appendectomy? Timing of appendectomy. (Speaker in Jerusalem CC Dr. M.D. Kelly)

The management of most intra-abdominal acute surgical conditions has evolved significantly over time and many are now managed without emergency operation. Since the 1880s, when Fitz and McBurney described emergency appendectomy, it has been the standard of care for suspected appendicitis. This is based on the traditional model of appendicitis where initial obstruction causes inflammation and infection, and delay to operation allows increasing tension in the wall with ischemia, necrosis and perforation. This pathophysiology probably does not fit with all cases of appendicitis, as discussed below, and emergency operation is not always needed.

Delay to appendectomy may be needed for various reasons, including a trial of conservative treatment with antibiotics, diagnostic tests to confirm the clinical diagnosis or to allow safe service provision and effective use of resources as not all hospitals are staffed or set up for 24 h operating room availability. Whatever the cause for delay, the real issue is if it will lead to more complications: there are numerous studies looking at the question of in-hospital delay and indirect evidence can be obtained from randomised trials of antibiotics versus surgery, however controversy persists.

A recent publication had a 27 % negative appendectomy rate and the authors justify their low threshold to operate by stating that it avoids perforation [73]. Others disagree and found that delaying surgical intervention did not put the patient at risk and may have actually improved patient outcomes [74]. The current diversity in practice appears to be caused by lack of high-level evidence although this is beginning to change. It should be noted that the danger of perforation is possibly overstated and that negative exploration is not benign [36].

Conservative management decreases the number of negative explorations and saves a number of patients with resolving appendicitis from an unnecessary operation. Andersson has shown that this leads to a high proportion of perforations among the operated patients but the number of perforations is not increased. The perforation rate, therefore, should not be used as a quality measure of the management of patients with suspected appendicitis [36]. He also notes that the increasing proportion of perforations over time is explained by an increase in the number of perforations according to the traditional model and mainly by selection due to resolution of non-perforated appendicitis according to the alternative model. According to the second model, only a few perforations can be prevented by a speedy operation after the patients have arrived at the hospital. Neither of these models can be proved, but the second model is more consistent with the available data [36].

Similarly, others have found that the trends for non-perforating and perforating appendicitis radically differ and it is unlikely that perforated appendicitis is simply the progression of appendicitis resulting from delayed treatment [75].

There are numerous retrospective single institution reviews with contradictory results.

Teixeira et al. found only increased rates of surgical site infection. They studied 4529 patients who were admitted with appendicitis over 8 years and 4108 (91 %) patients underwent appendectomy with perforation found in 942 (23 %). There were three independent predictors of perforation: age > 55 years, WBC count >16,000 and female sex, but delay to appendectomy was not associated with higher perforation rate [76]. However, Ditillo et al. found that increased patient and hospital intervals to operation were associated with advanced pathology, although patient delay was more significant. The risk of developing advanced pathology increased with time and it was associated with longer length of hospital stay and antibiotic treatment as well as postoperative complications [77].

In a large retrospective cohort study of 32,782 patients who underwent appendectomy for acute appendicitis (available through the American College of Surgeons National Quality Improvement Program), 75 % of patients underwent operation within 6 h, 15 % between 6 and 12 h and 10 % of patients experienced a delay of more than 12 h (mean 26.07 h (SD 132.62)). The patient characteristics were similar in all three groups. No clinically significant difference was found in outcome measures, including overall morbidity and serious morbidity or mortality. The authors concluded that the results did not change when disease severity was excluded from the model suggesting that there is no relationship between time from surgical admission and negative outcomes after appendectomy [78].

Busch et al. reported a prospective multicentre observational study on whether in-hospital delay negatively influences outcome after appendectomy. In-hospital delay of more than 12 h, age over 65 years, time of admission during regular hours, and the presence of co-morbidity are all independent risk factors for perforation. Perforation was associated with a higher re-intervention rate and increased hospital length of stay. They concluded that in elderly patients with co-morbidity and suspected appendicitis, a delay of surgery of more than 12 h should be avoided [79].

As can be seen, the evidence is conflicting but recently higher level evidence has become available in the study by Bhangu et al. This was a prospective, multicentre cohort study of 2510 patients with acute appendicitis, of whom 812 (32.4 %) had complex findings. They found that timing of operation was not related to risk of complex appendicitis. At 12–24 h, the odds ratio (OR) was 0.98 ($P = 0.869$), 24–48 h OR 0.88 ($P = 0.329$) and 48+ hours OR 0.82 ($P = 0.317$). After 48 h, the risk of surgical site infection and 30-day adverse events both increased [adjusted ORs 2.24 ($P = 0.039$) and 1.71 ($P = 0.024$), respectively]. They also did a meta-analysis of 11 nonrandomized studies (8858 patients) which showed that a delay of 12 to 24 h after admission did not increase the risk of complex appendicitis (OR 0.97, $P = 0.750$) [34].

In some jurisdictions, after hours surgery (especially night time surgery) is restricted to life or limb-threatening conditions as not all hospitals are staffed or equipped for safe 24-h operating room availability. In addition, especially in state funded health systems, where all expenditure has to be based on evidence, it is hard to justify after hours surgery for uncomplicated appendicitis.

There are now many randomised studies of initial antibiotic treatment for appendicitis. While not designed to look at delay to operation, they give indirect evidence of its safety in patients with uncomplicated appendicitis [2, 71, 80].

In summary, in the absence of level 1 evidence, the question of whether in-hospital delay is safe and not associated with more perforations cannot be answered with certainty. What can be said is that in most cases of uncomplicated appendicitis emergency operation is not necessary and a short delay of up to 12–24 h is not likely to be associated with a poorer outcome. However, delays should be minimised wherever possible to relieve pain, to enable quicker recovery and decrease costs.

Statement 4.1 Short, in-hospital surgical delay up to 12/24 h is safe in uncomplicated acute appendicitis and does not increase complications and/or perforation rate. (EL 2, GoR B)]

Statement 4.2 Surgery for uncomplicated appendicitis can be planned for next available list minimizing delay wherever possible (patient comfort etc.). (EL 2, GoR B)

Surgical treatment

- *Open or Laparoscopic?*
- *Lavage or Aspiration of pus?*
- *Mesoappendix dissection: endoclip, endoloop, electrocoagulation, Harmonic Scalpel or LigaSure?*
- *Stump Closure: Stapler or endoloop? Ligation or invagination of the stump?*
- *Drains?*
- *Primary or secondary closure of the wound?*

(Speaker in Jerusalem CC Dr. S. Di Saverio)

The most recent meta-analysis reported that the laparoscopic approach of appendicitis is often associated with longer operative times and higher operative costs, but it leads to less postoperative pain, shorter length of stay (LOS) and earlier return to work and physical activity [81] therefore lowering overall hospital and social costs [82], improved cosmesis, significantly fewer complications in terms of wound infection. A trend towards higher incidence of intra-abdominal infection (IAA) and organ space collections was seen [83], although this effect seems decreased or even inverted in the last decade [84] and in more recent randomised controlled trials (RCTs), being probably related to surgical expertise [85].

According to Sauerland et al., wound infections are less likely after laparoscopic appendectomy (LA) than after open appendectomy (OA) (OR 0.43; CI 0.34 to 0.54), pain on day 1 after surgery is reduced after LA by 8 mm (CI 5 to 11 mm) on a 100 mm visual analogue scale, hospital stay was shortened by 1.1 day (CI 0.7 to 1.5), return to normal activity, work, and sport occurred earlier after LA than after OA. However, as we said, the incidence of IAA is increased (OR 1.87; CI 1.19 to 2.93). In addition, the operation time is 10 min (CI 6 to 15) longer and more expensive. Seven studies on children were included, but the results do not seem to be much different when compared to adults. Diagnostic laparoscopy reduces the risk of a negative appendectomy, but this effect was stronger in fertile women (RR 0.20; CI 0.11 to 0.34) as compared to unselected adults. The authors conclude the in those clinical settings where surgical expertise and equipment are available and affordable, diagnostic laparoscopy and LA (either in combination or separately) seem to have numerous advantages over OA [83].

The overview by Jaschinski et al. included nine systematic reviews. The duration of surgery pooled by eight reviews was 7.6 to 18.3 min shorter using the open approach and the risk of abdominal abscesses was higher for laparoscopic surgery in half of six meta-analyses. The laparoscopic approach shortened hospital stay from 0.16 to 1.13 days in seven out of eight meta-analyses, pain scores on the first postoperative day were lower after LA in two out of three reviews and the occurrence of wound infections pooled by all reviews was lower after LA. One review showed no difference in mortality [86].

Although LA is extremely useful especially as a diagnostic tool in fertile women, in can be used also in male patients, even if advantages over OA in this group are not clearly demonstrated [87].

Recent database studies on more than 250,000 patients aged > 65 years entail improved clinical outcomes for laparoscopic appendectomy compared with OA [88] in terms of length of stay (LOS), mortality and overall morbidity. Patients older than 65 years, patients with comorbidities [89] and with complicated appendicitis [90] seem to benefit more from the laparoscopic approach, particularly in terms of hospital costs and reduced LOS but also for decreased postoperative mortality and overall morbidity [91].

A meta-analysis of prospective and retrospective comparative series evidences superiority of LA vs. OA also in obese (BMI >30) patients [92]. Dasari et al. reported the same encouraging results also in a recent Systematic Review [93].

Despite evidence which considers LA safe in pregnancy [94], advantages are minor (less pain, less infections, less early deliveries) if compared to the risk of fetal loss; more recent data from EL 2 reviews of comparative studies (599 LA vs. 2816 OA) show an increased fetal loss for LA, without significant advantages [95]; a database study on 859 pregnant women with appendicitis confirms a better outcome for those treated surgically vs. non-operative management, while it did find no difference in maternal complications between LA and OA [96]. While fetal events are unknown, LA in pregnant patients demonstrated shorter OR times, LOS, and reduced complications and were performed more frequently over time. Even in perforated cases, laparoscopy appears safe in pregnant patients [97]. In conclusion, there is no strong current evidence as to the preferred modality of appendectomy, open or laparoscopic, during pregnancy from the prospect of foetal or maternal safety. However, low grade evidence shows that laparoscopic appendectomy during pregnancy might be associated with higher rates of foetal loss [98]. The literature does not clearly define the balance between advantages and disadvantages in this particular setting and the choice of the approach should be taken by the attending surgeon after a thorough discussion with the patient, balancing the advantages of laparoscopy vs. the theoretical risk of fetal loss and making clear the current lack of literature defining balance between advantages and disadvantages of laparoscopic appendectomy in pregnancy.

A recent systematic review including more than 100.000 appendectomies in children found that laparoscopic appendectomy in uncomplicated acute appendicitis is associated with a reduced hospital stay (weighted mean difference 0–1.18; 95 % CI0 – 1.61 to –0.74; $P < 0.05$), but broad equivalence in postoperative morbidity when compared with the conventional approach. On the other hand, in cases of complicated acute appendicitis, although the overall morbidity is reduced (pooled odds ratio [POR] = 0.53; $P < 0.05$), wound infections (POR = 0.42; $P < 0.05$), length of hospital stay (WMD = –0.67; $P < 0.05$), and bowel obstruction episodes (POR = 0.8; $P < 0.05$), in the laparoscopic group the risk of intra-abdominal abscess is increased [99].

Complicated appendicitis can be approached laparoscopically by experienced surgeons [100], with significant advantages, including lower overall complications, readmission rate, small bowel obstruction rate, infections of the surgical site (minor advantage following Clavien's criteria) and faster recovery [89, 101, 102]. Regarding the costs, LA for complicated appendicitis can be performed with low cost equipment, allowing significantly lower overall costs (operative plus LOS) compared to open surgery [103].

Statement 5.1.1:

Laparoscopic appendectomy should represent the first choice where laparoscopic equipment and skills are available, since it offers clear advantages in terms of less pain, lower incidence of SSI, decreased LOS, earlier return to work and overall costs. (EL 1, GoR A)

Statement 5.1.2:

Laparoscopy offers clear advantages and should be preferred in obese patients, older patients and patients with comorbidities. (EL 2, GoR B)

Statement 5.1.3:

Laparoscopy is feasible and safe in young male patients although no clear advantages can be demonstrated in such patients. (EL 2, GoR B)

Statement 5.1.4:

Laparoscopy should not be considered as a first choice over open appendectomy in pregnant patients. (EL 1, GoR B)

Statement 5.1.5:

No major benefits have also been observed in laparoscopic appendectomy in children, but it reduces hospital stay and overall morbidity. (EL 1, GoR A)

Statement 5.1.6:

In experienced hands, laparoscopy is more beneficial and cost-effective than open surgery for complicated appendicitis. (EL 3, GoR B)

Peritoneal lavage and aspiration have been suggested by a low-powered study to be detrimental, but these conclusions are based on low-volume lavage and small numbers [104]; a definitive conclusion cannot be drawn, even though a LE 2 study in children [105] has not demonstrated advantages in terms of intra-abdominal abscesses (IAA) of >500 ml, although >6–8lt are needed to significantly lower the bacterial load [106].

Peritoneal irrigation is a practice traditionally used in case of localized or diffuse peritonitis and considered beneficial. However, either in the past decades for open appendectomy or in the latest years for laparoscopic appendectomy, many others argued the efficacy of irrigation for cleansing purposes. The most recent studies, retrospective [104] or RCTs, in laparoscopic or open appendectomy [107], did not show any advantages in favour of intraoperative irrigation for prevention of postoperative IAA. Instead, irrigation usually adds some extra-time to the overall duration of surgery [105]. Nonetheless, a non-significant trend to leave a drain when irrigation is not used can be noticed (52 % in the group of suction only vs. 40 % in the irrigation group). Furthermore, practice patterns may vary widely with regard to the amount and extent of irrigation and probably the common sense would suggest to avoid copious irrigation before achieving a careful suction first from every quadrant having purulent collections and to wash using small amounts of saline and repeated suction in order to avoid diffuse spreading of the infected matter into the remaining abdominal cavity, without forgetting to suck out as much as possible of the lavage fluid [108].

Statement 5.2:

Peritoneal irrigation does not have any advantages over suction alone in complicated appendicitis. (EL2, GoR B)

Simplified and cost effective techniques for LA have been described [109]. They use either two endoloops, securing the blood supply, or a small number of endoclips, appearing to be really useful in case of mobile cecum avoiding the need of an additional port. In addition, potential hazards of diathermy are avoided, the appendicular artery can be ligated under direct vision, and smoke is not created [110]. With clips, anonabsorbable foreign body is left in the peritoneal cavity and may slip or become detached. Moreover, it requires more experience especially in case of inflamed appendix with the risk of bleeding [111–113].

In case of inflamed and oedematous mesoappendix it has been suggested the use of LigaSure™, especially in case of gangrenous tissue [112, 113]. No significant hospital stay and complication rates were found between endoclip and LigaSure™. On the other hand, significant differences are present in surgical time and conversion to open rate [111]. Despite the potential advantages, Ligasure™ represents a high cost option and it may be logical using endoclip if the mesoappendix is not oedematous [111–113]. Diamantis et al. compared Ligasure™ and Harmonic Scalpel with monopolar electrocoagulation and bipolar coagulation: the first two caused more minimal thermal injury of the surrounding tissue than other techniques [114]. Between monopolar electrocoagulation, endoclip and Harmonic Scalpel no clinically significant differences were found in surgical time. All three methods gave acceptable complication rates. Because monopolar electrocoagulation requires no additional instruments, it may be the most cost-effective method for mesoappendix dissection in LA [115]. However, the need of evacuate of the smoke could affect the pneumoperitoneum [111].

Statement 5.3.1:

There are no clinical differences in outcomes, LOS and complications rates between the different techniques described for mesentery dissection (monopolar electrocoagulation, bipolar energy, metal clips, endoloops, Ligasure, Harmonic Scalpel etc.). (EL3, GoR B)

Statement 5.3.2:

Monopolar electrocoagulation and bipolar energy are the most cost-effective techniques, even if more experience and technical skillsis required to avoid potential complications (e.g. bleeding) and thermal injuries. (EL3, GoR B)

As for appendicular stump closure, stapler reduces operative time and superficial wound infections [116], but higher costs (6 to 12 fold) and no significant differences in IAA [117], suggest the preference of loop-closure. In perforated appendicitis the issue of using endoloops or stapler for appendicular stump closure needs further studies [118].

The stump closure may vary widely in practice and the associated costs can be significant. Whilst earlier studies initially reported advantages with routine use of endostaplers in terms of complication and operative times [116], more recent studies have repeatedly demonstrated no differences in intra- or post-operative complications incidence between either endostapler or endoloops stump closure [119]. Although operative times maybe longer (but it is probably biased by the learning curve) [120], the operative costs were invariably and significantly lower when endoloops are used [103, 121]. A metanalysis confirmed that use of endo-loop to secure the appendicular stump during LA takes longer than endo-GIA but it is associated with equal hospital stay, perioperative complication rate, and incidence of intra-abdominal abscess [122]. Endoloops were at least as safe and effective as endostapler also in paediatric population, without stump leaks nor differences in SSI and IAA in the group of non perforated appendicitis, whereas for perforated appendicitis, endoloops were perhaps safer than endostapler (IAA incidence 12.7 % vs. 50 %, OR 7.09) [123].

Many studies compared the simple ligation and the stump inversion and no significant differences were found [103, 124–127].

Statement 5.4.1:

There are no clinical advantages in the use of endostapler over endoloops for stump closure for both adults and children. (EL 1, GoR A)

Statement 5.4.2:

Endoloops might be preferred for lowering the costs when appropriate skills/learning curve are available. (EL 3, GoR B)

Statement 5.4.3: There are no advantages of stump inversion over simple ligation, either in open or laparoscopic surgery. (EL 2, GoR B)

Routine drainage has not proven its utility, with the exception of generalized peritonitis, and seems to cause more complications, LOS and transit recovery time [128], despite the widespread opinion that aspiration of the residual fluid after peritoneal lavage in the first 24 h postoperatively might lower the incidence of IAA in case of insufficient lavage [118].

The practice of leaving intra-abdominal drains is also widely used when complicated/perforated appendicitis is found. Mostly from paediatric experiences, it seems that the use of drainage and irrigation is associated with significantly longer operative times and LOS, without a decrease in post-operative infectious complications (instead a non-significant trend to more frequent wound infection and dehiscence, more IAA and longer postoperative ileus) [107].

Previous studies in children with perforated appendicitis have already reported a significantly lower incidence of SSI and IAA and better postoperative course in the group treated without peritoneal drainage [129].

This year, the meta-analyses by Cheng et al. included five trials involving 453 patients with complicated appendicitis who were randomised to the drainage group ($n = 228$) and the no drainage group ($n = 225$) after emergency open appendectomies and found no significant differences between the two groups in the rates of intra-peritoneal abscess or wound infection. The hospital stay was longer in the drainage group than in the no drainage group (MD 2.04 days; 95 % CI 1.46 to 2.62) (34.4 % increase of an 'average' hospital stay) [96].

Statement 5.5.1:

Drains are not recommended in complicated appendicitis in paediatric patients. (EL3, GoR B)

Statement 5.5.2:

In adult patients, drain after appendectomy for perforated appendicitis and abscess/peritonitis should be used with judicious caution, given the absence of good evidence from the literature. Drains did not prove any efficacy in preventing intra-abdominal abscess and seem to be associated with delayed hospital discharge. (EL1, GoR A)

In the most recent metanalysis investigating the advantages of delayed primary wound closure (DPC) vs. primary closure (PC) in contaminated abdominal operations DPC had a significantly longer length of stay than PC (1.6 days, 95 % CI: 1.41, 1.79). Two meta-analysis failed to prove the superiority of delayed primary skin closure in significantly reducing SSI (odds ratio 0.65; 95 % CI, 0.25–1.64; $P = .36$) [64] (risk ratio 0.89; 95 % CI: 0.46, 1.73) [130]. Similar result were achieved also in the paediatric population [131]. In addition, there is no evidence for any short-term or long-term advantage in peritoneal closure for non-obstetric operations [132].

Statement 5.6:

Delayed primary skin closure does not seem beneficial for reducing the risk of SSI and increase LOS in open appendectomies with contaminated/dirty wounds. (EL1, GoR A)

Scoring systems for intra-operative grading of appendicitis and their clinical usefulness

What are the histopathological criteria for appendicitis of clinical importance? Minor inflammatory changes, early appendicitis, catarrhal appendicitis. The criteria used will have an influence on the proportion of negative appendectomy, and also on evaluation of diagnostic performance. (Speaker in Jerusalem CC Dr. C. A. Gomes)

The systematic review by Swank et al. reported the incidence of unexpected findings in the histopathological examination of the surgical specimen after appendectomy as 0.5 % of benign neoplasm, 0.2 % of malignant neoplasms, 0–19 % of parasitic infection, endometriosis in 0 % and granulomatosis in 0–11 % of cases. Most patients with malignant neoplasms, parasite infection and granulomatosis underwent additional investigation or treatment [133].

Apart from the unexpected findings, there is a lack of validated system for histological classification of acute appendicitis and controversies exist on this topic. The paper by Carr proposes basic and classical but practical findings about the histological diagnosis of acute appendicitis. The author assesses three important disease aspects: appendix gross appearance, microscopic findings and clinical significance. The most important concept in the diagnosis of acute appendicitis is the transmural inflammation. "Endoappendicitis" is a histological finding, but its clinical significance is not clear. The term "periappendicitis" refers to inflammation outside the appendix and its most common causes are gynaecological disorders like salpingitis and pelvic peritonitis [134].

The issue of the removal indication in case of "normal-looking" appendices is still under debate and there are conflicting studies showing the pros and cons of the appendectomy. According to the retrospective study by Grimes et al., including 203 appendectomies performed with normal histology, appendicular faecaliths may be a cause of right iliac fossa pain in the absence of obvious appendicular inflammation. In this study, the policy of routine removal of a normal-looking appendix at laparoscopy in the absence of any other obvious pathology appeared to be an effective treatment for recurrent symptoms in those cases with a faecalith [135]. The study by Van den Broek et al. concluded that it is safe to leave a normal looking appendix in place when a diagnostic laparoscopy for suspected appendicitis is performed, even if another diagnosis cannot be found at laparoscopy [136]. On the other hand, in the retrospective study by Phillips et al., almost one-third of apparently normal appendices being inflamed histologically. For this reason the authors would advocate the removal of a normal looking appendix in the absence of other explanatory pathology [137]. Recently, Lee et al. compared the postoperative complications after removal of an inflamed or non-inflamed appendix and found no difference between the two groups. The authors conclude that negative appendectomy should not be undertaken routinely during laparoscopy for right iliac fossa pain [138]. In the Multicentre Appendectomy Audit by Strong et al., 138 out of 496 specimens (27.8 %) judged as normal by the operating surgeon were found to be inflamed at the histopathological assessment [139].

In order to evaluate the appendix during diagnostic laparoscopy, in 2013 Hamminga et al. proposed the LAPP (Laparoscopic APPpendicitis) score (six criteria), with a single-centre prospective pilot study (134 patients), reporting high positive and negative predictive values, 99 and 100 %, respectively. However, the score still needs to be validated within a multicentre study [140].

In 2014 also the AAST proposed a system for grading severity of emergency general surgery diseases based on several criteria encompassing clinical, imaging, endoscopic, operative, and pathologic findings, for eight commonly encountered gastrointestinal conditions, including acute appendicitis, ranging from Grade I (mild) to Grade V (severe) [141].

In the recent multicentre cohort study by Strong et al. involving 3138 patients from five centres, the overall disagreement between the surgeon and the pathologist was reported in 12.5 % of cases (moderate reliability, k 0.571). In particular, 27.8 % of appendices assessed as normal by the surgeon revealed a pathology at histopathological assessment, while in 9.6 % of macroscopically appearing inflamed appendicitis revealed to be normal. Interestingly, the surgeon's experience did not affect the disagreement rate. These findings suggest that surgeons' judgements of the intra-operative macroscopic appearance of the appendix is inaccurate and does not improve with seniority and therefore supports removal at the time of surgery [139]. Nonetheless, the clinical significance of these early and/or mild forms of microscopic appendicitis is still unclear at present.

The prospective study by Gomes et al. enrolled 186 patients with presumed acute appendicitis underwent appendectomy if diagnostic laparoscopy showed appendicitis or normal-looking appendix without any other intra-abdominal disease. The appendix was graded by the surgeon upon its visual appearance: grade 0 (normal looking), 1 (redness and oedema), 2 (fibrin), 3A (segmental necrosis), 3B (base necrosis), 4A (abscess), 4B (regional peritonitis), and 5 (diffuse peritonitis). This was then compared with a biochemical-histologic assessment of the removed appendix. The sensitivity, specificity, and accuracy of the laparoscopic grading system were 63, 83.3, and 80.1 %, respectively, and presented moderate concordance [k = 0.39 (95 % confidence interval, 0.23–0.55)]. The biochemical-histological diagnosis changed for 48 (25.8 %) patients who had been previously classified by surgeons during laparoscopy. Most incorrect grading occurred in grades 0 and 1 appendicitis [142]. The Gomes intraoperative grading score system is able to distinguish complicated appendicitis from uncomplicated cases has been externally validated [103] and may be useful for guiding postoperative management (e.g. use of antibiotics, antibiotic duration, LOS) and comparing therapeutic outcomes [143].

Statement 6.1: The incidence of unexpected findings in appendectomy specimens is low but the intra-operative diagnosis alone is insufficient for identifying unexpected disease. From the current available evidence, routine histopathology is necessary. (EL 2, GoR B)

Statement 6.2: There is a lack of validated system for histological classification of acute appendicitis and controversies exist on this topic. (EL 4, GoR C)

Statement 6.3: Surgeon's macroscopic judgement of early grades of acute appendicitis is inaccurate. (EL 2, GoR B)

Statement 6.4: If the appendix looks "normal" during surgery and no other disease is found in symptomatic patient, we recommend removal in any case. (EL 4, GoR C)

Statement 6.5: We recommend adoption of a grading system for acute appendicitis based on clinical, imaging and operative findings, which can allow identification of homogeneous groups of patients, determining optimal grade disease management and comparing therapeutic modalities. (EL 2, GoR B)

Non-surgical treatment for complicated appendicitis: abscess or phlegmone

Role of percutaneous drainage and Interval Appendectomy or immediate surgery. (Speaker in Jerusalem CC Dr. M. De Moya)

The study with highest level of evidence about the conservative treatment of complicated appendicitis with abscess or phlegmon is the meta-analysis by Simillis et al., published in 2010. It included 17 studies (16 nonrandomized retrospective and one non-randomized prospective) for a total of 1572 patients (847 treated with conservative treatment and 725 with appendectomy). Data revealed that conservative treatment was associated with significantly less overall complications (wound infections, abdominal/pelvic abscesses, ileus/bowel obstructions, and re-operations) if compared to immediate appendectomy. No significant difference was found in the duration of the first hospitalization, the overall hospital stay and the duration of intravenous antibiotics [144].

On the other hand, the recent randomized controlled trial by Mentula et al. compared the results from 60 patients with appendicular abscess treated either with immediate laparoscopic surgery (30 patients) or with conservative treatment (30 patients). The results showed that there was no difference in hospital stay between the two groups. In the laparoscopy group there were significantly fewer unplanned readmissions (3 % versus 27 %, $P = 0.026$), even if this group had 10 % risk for bowel resection and 13 % risk for incomplete appendectomy. The conservative group, instead, required more additional interventions (surgery or percutaneous drainage) (30 % versus 7 %, $P = 0.042$). Open surgery was required in three (10 %) patients in the laparoscopy group and in four (13 %) patients in the conservative group. The rate of uneventful recovery was 90 % in the laparoscopy group versus 50 % in the conservative group ($P = 0.002$). These data brought to the conclusion that several factors support the use of immediate surgery in patients with appendicular abscess [145]. However, it should be highlighted that laparoscopic appendectomy as first line approach, is a feasible and safe alternative to non-operative management +/- percutaneous drain only in presence of specific laparoscopic experience and advanced skills [146].

In the systematic review and meta-analysis by Andersson et al., including 61 studies (mainly retrospective studies, three randomized controlled trials), immediate surgery was associated with a higher morbidity if compared with conservative treatment (OR 3.3; CI: 1.9–5.6; $P < 0.001$), while the non-surgical treatment of appendicular abscess or phlegmon has been reported to succeed in over 90 % of patients, with an overall risk of recurrence of 7.4 % (CI: 3.7–11.1) and only 19.7 % of cases of abscess percutaneous drainage [3]. Other single-centre studies including complicated appendicitis reported higher rates of recurrence after non-surgical treatment of 14 % after 2 years [69], 27 % within 2 months [145], up to 38 % after 12 months [70]. In order to avoid this quite high chance of recurrence, some authors recommend routine elective interval appendectomy following the conservative management. However, this procedure is associated with morbidity in 12.4 % of patients (CI 0.3–24.5) [3]. The systematic review by Hall et al. included three retrospective studies for a total of 127 cases of non-surgical treatment of appendix mass in children: after successful non-operative treatment, the risk of recurrent appendicitis was found to be 20.5 % (95 % confidence interval [CI], 14.3 %–28.4 %). However, this means that 80 % of children may not need interval appendectomy. In addition, the results showed 0.9 % of carcinoid tumor (95 % CI, 0.5–1.8) and 3.4 % of complications after interval appendectomy (95 % CI, 2.2–5.1). Overall, the complications reported included wound infection, prolonged postoperative ileus, hematoma formation, and small bowel obstruction, but the incidence of any individual complication was not determined [147].

Because of its consistent morbidity, after successful conservative management, the routine indication to interval appendectomy is justified only in case of persistent or recurrent symptoms, and should be avoided in asymptomatic patients [148]. Some authors recommend routine interval appendectomy, not to avoid the risk of recurrence, but to rule out possible appendicular neoplasia. In the retrospective study by Carpenter et al., including 315 patients with AA, 18 out of 24 patients with complicated appendicitis (7.6 % of the total series) that were treated conservatively, underwent interval appendectomy. The incidence of neoplasms was significantly higher in the patients underwent interval appendectomy than in the immediate appendectomy group (five patients, 28 % vs. three patients, 1 % $P < 0.0001$). Appendicular or colonic neoplasms should be investigated after nonoperative management of AA, especially in patients older than 40 years [149].

Statement 7.1: Percutaneous drainage of a periappendicular abscess, if accessible, is an appropriate treatment in addition to antibiotics for complicated appendicitis. (EL 2, GOR B)

Statement 7.2: Non-operative management is a reasonable first line treatment for appendicitis with phlegmon or abscess. (EL 1, GOR A)

Statement 7.3: Operative management of acute appendicitis with phlegmon or abscess is a safe alternative to non-operative management in experienced hands. (EL 2, LOR B)

Statement 7.4: Interval appendectomy is not routinely recommended both in adults and children. (EL 1, LOR A)

Statement 7.5: Interval appendectomy is recommended for those patients with recurrent symptoms. (EL 2, LOR B)

Statement 7.6: Colonic screening should be performed in those patients with appendicitis treated non-operatively if >40y/o. (EL 3, LoR C)

Preoperative and postoperative antibiotics

Should Preoperative antibiotics prophylaxis be given? What antibiotics? When should postoperative antibiotics be given? What antibiotics? Duration? (Speaker in Jerusalem CC Dr. M. Sartelli)

In the last years use of antibiotics in patients undergoing appendectomy has been debated [150, 151].

In 2005 a Cochrane meta-analysis supported that broad-spectrum antibiotics given preoperatively are effective in decreasing wound infection and abscesses. Randomised Controlled Trials (RCTs) and Controlled Clinical Trials (CCTs) in which any antibiotic regime were compared to placebo in patients suspected of having appendicitis, and undergoing appendectomy were analysed. Forty-five studies including 9576 patients were included in this review. Antibiotics were superior to placebo for preventing wound infection and intra-abdominal abscess, with no apparent difference in the nature of the removed appendix [152].

In 2005 a randomized controlled trial on 269 patients, aged 15–70 years, with non-perforated appendicitis undergoing open appendectomy was published. 92 patients received single dose preoperative (group A), 94 received three-dose (group B) and 83 received 5-day perioperative (group C) regimens of cefuroxime and metronidazole. The rate of postoperative infective complication was not significantly different among the groups (6.5 % group A, 6.4 % group B, 3.6 % group C). The duration of antibiotic therapy had no significant effect on the length of hospital stay. Complications related to antibiotic treatment were significantly more common for 5-day perioperative antibiotic group (C) compared with single dose preoperative antibiotic group (A) ($P = 0.048$) [153].

Some prospective trials demonstrated that patients with perforated appendicitis should have postoperative antibiotic treatment [154, 155]. The major pathogens involved in community-acquired appendicitis are Enterobacteriaceae, Streptococcus species, and anaerobes (especially *B. fragilis*) [156].

In 2013 the World Society of Emergency Surgery published their guidelines for management of intra-abdominal infections (IAIs) stratifying the antimicrobial regimen according to patient's condition (Sepsis Vs. severe sepsis and septic shock), the pathogens presumed to be involved, and the risk factors indicative of major resistance patterns [157].

Many studies compared duration of antibiotic regimens for perforated appendicitis and they showed a variation in the duration of treatment [154, 155, 158].

In 2000 Taylor et al. published a prospective trial comparing a minimum IV 5-days antibiotic regimen versus no minimum IV regimen. Infectious complications were not statistically different between the two groups. Average hospital stay was also not statistically different between the two groups. The study demonstrated that an antimicrobial regimen with no minimum IV antibiotic requirement in patients with complicated appendicitis did not increase morbidity. Furthermore, the protocol arm with no minimum IV antibiotic requirement led to less IV antibiotic use but did not significantly decrease hospital stay [159].

Recently, a prospective randomized trial on 518 patients with complicated intra-abdominal infection, including also complicated appendicitis, undergoing adequate source control demonstrated the outcomes after fixed-duration antibiotic therapy (approximately 4 days) were similar to those after a longer course of antibiotics (approximately 8 days) that extended until after the resolution of physiological abnormalities [160].

Although discontinuation of antimicrobial treatment should be based on clinical and laboratory criteria, a period of 3–5 days for adult patients is generally sufficient to treat complicated acute appendicitis.

Statement 8.1: In patients with acute appendicitis preoperative broad-spectrum antibiotics are always recommended. (EL 1, GoR A)

Statement 8.2: For patients with uncomplicated appendicitis, post-operative antibiotics are not recommended .(EL 2, GoR B)

Statement 8.3: In patients with complicated acute appendicitis, postoperative, broad-spectrum antibiotics are always recommended. (EL 2, GoR B)

Statement 8.4: Although discontinuation of antimicrobial treatment should be based on clinical and laboratory criteria such as fever and leucocytosis, a period of 3–5 days for adult patients is generally recommended. (EL 2, GoR B)

Conclusions

The current evidence-based Guidelines represent to the best of our knowledge, the first international Comprehensive Clinical Guidelines for diagnosis and management of Acute Appendicitis. During the 3rd World Congress of the WSES, held in Jerusalem (Israel) in July 2015, a panel of experts including an Organizational Committee and Scientific Committee and Scientific Secretariat, participated to a Consensus Conference where eight panelists (SDS, MDK, FC, DW, MiSu, MaSa, MDM, CAG) presented a number of statements, which were developed for each of the eight main questions about diagnosis and management of AA (Appendix). The statements were then voted, eventually modified and finally approved by the participants to The Consensus Conference and subsequently by the board of co-authors. The current paper is reporting the definitive Guidelines Statements and Clinical Recommendations on each of the following topics: 1) Diagnostic efficiency of clinical scoring systems, 2) Role of Imaging, 3) Non-operative treatment for uncomplicated appendicitis, 4) Timing of appendectomy and in-hospital delay, 5) Surgical treatment 6) Scoring systems for intra-operative grading of appendicitis and their clinical usefulness 7) Non-surgical treatment for complicated appendicitis: abscess or phlegmon 8) Pre-operative and post-operative antibiotics. In summary, The Alvarado score (with cut-off score < 5) is sufficiently sensitive to exclude acute appendicitis, nonetheless the ideal (highly sensitive and specific), clinically applicable, diagnostic scoring system/clinical rule remains currently out of reach. Imaging should be linked to Risk Stratification such as AIR or Alvarado score, low-risk patients being admitted to hospital and not clinically improving or reassessed score could have appendicitis ruled in or out by abdominal CT, in high-risk and young pre-operative imaging may be avoided, MRI is recommended in pregnant patients with suspected appendicitis. Regarding non-operative treatment of AA, antibiotic therapy can be successful in selected patients with uncomplicated appendicitis who wish to avoid surgery and accept the risk up to 38 % recurrence. The timing of performing an appendectomy is a great matter of debate and our recommendations are that a short, in-hospital surgical delay up to 12/24 h is safe in uncomplicated acute appendicitis and does not increase complications and/or perforation rate, however surgery for uncomplicated appendicitis should be planned for next available list minimizing delay wherever possible. When analysing the surgical treatment, laparoscopic appendectomy should represent the first choice where laparoscopic equipment and skills are available, since it offers clear advantages in terms of less pain, lower incidence of SSI, decreased LOS, earlier return to work and overall costs. In particular, laparoscopy offers clear advantages and should be preferred in obese patients, older patients and patients with comorbidities. In experienced hands, laparoscopy is more beneficial and cost-effective than open surgery for complicated appendicitis. Laparoscopy should not be considered as a first choice over open appendectomy in pregnant patients. No major benefits have also been observed in laparoscopic appendectomy in children, but it reduces hospital stay and overall morbidity. Analysing the technical issues in performing an appendectomy, peritoneal irrigation does not have any advantages over suction alone in complicated appendicitis; there are no clinical differences in outcomes, LOS and complications rates between the different techniques described for mesentery dissection (monopolar electrocoagulation, bipolar energy, metal clips, endoloops, Ligasure, Harmonic Scalpel etc.). There are no clinical advantages in the use of endostapler over endoloops for stump closure for both adults and children, but Endoloops might be preferred for lowering the costs when appropriate skills/learning curve are available. Finally, drains are not recommended in complicated appendicitis in paediatric patients, in adult patients, drain after appendectomy for perforated appendicitis and abscess/peritonitis should be used with judicious caution, given the absence of good evidence from the literature. Drains did not prove any efficacy in preventing intra-abdominal abscesses and seem to be associated with delayed hospital discharge.

Delayed primary skin closure does not seem beneficial for reducing the risk of SSI and increase LOS in open appendectomies with contaminated/dirty wounds. When a "normal" looking appendix is found at surgery and no other disease is found in a symptomatic patient, we recommend its removal. Percutaneous drainage of a periappendiceal abscess, if accessible, is an appropriate treatment in addition to antibiotics for complicated appendicitis. Non-operative management is a reasonable first line treatment for appendicitis with phlegmon or abscess. Operative management of acute appendicitis with phlegmon or abscess can be a safe alternative to non-operative management but only in experienced hands. Interval appendectomy is not routinely recommended both in adults and children, but it can be recommended for those patients with recurrent symptoms. Important is to recommend colonic screening in patients >40 y/o with appendicitis treated non-operatively. Finally, in patients with acute appendicitis preoperative broad spectrum antibiotics are recommended, for patients with uncomplicated appendicitis postoperative antibiotics are not recommended, whereas in those with complicated acute appendicitis postoperative, broad spectrum antibiotics are always recommended, usually for a period of 3–5 days.

After reaching consensus on each of the above mentioned statements proposed by every one of the Speakers of the Panel (see Appendix), the participants to the Consensus Conference in Jerusalem and the Scientific Committee members, developed and shared the WSES algorithm for diagnosis and management of Acute Appendicits, reported in Fig. 1.

Appendix

Table 3: Guidelines Statements

	LE	GoR	Statement
1) Diagnostic efficiency of clinical scoring systems			
1.1	1	A	The Alvarado score (with cutoff score < 5) is sufficiently sensitive to exclude acute appendicitis.
1.2	1	A	The Alvarado score is not sufficiently specific in diagnosing acute appendicitis.
1.3	1	B	An ideal (high sensitivity and specificity), clinically applicable, diagnostic scoring system/clinical rule remains outstanding. This remains an area for future research
2) Role of imaging			
2.1	2	B	In patients with suspected appendicitis a tailored individualised approach is recommended, depending on disease probability, sex and age of the patient
2.2	2	B	Imaging should be linked to Risk Stratification such as AIR or Alvarado score
2.3	2	B	Low risk patients being admitted to hospital and not clinically improving or reassessed score could have appendicitis ruled-in or out by abdominal CT
2.4	2	B	Intermediaterisk classification identifies patients likely to benefit from observation and systematic diagnostic imaging.
2.5	2	B	Highrisk patients (younger than 60 yearsold) may not require preoperative imaging.
2.6	3	B	US Standard reporting templates for ultrasound and US three step sequential positioning may enhance over accuracy .
2.7	2	B	MRI is recommended in pregnant patients with suspected appendicitis, if this resource is available
3) Nonoperative treatment for uncomplicated appendicitis			
3.1	1	A	Antibiotic therapy can be successful in selected patients with uncomplicated appendicitis who wish to avoid surgery and accept the risk up to 38 % recurrence.
3.2	2	B	Current evidence supports initial intravenous antibiotics with subsequent conversion to oral antibiotics.
3.3	2	B	In patients with normal investigations and symptoms unlikely to be appendicitis but which do not settle: • Cross-sectional imaging is recommended before surgery • Laparoscopy is the surgical approach of choice • There is inadequate evidence to recommend a routine approach at present
4) Timing of appendectomy and in-hospital delay			
4.1	2	B	Short, in-hospital surgical delay up to 12/24 h is safe in uncomplicated acute appendicitis and does not increase complications and/or perforation rate.
4.2	2	B	Surgery for uncomplicated appendicitis can be planned for next available list minimizing delay wherever possible (patient comfort etc.).
5) Surgical treatment			
5.1.1	1	A	Laparoscopic appendectomy should represent the first choice where laparoscopic equipment and skills are available, since it offers clear advantages in terms of less pain, lower incidence of SSI, decreased LOS, earlier return to work and overall costs.
5.1.2	2	B	Laparoscopy offers clear advantages and should be preferred in obese patients, older patients and patients with comorbidities
5.1.3	2	B	Laparoscopy is feasible and safe in young male patients although no clear advantages can be demonstrated in such patients.
5.1.4	I	B	Laparoscopy should not be considered as a first choice over open appendectomy in pregnant patients
5.1.5	1	A	No major benefits have also been observed in laparoscopic appendectomy in children, but it reduces hospital stay and overall morbidity

Table 3: Guidelines Statements *(Continued)*

5.1.6	3	B	In experienced hands, laparoscopy is more beneficial and cost-effective than open surgery for complicated appendicitis
5.2	2	B	Peritoneal irrigation does not have any advantages over suction alone in complicated appendicitis
5.3.1	3	B	There are no clinical differences in outcomes, LOS and complications rates between the different techniques described for mesentery dissection (monopolar electrocoagulation, bipolar energy, metal clips, endoloops, Ligasure, Harmonic Scalpel etc.).
5.3.2	3	B	Monopolar electrocoagulation and bipolar energy are the most cost-effective techniques, even if more experience and technical skills is required to avoid potential complications (e.g. bleeding) and thermal injuries.
5.4.1	1	A	There are no clinical advantages in the use of endostapler over endoloops for stump closure for both adults and children
5.4.2	3	B	Endoloops might be preferred for lowering the costs when appropriate skills/learning curve are available
5.4.3	2	B	There are no advantages of stump inversion over simple ligation, either in open or laparoscopic surgery
5.5.1	3	B	Drains are not recommended in complicated appendicitis in paediatric patients
5.5.2	1	A	In adult patients, drain after appendectomy for perforated appendicitis and abscess/peritonitis should be used with judicious caution, given the absence of good evidence from the literature. Drains did not prove any efficacy in preventing intraabdominal abscess and seem to be associated with delayed hospital discharge.
5.6	1	A	Delayed primary skin closure does not seem beneficial for reducing the risk of SSI and increase LOS in open appendectomies with contaminated/dirty wounds
6) Scoring systems for intraoperative grading of appendicitis and their clinical usefulness			
6.1	2	B	The incidence of unexpected findings in appendectomy specimens is low but the intraoperative diagnosis alone is insufficient for identifying unexpected disease. From the current available evidence, routine histopathology is necessary
6.2	4	C	There is a lack of validated system for histological classification of acute appendicitis and controversies exist on this topic.
6.3	2	B	Surgeon's macroscopic judgement of early grades of acute appendicitis is inaccurate
6.4	4	C	If the appendix looks "normal" during surgery and no other disease is found in symptomatic patient, we recommend removal in any case.
6.5	2	B	We recommend adoption of a grading system for acute appendicitis based on clinical, imaging and operative findings, which can allow identification of homogeneous groups of patients, determining optimal grade disease management and comparing therapeutic modalities
7) Nonsurgical treatment for complicated appendicitis :abscess or phlegmone			
7.1	2	B	Percutaneous drainage of a periappendiceal abscess, if accessible, is an appropriate treatment in addition to antibiotics for complicated appendicitis.
7.2	1	A	Nonoperative management is a reasonable first line treatment for appendicitis with phlegmon or abscess
7.3	2	B	Operative management of acute appendicitis with phlegmon or abscess is a safe alternative to nonoperative management in experienced hands
7.4	1	A	Interval appendectomy is not routinely recommended both in adults and children.
7.5	2	B	Interval appendectomy is recommended for those patients with recurrent symptoms.
7.6	3	C	Colonic screening should be performed in those patients with appendicitis treated non-operatively if >40y/o

Table 3: Guidelines Statements *(Continued)*

8) Preoperative and Postoperative Antibiotics			
8.1	1	A	In patients with acute appendicitis preoperative broad-spectrum antibiotics are always recommended
8.2	2	B	For patients with uncomplicated appendicitis, postoperative antibiotics are not recommended
8.3	2	B	In patients with complicated acute appendicitis, postoperative, broad-spectrum antibiotics are always recommended
8.4	2	B	Although discontinuation of antimicrobial treatment should be based on clinical and laboratory criteria such as fever and leucocytosis, a period of 3–5 days for adult patients is generally recommended

Abbreviations

AA, acute appendicitis; AAS score, Adult Appendicitis Score; AIR, Appendicitis Inflammatory Response Score; AS, Alvarado Score; ASA, American Society of Anaesthesiology; CC, Consensus Conference; CCT, Controlled Clinical Trials; CT, computed tomography; GoR, grade of recommendation; IAA, Intra-abdominal abscess; LA, Laparoscopic Appendectomy; LoE or EL, level of evidence; LOS, length of stay; MRI, magnetic resonance imaging; OA, open appendectomy; OC, Organization Committee; OR, odds ratio; POR, pooled odds ratio; RCT, randomised controlled trials; RIPASA score, Raja Isteri Pengiran Anak Saleha Appendicitis; SC, Scientific Committee; SD, standard deviation; SS, Scientific Secretariat; SSI, surgical site infection; US, ultrasound; WSES, World Society of Emergency Surgery; RIF, right iliac fossa

Acknowledgements

Not applicable.

Funding

No authors received any funding resource. The paper received a WSES Institutional waiver for this publication.

Authors' contributions

The WSES president was supported by the Scientific Secretariat in establishing the timetable of the CC and choosing the eight plus eight experts who were asked to participate respectively to Organization Committee and Scientific Committee: the Organization Committee had the task to support the Scientific Secretariat in building the framework for the Consensus and to support the Scientific Committee for the strict scientific part; the Scientific Committee had the assignment to select the literature and to elaborate, in co-working to Scientific Secretariat and Organization Committee, the statements. The Scientific Secretariat supported the WSES President, establishing the agenda, choosing the working tools and finally collaborating with Organization Committee and Scientific Secretariat. Consequently each question was assigned to one team consisting of one member of Organization Committee, one member of Scientific Committee and one member of Scientific Secretariat (each member of Scientific Secretariat covered two questions). Each team reviewed, selected and analyzed the literature, wrote and proposed the statement's drafts for one of the eight questions. WSES board reviewed the draft and made critical appraisals. All the statements were discussed and approved during the 3rd WSES World Congress, held in Jerusalem on 6th July 2015. The manuscript was further reviewed by Scientific Secretariat, Organization Committee and Scientific Committee according to congress comments and was then approved by the WSES board. SDS, AB, MDK, FC, DW, MiSu, CAG, MDM, MaSa, RA: conception, design and coordination of the study; data acquisition, analysis and interpretation; draft the manuscript. All authors read and approved the final manuscript.

Authors' information

Component of the teams for the Consensus Conference and the WSES Guidelines Development
President: Salomone Di Saverio
Scientific Secretariat members: Salomone Di Saverio, Arianna Birindelli, Dieter Weber, Michael Denis Kelly, Fausto Catena, Massimo Sartelli
Organization Committee members: Salomone Di Saverio, Fausto Catena, Micheal D. Kelly, Dieter Weber, Federico Coccolini, Massimo Sartelli, Luca Ansaloni, Ernest E Moore, Jeffry Kashuk, Yoram Kluger
Scientific Committee members: Salomone Di Saverio, Dieter Weber, Michael Denis Kelly, Michael Sugrue, Fausto Catena, Arianna Birindelli, Aneel Bhangu, Kjetil Soreide, Ferdinando Agresta, Marc De Moya, Massimo Sartelli, Carlos Augusto Gomes, Ewen Griffths, Steve De Castro, Osvaldo Chiara, Fabio Cesare Campanile, Walt Biffl, George Velmahos, Raul Coimbra, Ari Leppaniemi, Ernest E Moore, Roland Andersson.

Competing interests

The authors declare that they have no competing interests.

Author details

[1]Emergency and Trauma Surgery – Maggiore Hospital, AUSL, Bologna, Italy. [2]S. Orsola Malpighi University Hospital – University of Bologna, Bologna, Italy. [3]Locum Surgeon, Acute Surgical Unit, Canberra Hospital, Canberra, ACT, Australia. [4]Emergency and Trauma Surgery Department, Maggiore Hospital of Parma, Parma, Italy. [5]Trauma and General Surgeon Royal Perth Hospital & The University of Western Australia, Perth, Australia. [6]Macerata Hospital, Macerata, Italy. [7]Letterkenny Hospital, Donegal, Ireland. [8]Harvard Medical School - Massachusetts General Hospital, Boston, USA. [9]Department of Surgery Hospital Universitario, Universidade General de Juiz de Fora, Juiz de Fora, Brazil. [10]Academic Department of Surgery, University Hospitals Birmingham NHS Foundation Trust, Edgabaston, Birmingham, UK. [11]General Surgery, Civil Hospital - ULSS19, Veneto, Adria, RO, Italy. [12]Denver Health System – Denver Health Medical Center, Denver, USA. [13]Department of Gastrointestinal Surgery, Stavanger University Hospital, Stavanger, Norway. [14]University Hospitals Birmingham NHS Foundation Trust Queen Elizabeth Hospital, Birmingham, UK. [15]Department of Surgery, OLVG, Amsterdam, The Netherlands. [16]Department of Surgery, University of Jerusalem, Jerusalem, Israel. [17]Division of General Surgery, Rambam Health Care Campus, Haifa, Israel. [18]Abdominal Center, University of Helsinki, Helsinki, Finland. [19]General Surgery I, Papa Giovanni XXIII Hospital, Bergamo, Italy. [20]Department of Surgery, Linkoping University, Linkoping, Sweden. [21]UCSD Health System - Hillcrest Campus Department of Surgery Chief Division of Trauma, Surgical Critical Care, Burns, and Acute Care Surgery, San Diego, CA, USA. [22]Royal Free Campus, University College London, London, UK. [23]Department of Surgery, San Giovanni Decollato Andosilla Hospital, Viterbo, Italy. [24]Queen's Medical Center, University of Hawaii, Honolulu, HI, USA. [25]Niguarda Hospital, Milan, Italy. [26]University of Florida, Gainesville, USA. [27]Department of Surgery, University of Pittsburgh School of Medicine, UPMC-Presbyterian, Pittsburgh, USA. [28]Faculdade de Ciências Médicas (FCM) - Unicamp, Campinas, SP, Brazil. [29]Alicante, Spain. [30]Department of Surgery, University of Washington, Harborview Medical Center, Seattle, WA, USA. [31]St. Michael Hospital, Toronto, Canada. [32]Department of Traumatology, John Hunter Hospital and University of Newcastle, Newcastle, NSW, Australia. [33]Department of Surgery, Terni Hospital, University of Perugia, Terni, Italy. [34]Trauma Surgery Unit - Maggiore Hospital AUSL, Bologna, Italy. [35]Department of Surgery, Maggiore Hospital

AUSL, Bologna, Italy. [36]Catholic University, A. Gemelli University Hospital, Rome, Italy. [37]Department of Surgery, University of Catania, Catania, Italy. [38]R. Adams Cowley Trauma Center, Baltimore, MD, USA. [39]Professor Emeritus Virginia Commonwealth University, Richmond, VA, USA. [40]Harvard Medical School - Chief of Trauma, Emergency Surgery, and Surgical Critical Care, Massachusetts General Hospital, Boston, USA.

References

1. Addiss DG, et al. The epidemiology of appendicitis and appendectomy in the United States. Am J Epidemiol. 1990;132(5):910–25.
2. Varadhan KK, Neal KR, Lobo DN. Safety and efficacy of antibiotics compared with appendicectomy for treatment of uncomplicated acute appendicitis: meta-analysis of randomised controlled trials. BMJ. 2012;344, e2156.
3. Andersson RE, Petzold MG. Nonsurgical treatment of appendiceal abscess or phlegmon: a systematic review and meta-analysis. Ann Surg. 2007;246(5): 741–8.
4. Alvarado A. A practical score for the early diagnosis of acute appendicitis. Ann Emerg Med. 1986;15(5):557–64.
5. Samuel M. Pediatric appendicitis score. J Pediatr Surg. 2002;37(6):877–81.
6. Andersson M, Andersson RE. The appendicitis inflammatory response score: a tool for the diagnosis of acute appendicitis that outperforms the Alvarado score. World J Surg. 2008;32(8):1843–9.
7. Chong CF, et al. Development of the RIPASA score: a new appendicitis scoring system for the diagnosis of acute appendicitis. Singapore Med J. 2010;51(3):220–5.
8. Sammalkorpi HE, Mentula P, Leppaniemi A. A new adult appendicitis score improves diagnostic accuracy of acute appendicitis–a prospective study. BMC Gastroenterol. 2014;14:114.
9. Atema JJ, et al. Scoring system to distinguish uncomplicated from complicated acute appendicitis. Br J Surg. 2015;102(8):979–90.
10. Debnath J, et al. Alvarado score: is it time to develop a clinical-pathological-radiological scoring system for diagnosing acute appendicitis? Am J Emerg Med. 2015;33(6):839–40.
11. Ohle R, et al. The Alvarado score for predicting acute appendicitis: a systematic review. BMC Med. 2011;9:139.
12. McKay R, Shepherd J. The use of the clinical scoring system by Alvarado in the decision to perform computed tomography for acute appendicitis in the ED. Am J Emerg Med. 2007;25(5):489–93.
13. Gwynn LK. The diagnosis of acute appendicitis: clinical assessment versus computed tomography evaluation. J Emerg Med. 2001;21(2):119–23.
14. de Castro SM, et al. Evaluation of the appendicitis inflammatory response score for patients with acute appendicitis. World J Surg. 2012;36(7):1540–5.
15. Kollar D, et al. Predicting acute appendicitis? A comparison of the Alvarado score, the Appendicitis Inflammatory Response Score and clinical assessment. World J Surg. 2015;39(1):104–9.
16. Scott AJ, et al. Risk stratification by the Appendicitis Inflammatory Response score to guide decision-making in patients with suspected appendicitis. Br J Surg. 2015;102(5):563–72.
17. Ebell MH, Shinholser J. What are the most clinically useful cutoffs for the Alvarado and Pediatric Appendicitis Scores? A systematic review. Ann Emerg Med. 2014;64(4):365–72. e2.
18. Kharbanda AB, et al. Interrater reliability of clinical findings in children with possible appendicitis. Pediatrics. 2012;129(4):695–700.
19. Kulik DM, Uleryk EM, Maguire JL. Does this child have appendicitis? A systematic review of clinical prediction rules for children with acute abdominal pain. J Clin Epidemiol. 2013;66(1):95–104.
20. Andersson RE. Meta-analysis of the clinical and laboratory diagnosis of appendicitis. Br J Surg. 2004;91(1):28–37.
21. Hallan S, Asberg A. The accuracy of C-reactive protein in diagnosing acute appendicitis–a meta-analysis. Scand J Clin Lab Invest. 1997;57(5): 373–80.
22. Velanovich V, Satava R. Balancing the normal appendectomy rate with the perforated appendicitis rate: implications for quality assurance. Am Surg. 1992;58(4):264–9.
23. Kirkil C, et al. Appendicitis scores may be useful in reducing the costs of treatment for right lower quadrant pain. Ulus Travma Acil Cerrahi Derg. 2013;19(1):13–9.
24. Bongard F, Landers DV, Lewis F. Differential diagnosis of appendicitis and pelvic inflammatory disease. A prospective analysis. Am J Surg. 1985;150(1): 90–6.
25. Webster DP, et al. Differentiating acute appendicitis from pelvic inflammatory disease in women of childbearing age. Am J Emerg Med. 1993;11(6):569–72.
26. Arnbjornsson E. Varying frequency of acute appendicitis in different phases of the menstrual cycle. Surg Gynecol Obstet. 1982;155(5):709–11.
27. Rothrock SG, et al. Misdiagnosis of appendicitis in nonpregnant women of childbearing age. J Emerg Med. 1995;13(1):1–8.
28. Dahlberg DL, et al. Differential diagnosis of abdominal pain in women of childbearing age. Appendicitis or pelvic inflammatory disease? Adv Nurse Pract. 2004;12(1):40–5. quiz 45–6.
29. Morishita K, et al. Clinical prediction rule to distinguish pelvic inflammatory disease from acute appendicitis in women of childbearing age. Am J Emerg Med. 2007;25(2):152–7.
30. Albiston E. The role of radiological imaging in the diagnosis of acute appendicitis. Can J Gastroenterol. 2002;16(7):451–63.
31. Smith MP, et al. ACR Appropriateness Criteria(R) Right Lower Quadrant Pain–Suspected Appendicitis. Ultrasound Q. 2015;31(2):85–91.
32. Gaitan HG, et al. Laparoscopy for the management of acute lower abdominal pain in women of childbearing age. Cochrane Database Syst Rev. 2014;5, CD007683.
33. Peery AF, et al. Burden of gastrointestinal disease in the United States: 2012 update. Gastroenterology. 2012;143(5):1179–87 e1-3.
34. United Kingdom National Surgical Research C, Bhangu A. Bhangu, *Safety of short, in-hospital delays before surgery for acute appendicitis: multicentre cohort study, systematic review, and meta-analysis.* Ann Surg. 2014;259(5):894–903.
35. Krajewski S, et al. Impact of computed tomography of the abdomen on clinical outcomes in patients with acute right lower quadrant pain: a meta-analysis. Can J Surg. 2011;54(1):43–53.
36. Andersson RE. The natural history and traditional management of appendicitis revisited: spontaneous resolution and predominance of prehospital perforations imply that a correct diagnosis is more important than an early diagnosis. World J Surg. 2007;31(1):86–92.
37. Kotagal M, et al. Use and accuracy of diagnostic imaging in the evaluation of pediatric appendicitis. J Pediatr Surg. 2015;50(4):642–6.
38. Kotagal M, et al. Improving ultrasound quality to reduce computed tomography use in pediatric appendicitis: the Safe and Sound campaign. Am J Surg. 2015;209(5):896–900. discussion 900.
39. Kim ME, et al. Performance of CT examinations in children with suspected acute appendicitis in the community setting: a need for more education. AJR Am J Roentgenol. 2015;204(4):857–60.
40. Nielsen JW, et al. Reducing computed tomography scans for appendicitis by introduction of a standardized and validated ultrasonography report template. J Pediatr Surg. 2015;50(1):144–8.
41. Freeland M, et al. Diagnosis of appendicitis in pregnancy. Am J Surg. 2009; 198(6):753–8.
42. Spalluto LB, et al. MR imaging evaluation of abdominal pain during pregnancy: appendicitis and other nonobstetric causes. Radiographics. 2012;32(2):317–34.
43. Theilen LH, et al. Utility of magnetic resonance imaging for suspected appendicitis in pregnant women. Am J Obstet Gynecol. 2015;212(3): 345 e1–6.
44. Heineman J. Towards evidence based emergency medicine: Best BETs from the Manchester Royal Infirmary. BET 1: An evaluation of the Alvarado score as a diagnostic tool for appendicitis in children. Emerg Med J. 2012;29(12): 1013–4.
45. Trout AT, Sanchez R, Ladino-Torres MF. Reevaluating the sonographic criteria for acute appendicitis in children: a review of the literature and a retrospective analysis of 246 cases. Acad Radiol. 2012;19(11):1382–94.
46. Dingemann J, Ure B. Imaging and the use of scores for the diagnosis of appendicitis in children. Eur J Pediatr Surg. 2012;22(3):195–200.
47. Andersson RE. Short and long-term mortality after appendectomy in Sweden 1987 to 2006. Influence of appendectomy diagnosis, sex, age, co-morbidity, surgical method, hospital volume, and time period. A national population-based cohort study. World J Surg. 2013;37(5):974–81.
48. Omari AH, et al. Acute appendicitis in the elderly: risk factors for perforation. World J Emerg Surg. 2014;9(1):6.
49. Jones RP, et al. Journal Club: the Alvarado score as a method for reducing the number of CT studies when appendiceal ultrasound fails to visualize the appendix in adults. AJR Am J Roentgenol. 2015;204(3):519–26.

50. Soreide K. The research conundrum of acute appendicitis. Br J Surg. 2015; 102(10):1151–2.
51. National Surgical Research, C. Multicentre observational study of performance variation in provision and outcome of emergency appendicectomy. Br J Surg. 2013;100(9):1240–52.
52. Brockman SF, et al. Does an Acute Surgical Model increase the rate of negative appendicectomy or perforated appendicitis? ANZ J Surg. 2013; 83(10):744–7.
53. Tan WJ, et al. Alvarado score: a guide to computed tomography utilization in appendicitis. ANZ J Surg. 2013;83(10):748–52.
54. Poortman P, et al. Improving diagnosis of acute appendicitis: results of a diagnostic pathway with standard use of ultrasonography followed by selective use of CT. J Am Coll Surg. 2009;208(3):434–41.
55. Chang ST, Jeffrey RB, Olcott EW. Three-step sequential positioning algorithm during sonographic evaluation for appendicitis increases appendiceal visualization rate and reduces CT use. AJR Am J Roentgenol. 2014;203(5):1006–12.
56. Schuh S, et al. Properties of serial ultrasound clinical diagnostic pathway in suspected appendicitis and related computed tomography use. Acad Emerg Med. 2015;22(4):406–14.
57. Mallin M, et al. Diagnosis of appendicitis by bedside ultrasound in the ED. Am J Emerg Med. 2015;33(3):430–2.
58. Kepner AM, Bacasnot JV, Stahlman BA. Intravenous contrast alone vs intravenous and oral contrast computed tomography for the diagnosis of appendicitis in adult ED patients. Am J Emerg Med. 2012;30(9):1765–73.
59. Kessler N, et al. Appendicitis: evaluation of sensitivity, specificity, and predictive values of US, Doppler US, and laboratory findings. Radiology. 2004;230(2):472–8.
60. Terasawa T, et al. Systematic review: computed tomography and ultrasonography to detect acute appendicitis in adults and adolescents. Ann Intern Med. 2004;141(7):537–46.
61. Koseekriniramol V, Kaewlai R. Abdominal wall thickness is not useful to predict appendix visualization on sonography in adult patients with suspected appendicitis. J Clin Ultrasound. 2015;43(5):269–76.
62. Leeuwenburgh MM, et al. Accuracy of MRI compared with ultrasound imaging and selective use of CT to discriminate simple from perforated appendicitis. Br J Surg. 2014;101(1):e147–55.
63. Carroll PJ, et al. Surgeon-performed ultrasound at the bedside for the detection of appendicitis and gallstones: systematic review and meta-analysis. Am J Surg. 2013;205(1):102–8.
64. Bhangu A, et al. Systemic review and meta-analysis of randomized clinical trials comparing primary vs delayed primary skin closure in contaminated and dirty abdominal incisions. JAMA Surg. 2013;148(8):779–86.
65. Collaborative S, et al. Negative appendectomy and imaging accuracy in the Washington State Surgical Care and Outcomes Assessment Program. Ann Surg. 2008;248(4):557–63.
66. Singh P, et al. Safety assessment of resident grade and supervision level during emergency appendectomy: analysis of a multicenter, prospective study. Surgery. 2014;156(1):28–38.
67. Bhangu A, et al. Acute appendicitis: modern understanding of pathogenesis, diagnosis, and management. Lancet. 2015;386(10000):1278–87.
68. Di Saverio S, Piccinini BA, Catena F, Biscardi A, Tugnoli G. How reliable is Alvarado score and its subgroups in ruling out acute appendicitis and suggesting the opportunity of nonoperative management or surgery? Annals of Surgery. 2016. June 8, 2016 published ahead of print.
69. Di Saverio S, et al. The NOTA Study (Non Operative Treatment for Acute Appendicitis): prospective study on the efficacy and safety of antibiotics (amoxicillin and clavulanic acid) for treating patients with right lower quadrant abdominal pain and long-term follow-up of conservatively treated suspected appendicitis. Ann Surg. 2014;260(1):109–17.
70. Svensson JF, et al. Nonoperative treatment with antibiotics versus surgery for acute nonperforated appendicitis in children: a pilot randomized controlled trial. Ann Surg. 2015;261(1):67–71.
71. Salminen P, et al. Antibiotic Therapy vs Appendectomy for Treatment of Uncomplicated Acute Appendicitis: The APPAC Randomized Clinical Trial JAMA. 2015;313(23):2340–8.
72. Flum DR. Clinical practice. Acute appendicitis–appendectomy or the "antibiotics first" strategy. N Engl J Med. 2015;372(20):1937–43.
73. Teo AT, et al. Institutional review of patients presenting with suspected appendicitis. ANZ J Surg. 2015;85(6):420–4.
74. Stahlfeld K, et al. Is acute appendicitis a surgical emergency? Am Surg. 2007; 73(6):626–9. discussion 629–30.
75. Livingston EH, et al. Disconnect between incidence of nonperforated and perforated appendicitis: implications for pathophysiology and management. Ann Surg. 2007;245(6):886–92.
76. Teixeira PG, et al. Appendectomy timing: waiting until the next morning increases the risk of surgical site infections. Ann Surg. 2012; 256(3):538–43.
77. Ditillo MF, Dziura JD, Rabinovici R. Is it safe to delay appendectomy in adults with acute appendicitis? Ann Surg. 2006;244(5):656–60.
78. Ingraham AM, et al. Effect of delay to operation on outcomes in adults with acute appendicitis. Arch Surg. 2010;145(9):886–92.
79. Busch M, et al. In-hospital delay increases the risk of perforation in adults with appendicitis. World J Surg. 2011;35(7):1626–33.
80. Ansaloni L, et al. Surgery versus conservative antibiotic treatment in acute appendicitis: a systematic review and meta-analysis of randomized controlled trials. Dig Surg. 2011;28(3):210–21.
81. Liu Z, et al. Laparoscopy or not: a meta-analysis of the surgical effects of laparoscopic versus open appendicectomy. Surg Laparosc Endosc Percutan Tech. 2010;20(6):362–70.
82. Wei B, et al. Laparoscopic versus open appendectomy for acute appendicitis: a metaanalysis. Surg Endosc. 2011;25(4):1199–208.
83. Sauerland S, Jaschinski T, Neugebauer EA. Laparoscopic versus open surgery for suspected appendicitis. Cochrane Database Syst Rev. 2010; 10, CD001546.
84. Li X, et al. Laparoscopic versus conventional appendectomy–a meta-analysis of randomized controlled trials. BMC Gastroenterol. 2010;10:129.
85. Wei HB, et al. Laparoscopic versus open appendectomy: a prospective randomized comparison. Surg Endosc. 2010;24(2):266–9.
86. Jaschinski T, et al. Laparoscopic versus open appendectomy in patients with suspected appendicitis: a systematic review of meta-analyses of randomised controlled trials. BMC Gastroenterol. 2015;15:48.
87. Tzovaras G, et al. Laparoscopic versus open appendectomy in men: a prospective randomized trial. Surg Endosc. 2010;24(12):2987–92.
88. Ward NT, Ramamoorthy SL, Chang DC, Parsons JK. Laparoscopic appendectomy is safer than open appendectomy in an elderly population. JSLS. 2014;18(3):e2014. doi:10.4293/JSLS.2014.00322.
89. Yeh CC, et al. Laparoscopic appendectomy for acute appendicitis is more favorable for patients with comorbidities, the elderly, and those with complicated appendicitis: a nationwide population-based study. Surg Endosc. 2011;25(9):2932–42.
90. Tiwari MM, et al. Comparison of outcomes of laparoscopic and open appendectomy in management of uncomplicated and complicated appendicitis. Ann Surg. 2011;254(6):927–32.
91. Southgate E, et al. Laparoscopic vs open appendectomy in older patients. Arch Surg. 2012;147(6):557–62.
92. Ciarrocchi A, Amicucci G. Laparoscopic versus open appendectomy in obese patients: A meta-analysis of prospective and retrospective studies. J Minim Access Surg. 2014;10(1):4–9.
93. Dasari BV, et al. Laparoscopic appendicectomy in obese is associated with improvements in clinical outcome: systematic review. Int J Surg. 2015;13: 250–6.
94. Jackson H, et al. Diagnosis and laparoscopic treatment of surgical diseases during pregnancy: an evidence-based review. Surg Endosc. 2008;22(9):1917–27.
95. Wilasrusmee C, et al. Systematic review and meta-analysis of safety of laparoscopic versus open appendicectomy for suspected appendicitis in pregnancy. Br J Surg. 2012;99(11):1470–8.
96. Cheng HT, et al. Laparoscopic appendectomy versus open appendectomy in pregnancy: a population-based analysis of maternal outcome. Surg Endosc. 2015;29(6):1394–9.
97. Cox TC, et al. Laparoscopic appendectomy and cholecystectomy versus open: a study in 1999 pregnant patients. Surg Endosc. 2016;30(2):593–602.
98. Walker HG, et al. Laparoscopic appendicectomy in pregnancy: a systematic review of the published evidence. Int J Surg. 2014;12(11):1235–41.
99. Markar SR, et al. Laparoscopic versus open appendectomy for complicated and uncomplicated appendicitis in children. J Gastrointest Surg. 2012;16(10): 1993–2004.
100. Wang CC, et al. Outcome comparison between laparoscopic and open appendectomy: evidence from a nationwide population-based study. PLoS One. 2013;8(7), e68662.
101. Masoomi H, et al. Comparison of outcomes of laparoscopic versus open appendectomy in adults: data from the Nationwide Inpatient Sample (NIS), 2006–2008. J Gastrointest Surg. 2011;15(12):2226–31.

102. Isaksson K, et al. Long-term follow-up for adhesive small bowel obstruction after open versus laparoscopic surgery for suspected appendicitis. Ann Surg. 2014;259(6):1173–7.
103. Di Saverio S, et al. A cost-effective technique for laparoscopic appendectomy: outcomes and costs of a case–control prospective single-operator study of 112 unselected consecutive cases of complicated acute appendicitis. J Am Coll Surg. 2014;218(3):e51–65.
104. Moore CB, et al. Does use of intraoperative irrigation with open or laparoscopic appendectomy reduce post-operative intra-abdominal abscess? Am Surg. 2011;77(1):78–80.
105. St Peter SD, et al. Irrigation versus suction alone during laparoscopic appendectomy for perforated appendicitis: a prospective randomized trial. Ann Surg. 2012;256(4):581–5.
106. Ohno Y, Furui J, Kanematsu T. Treatment strategy when using intraoperative peritoneal lavage for perforated appendicitis in children: a preliminary report. Pediatr Surg Int. 2004;20(7):534–7.
107. Akkoyun I, Tuna AT. Advantages of abandoning abdominal cavity irrigation and drainage in operations performed on children with perforated appendicitis. J Pediatr Surg. 2012;47(10):1886–90.
108. Schein M, Rogers P, Assalia A. Schein's Common Sense Emergency Abdominal Surgery: an Unconventional Book. 3rd ed. Springer; 2010. p. 456.
109. Motson RW, Kelly MD. Simplified technique for laparoscopic appendectomy. ANZ J Surg. 2002;72(4):294–5.
110. Naguib N. Simple technique for laparoscopic appendicectomy to ensure safe division of the mesoappendix. Scand J Surg. 2014;103(1):73–4.
111. Aydogan F, et al. A comparison of the adverse reactions associated with isosulfan blue versus methylene blue dye in sentinel lymph node biopsy for breast cancer. Am J Surg. 2008;195(2):277–8.
112. Yang HR, et al. Laparoscopic appendectomy using the LigaSure Vessel Sealing System. J Laparoendosc Adv Surg Tech A. 2005;15(4):353–6.
113. Sucullu I, et al. The effects of LigaSure on the laparoscopic management of acute appendicitis: "LigaSure assisted laparoscopic appendectomy". Surg Laparosc Endosc Percutan Tech. 2009;19(4):333–5.
114. Diamantis T, et al. Comparison of monopolar electrocoagulation, bipolar electrocoagulation, Ultracision, and Ligasure. Surg Today. 2006;36(10):908–13.
115. Lee JS, Hong TH. Comparison of various methods of mesoappendix dissection in laparoscopic appendectomy. J Laparoendosc Adv Surg Tech A. 2014;24(1):28–31.
116. Kazemier G, et al. Securing the appendiceal stump in laparoscopic appendectomy: evidence for routine stapling? Surg Endosc. 2006;20(9):1473–6.
117. Sahm M, et al. Current analysis of endoloops in appendiceal stump closure. Surg Endosc. 2011;25(1):124–9.
118. Lin HF, Lai HS, Lai IR. Laparoscopic treatment of perforated appendicitis. World J Gastroenterol. 2014;20(39):14338–47.
119. Swank HA, et al. Endostapler or endoloops for securing the appendiceal stump in laparoscopic appendectomy: a retrospective cohort study. Surg Endosc. 2014;28(2):576–83.
120. Lukish J, et al. Laparoscopic appendectomy in children: use of the endoloop vs the endostapler. Arch Surg. 2007;142(1):58–61. discussion 62.
121. Rakic M, et al. Analysis of endoloops and endostaples for closing the appendiceal stump during laparoscopic appendectomy. Surg Today. 2014; 44(9):1716–22.
122. Sajid MS, et al. Use of endo-GIA versus endo-loop for securing the appendicular stump in laparoscopic appendicectomy: a systematic review. Surg Laparosc Endosc Percutan Tech. 2009;19(1):11–5.
123. Safavi A, Langer M, Skarsgard ED. Endoloop versus endostapler closure of the appendiceal stump in pediatric laparoscopic appendectomy. Can J Surg. 2012;55(1):37–40.
124. Street D, et al. Simple ligation vs stump inversion in appendectomy. Arch Surg. 1988;123(6):689–90.
125. Niemineva K. The pioneer of operative gynecology in Finland. Nord Med. 1970;84(46):1449–52.
126. Lavonius MI, et al. Simple ligation vs stump inversion in appendicectomy. Ann Chir Gynaecol. 1996;85(3):222–4.
127. van der Graaf YOH. Simple ligation better than invagination of the appendix stump; a prospective randomized study. Ned Tijdschr Geneeskd. 1992; 136(31):1525.
128. Allemann P, et al. Prevention of infectious complications after laparoscopic appendectomy for complicated acute appendicitis–the role of routine abdominal drainage. Langenbecks Arch Surg. 2011; 396(1):63–8.
129. Narci A, et al. Is peritoneal drainage necessary in childhood perforated appendicitis?–a comparative study. J Pediatr Surg. 2007;42(11):1864–8.
130. Siribumrungwong B, et al. A systematic review and meta-analysis of randomised controlled trials of delayed primary wound closure in contaminated abdominal wounds. World J Emerg Surg. 2014;9(1):49.
131. Henry MC, Moss RL. Primary versus delayed wound closure in complicated appendicitis: an international systematic review and meta-analysis. Pediatr Surg Int. 2005;21(8):625–30.
132. Gurusamy KS, Cassar Delia E, Davidson BR. Peritoneal closure versus no peritoneal closure for patients undergoing non-obstetric abdominal operations. Cochrane Database Syst Rev. 2013;7, CD010424.
133. Swank HA, et al. Is routine histopathological examination of appendectomy specimens useful? A systematic review of the literature. Colorectal Dis. 2011; 13(11):1214–21.
134. Carr NJ. The pathology of acute appendicitis. Ann Diagn Pathol. 2000;4(1):46–58.
135. Grimes C, et al. Appendiceal faecaliths are associated with right iliac fossa pain. Ann R Coll Surg Engl. 2010;92(1):61–4.
136. van den Broek WT, et al. A normal appendix found during diagnostic laparoscopy should not be removed. Br J Surg. 2001;88(2):251–4.
137. Phillips AW, Jones AE, Sargen K. Should the macroscopically normal appendix be removed during laparoscopy for acute right iliac fossa pain when no other explanatory pathology is found? Surg Laparosc Endosc Percutan Tech. 2009;19(5):392–4.
138. Lee M, et al. The morbidity of negative appendicectomy. Ann R Coll Surg Engl. 2014;96(7):517–20.
139. Strong S, et al. How good are surgeons at identifying appendicitis? Results from a multi-centre cohort study. Int J Surg. 2015;15:107–12.
140. Hamminga JT, et al. Evaluation of the appendix during diagnostic laparoscopy, the laparoscopic appendicitis score: a pilot study. Surg Endosc. 2013;27(5):1594–600.
141. Shafi S, et al. Measuring anatomic severity of disease in emergency general surgery. J Trauma Acute Care Surg. 2014;76(3):884–7.
142. Gomes CA, et al. Laparoscopy grading system of acute appendicitis: new insight for future trials. Surg Laparosc Endosc Percutan Tech. 2012; 22(5):463–6.
143. Gomes CA, et al. Lessons learned with laparoscopic management of complicated grades of acute appendicitis. J Clin Med Res. 2014;6(4): 261–6.
144. Simillis C, et al. A meta-analysis comparing conservative treatment versus acute appendectomy for complicated appendicitis (abscess or phlegmon). Surgery. 2010;147(6):818–29.
145. Mentula P, Sammalkorpi H, Leppaniemi A. Laparoscopic Surgery or Conservative Treatment for Appendiceal Abscess in Adults? A Randomized Controlled Trial. Ann Surg. 2015;262(2):237–42.
146. Weber DG, Di Saverio S. Letter to the Editor: Laparoscopic Surgery or Conservative Treatment for Appendiceal Abscess in Adults? Ann Surg. 2015. [Epub ahead of print].
147. Hall NJ, et al. Is interval appendicectomy justified after successful nonoperative treatment of an appendix mass in children? A systematic review. J Pediatr Surg. 2011;46(4):767–71.
148. Deakin DE, Ahmed I. Interval appendicectomy after resolution of adult inflammatory appendix mass–is it necessary? Surgeon. 2007;5(1):45–50.
149. Carpenter SG, et al. Increased risk of neoplasm in appendicitis treated with interval appendectomy: single-institution experience and literature review. Am Surg. 2012;78(3):339–43.
150. Sartelli M, et al. 2013 WSES guidelines for management of intra-abdominal infections. World J Emerg Surg. 2013;8(1):3.
151. Daskalakis K, Juhlin C, Pahlman L. The use of pre- or postoperative antibiotics in surgery for appendicitis: a systematic review. Scand J Surg. 2014;103(1):14–20.
152. Andersen BR, Kallehave FL, Andersen HK. Antibiotics versus placebo for prevention of postoperative infection after appendicectomy. Cochrane Database Syst Rev. 2005;3, CD001439.
153. Mui LM, et al. Optimum duration of prophylactic antibiotics in acute non-perforated appendicitis. ANZ J Surg. 2005;75(6):425–8.
154. Allo MD, et al. Ticarcillin/clavulanate versus imipenem/cilistatin for the treatment of infections associated with gangrenous and perforated appendicitis. Am Surg. 1999;65(2):99–104.
155. Hopkins JA, Wilson SE, Bobey DG. Adjunctive antimicrobial therapy for complicated appendicitis: bacterial overkill by combination therapy. World J Surg. 1994;18(6):933–8.

156. Sartelli M, et al. Complicated intra-abdominal infections worldwide: the definitive data of the CIAOW Study. World J Emerg Surg. 2014;9:37.
157. Sartelli M, et al. Antimicrobial management of intra-abdominal infections: literature's guidelines. World J Gastroenterol. 2012;18(9):865–71.
158. Berne TV, et al. Meropenem versus tobramycin with clindamycin in the antibiotic management of patients with advanced appendicitis. J Am Coll Surg. 1996;182(5):403–7.
159. Taylor E, et al. Complicated appendicitis: is there a minimum intravenous antibiotic requirement? A prospective randomized trial. Am Surg. 2000;66(9): 887–90.
160. Sawyer RG, et al. Trial of short-course antimicrobial therapy for intraabdominal infection. N Engl J Med. 2015;372(21):1996–2005.
161. SMM de Castro, CUnlu, EP Steller, et al. Evaluation of the Appendicitis Inflammatory Response Score for Patients with Acute Appendicitis. World J Surg. 2012;36:1540–1545.

The role of red cell distribution width in the diagnosis of acute appendicitis

Huseyin Narci[1*], Emin Turk[2], Erdal Karagulle[2], Turhan Togan[3] and Keziban Karabulut[1]

Abstract

Purpose: The aim of this study was to seek whether red cell distribution width (RDW) has a role in the diagnosis of acute appendicitis. It was also aimed to show the relationship of RDW with leukocyte count and C-reactive protein (CRP) level.

Methods: This study was conducted via retrospective assessment of the hospital records of the adult patients who were operated for acute appendicitis between January 2010 and February 2013 and had a pathology report that confirmed the diagnosis of acute appendicitis. The patients in the control group were selected from healthy adults of similar age who applied to check-up clinic. Age, gender, leukocyte count, CRP, and RDW values were recorded. This study is a case controlled retrospective clinical study.

Results: A total of 590 patients in the acute appendicitis group and 121 patients in the control group were included, making up a total of 711 subjects. The mean RDW levels were 15.4 ± 1.5% in the acute appendicitis group, while 15.9 ± 1.4% in the control group. CRP, leukocyte count were significantly higher in the acute appendicitis group, and RDW level were significantly lower in the acute appendicitis group ($p < 0.001$, $p < 0.001$, $p = 0.001$, respectively). RDW, leukocyte count, and CRP had a sensitivity and specificity of 47% and 67%; 91% and 74%; and 97% and 41%, respectively in acute appendicitis. RDW was not correlated with CRP and leukocyte levels. However, we found a correlation between CRP and leukocyte levels.

Conclusion: RDW level was lower in patients with acute appendicitis. The magnitude of difference in RDW seen between acute appendicitis and controls was so slight as to be of no utility in diagnostic testing.

Keywords: Acute appendicitis, C-reactive protein, Leukocyte, Red cell distribution width

Introduction

Acute appendicitis (AA) is the most common surgical abdominal emergency [1]. Rapid diagnosis is important, because increased time between onset of symptoms and surgical intervention is associated with increased risk of appendiceal perforation and therefore potential peritonitis, sepsis, and death [2]. However, the rate of negative appendectomy (when appendectomy is performed, but the appendix is found to be normal on histological evaluation) ranges from 5% to 42%, and this can be associated with considerable morbidity [1-4]. Clinical diagnosis can be challenging, particularly in the early stages of appendicitis when clinical manifestations may be quite non-specific or atypical. Different elements of history, examination, and laboratory findings have varying predictive power in the diagnosis of appendicitis, and algorithms and scoring systems for clinical evaluation exist, but appendicitis can nevertheless be easily missed [1,3].

The preoperative laboratory tests can be performed easily in primary healthcare settings and often aid primary clinicians with decision making about patients with clinically suspected AA. Several parameters for the diagnosis of AA have been investigated in the literature [5]. RDW, a measure of heterogeneity in the size of circulating red blood cells, is a component of the standard complete blood count and calculated as a percentage of

* Correspondence: hsnnarci@gmail.com
[1]Department of Emergency Medicine, Baskent Universitesi Konya Hastanesi Hocacihan mah, Saray caddesi No: 1, Selcuklu, Konya 42080, Turkey
Full list of author information is available at the end of the article

the standard deviation of the red cell volume divided by the mean corpuscular volume. It has been reported that RDW level has clinical implications in various pathologies such as inflammatory bowel disease, celiac disease, pulmonary embolism, and coronary artery disease [6-10]. In addition, its predictive role has been shown in inflammatory and infectious pathological diseases including acute pancreatitis, bacteremia, sepsis, and septic shock [11-13]. In the present study we aimed to seek whether RDW level is important in the diagnosis of AA. No studies in literature have examined this subject before. In addition, it was aimed to show the relationship of RDW level with leukocyte count and CRP level.

Materials and method

The main analysis in this study was the comparison of the difference RDW measurements between acute appendicitis and control groups. In healthy individuals RDW levels have been reported as 11.6% and 15.5% with a standard deviation of approximately 1.3%. A 0.6% difference in the mean RDW values was determined to represent a significant difference between acute appendicitis and control groups. Given these assumptions and assuming that two-sample independent t test was to be used for comparison of means, it was determined that both groups had to include at least 123 test subjects to achieve a power level of 90%. Sample sizes were calculated by using the Minitab statistical package software (Release 14). This study was conducted via retrospective assessment of hospital records of the adult patients who were operated for acute appendicitis in Baskent University, Konya Research and Application Center, between January 2010 and February 2013 and had a pathology report that confirmed the diagnosis of acute appendicitis. A total of 590 patients were included in the AA group. The patients in the control group were selected from healthy adults of similar age who applied to check-up clinic and had no active complaint, chronic disease, or abnormal physical examination. Age, gender, leukocyte count, and CRP and RDW levels were recorded. This study is a case controlled retrospective clinical study.

Laboratory measurements

WBC counts were determined using an electronic cell counter (Cell-Dyne 3700, Abbott, Abbott Park, IL, USA). Serum CRP levels were measured by spectrophotometric methods (Abbott Aeroset, Tokyo, Japan). The expected RDW values in our laboratory ranged between 11.6% and 15.5%.

Statistical analysis

Statistical analyses were performed with SPSS software. The groups were compared using the *t* test for continuous variables and chi-square test for categorical variables. Mann–Whitney *U* test was used to compare nonhomogeneous groups in pairs. A simple correlation test (Spearman's test) was used to observe the correlation between the RDW and other variables. Numeric values were expressed as means ± SD. A *P* value less than .05 was considered statistically significant.

Results

A total of 590 patients were included in the AA group and 121 patients were included in the control group, making up a total of 711 subjects. No significant difference was observed between the AA and control groups with respect to age and gender $p > 0.05$ (Table 1). The mean leukocyte count was 13.5 ± 4.5 ($\times 10^3/mm^3$) in the AA group and 7.5 ± 2 ($\times 10^3/mm^3$) in the control group. The leukocyte count was significantly higher in the AA group ($p < 0.001$). The mean CRP level was 48.8 ± 73.6 mg/dL in the AA group and 4.6 ± 4.7 mg/dL in the control group. CRP level in the AA group was significantly higher compared with the control group ($p < 0.001$). The mean RDW level was 15.4 ± 1.5% in the AA group and 15.9 ± 1.4% in the control group. RDW level was significantly lower in the AA group compared with the control group ($p = 0.001$) (Table 1). Receiver operating characteristic curve analysis suggested that the best cutoff point for RDW in the diagnosis of AA was 15.6%, which had a sensitivity of 47% and a specificity of 67%, (area under curve [AUC]: 0,62; Figure 1). Receiver operating characteristic curve analysis suggested that the best cutoff point for leukocyte count in the diagnosis of AA was 10.4 ($\times 10^3/mm^3$), which had a sensitivity of 91% and a specificity of 74% (area under curve [AUC]: 0.9; Figure 1). Receiver operating characteristic curve analysis suggested the best cutoff point for CRP level in the diagnosis of AA was 27.1 mg/dL, which had a sensitivity of 97% and a specificity of 41% (area under curve [AUC]: 0.77; Figure 1). RDW was not correlated with CRP and leukocyte levels. However, we found a correlation between CRP and leukocyte levels (Table 2).

Table 1 Comparison of the demographic features and leukocyte count, CRP, and RDW levels of the subjects in the acute appendicitis and the control groups

	Acute appendicitis (n = 590)	Control group (n = 121)	*p*
Male/female	332/258	69/52	.82
Age (y)*	36.7 ± 12.2	35.2 ± 8.1	.67
Leukocyte (× 10^3/mm3)*	13.5 ± 4.5	7.5 ± 2	<0.01
CRP (mg/L)*	48.8 ± 73.6	4.6 ± 4.7	<0.01
RDW (%)*	15.4 ± 1.5	15.9 ± 1.4	0.01

*Values are means±standard deviation.
Abbreviations: *CRP* C-reactive protein, *RDW* red cell distribution width.

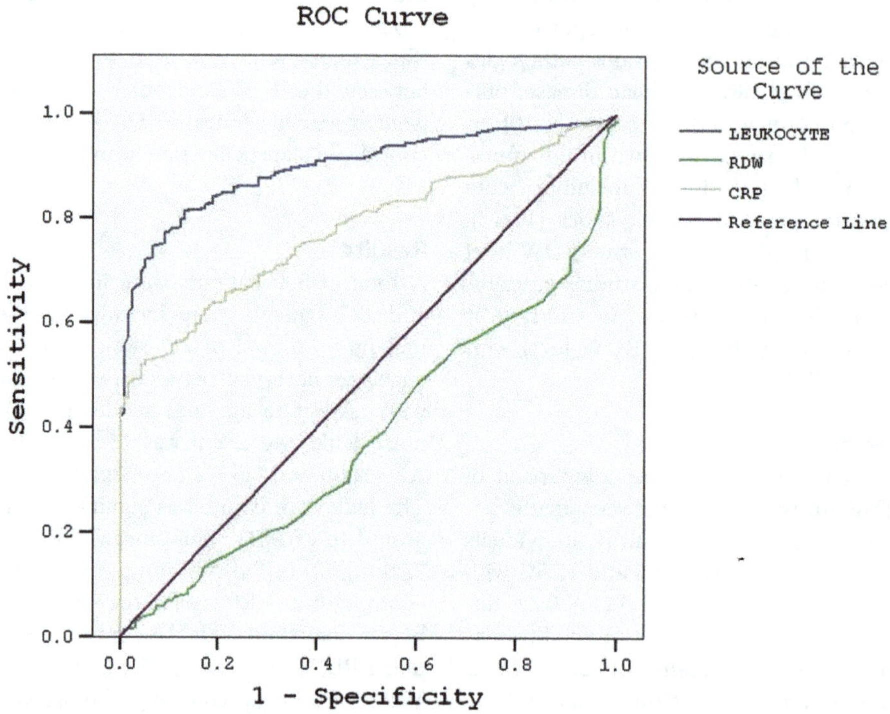

Figure 1 Receiver operating characteristic (ROC) curve of red cell distribution width (RDW), leukocyte, and C-reactive protein (CRP).

Discussion

A parameter with ability to establish the diagnosis of acute appendicitis has always been a center of attention for physicians. Many different parameters have been examined or are under active investigation for that purpose. The pathophysiology of acute appendicitis is characterized by the mucosal ischemia of the appendix that results from ongoing mucus secretion from the appendiceal mucosa distal to an obstruction of the lumen, elevating intraluminal and, in turn, venous pressures. Once luminal pressure exceeds 85 mmHg, venules that drain the appendix become thrombosed and, in the setting of continued arteriolar in flow, vascular congestion and engorgement of the appendix become manifest [5]. Infection is added to the inflammation of appendicitis.

WBC count is most frequently used to diagnose AA. Several reports have suggested that an elevated WBC count is usually the earliest laboratory measure to indicate inflammation of the appendix, and most patients with AA present with leukocytosis [14,15]. We found that WBC count was significantly higher in AA. In various studies, the range of sensitivity and specificity of WBC in the diagnosis of AA have been reported 67%-97.8% and 31.9%-80%, respectively [16]. Similar to the literature, the present study found that the sensitivity and specificity of leukocyte level were 91% and 74%, respectively.

Table 2 Correlation analysis of leukocyte, CRP, and RDW levels in patients with acute appendicitis

Parameters	Correlation coefficient (r)	*P value*
Leukocyte - RDW	−0.031	.44
Leukocyte - CRP	0.21	<0.01
CRP – RDW	−0.065	.11

Abbreviations: CRP C-reactive protein, *RDW* red cell distribution width.

CRP is a sensitive acute phase protein that lacks specificity due to increased levels in all acute inflammatory processes. Its concentration increases with the duration and extent of the inflammation. In a meta-analysis examining the accuracy of CRP level in the diagnosis of AA, Hallan and Asberg found a wide range of sensitivity (40%-99%) and specificity (27%-90%) [17]. Similar to the literature, this study found a sensitivity of 97% and a specificity of 41% for CRP in the diagnosis of acute appendicitis. Among the assessed parameters, CRP had the highest sensitivity and the lowest specificity.

RDW is commonly used to discriminate between microcytic anemia's due to iron deficiency and those due to thalassemia or hemoglobinopathies [7]. Increased RDW levels are related to impaired erythropoiesis or erythrocyte degradation [7]. The typical reference range spans between 11.6 and 15.5%. Recent studies have demonstrated that higher RDW levels, even within the normal reference range, were associated with unfavorable clinical outcomes in patients with heart failure, coronary artery disease, pulmonary hypertension, diabetes mellitus, and stroke independent of hemoglobin values [8-10,18,19]. Furthermore RDW has been studied as a surrogate marker in many pathological conditions such as rheumatoid arthritis, inflammatory bowel disease, colon cancer, and celiac disease [6,20,21]. Although the exact pathophysiological basis of this relationship is unclear, chronic inflammation, aging, malnutrition, and anemia are proposed underlying factors in this topic [10,22].

In a patient with acute pancreatitis, RDW level at the presentation has been reported to be an independent risk factor for mortality [12]. Similarly, RDW level has also been found to be a predictor for mortality in bacteremia and septic shock [11,13]. An increased RDW level has been reported in these inflammatory and infectious pathologies. Elevated RDW can result from any disease process that causes the premature release of reticulocytes into the circulation. Elevations in RDW have been shown to be associated with elevated inflammatory markers, such as CRP, erythrocyte sedimentation rate, and interleukin 6 [13,23,24]. Proinflammatory cytokines of sepsis (tumor necrosis factor A, interleukin 6, and interleukin 1b) have been shown to directly and negatively affect the survival of red blood cells in the circulation, promote deformability of the red blood cell membrane, and suppress erythrocyte maturation. These inflammatory mediators of sepsis can thus lead to newer, larger reticulocytes to enter the peripheral circulation, and thus increase RDW [13]. Unlike the above-mentioned studies, we found a significantly lower, albeit within normal limits, RDW level in patients with acute appendicitis compared with subjects in the control group. This finding may be the result of greater RDW level in chronic inflammatory diseases compared to that in acute conditions. A strong correlation of RDW with inflammatory markers, CRP and sedimentation rate has also been observed [13,23,24]. In our study, on the other hand, RDW was not correlated with CRP and leukocyte count.

In conclusion, RDW level was lower in patients with acute appendicitis. No studies in literature have examined RDW level in acute appendicitis before. The magnitude of difference in RDW seen between AA and controls was so slight as to be of no utility in diagnostic testing. We think that further prospective, multicenter studies with a large sample size are needed in this field.

Competing interests

The authors declare that they have no competing interests and no funding statement.

Authors' contributions

Study concept and design: HN, ET and EK. Analysis and interpretation of data: HN, ET, EK, TT and KK. Drafting of the manuscript: HN, ET and EK. All authors read and approved the final manuscript.

Acknowledgments

This study was approved by Baskent University Institutional Review Board and supported by Baskent University Research Fund.

Author details

[1]Department of Emergency Medicine, Baskent Universitesi Konya Hastanesi Hocacihan mah, Saray caddesi No: 1, Selcuklu, Konya 42080, Turkey. [2]Department of General Surgery, Baskent University Faculty of Medicine, Ankara, Turkey. [3]Department of Infectious Diseases and Clinical Microbiology, Baskent University Faculty of Medicine, Ankara, Turkey.

References

1. Humes DJ, Simpson J: **Acute appendicitis.** *BMJ* 2006, **333:**530–534.
2. Bickell NA, Aufses AH Jr, Rojas M, Bodian C: **How time affects the risk of rupture in appendicitis.** *J Am Coll Surg* 2006, **202:**401–406.
3. Shefki X, Lumturije GL, Kumrije X, Fahredin V, Besnik B, Fatos S, Avdyl K: **Correlation of serum C-reactive protein, white blood count and neutrophil percentage with histopathology findings in acute appendicitis.** *World J Emerg Surg* 2012, **7:**27.
4. Ashdown HF, D'Souza N, Karim D, Stevens RJ, Huang A, Harnden A: **Pain over speed bumps in diagnosis of acute appendicitis: diagnostic accuracy study.** *BMJ* 2012, **345:**e8012.
5. Karagulle E, Turk E, Ezer A, Nursal TZ, Kulaksızoglu S, Moray G: **Value of plasma viscosity in acute appendicitis: a preliminary.** *J Med Med Sci* 2010, **1:**423–425.
6. Harmanci O, Kav T, Sivri B: **Red cell distribution width can predict intestinal atrophy in selected patients with celiac disease.** *J Clin Lab Anal* 2012, **26:**497–502.
7. Öztürk ZA, Ünal A, Yiğiter R, Yesil Y, Kuyumcu ME, Neyal M, Kepekçi Y: **Is increased red cell distribution width (RDW) indicating the inflammation in Alzheimer's disease (AD)?** *Arch Gerontol Geriatr* 2013, **56:**50–54.
8. Felker GM, Allen LA, Pocock SJ, Shaw LK, McMurray JJ, Pfeffer MA, Swedberg K, Wang D, Yusuf S, Michelson EL, Granger CB, CHARM Investigators: **Red cell distribution width as a novel prognostic marker in heart failure: data from the CHARM Program and the Duke Databank.** *J Am Coll Cardiol* 2007, **50:**40–47.
9. Hampole CV, Mehrotra AK, Thenappan T, Gomberg-Maitland M, Shah SJ: **Usefulness of red cell distribution width as a prognostic marker in pulmonary hypertension.** *Am J Cardiol* 2009, **104:**868–872.
10. Tonelli M, Sacks F, Arnold M, Moye L, Davis B, Pfeffer M, for the Cholesterol and Recurrent Events (CARE) Trial Investigators: **Relation between red blood cell distribution width and cardiovascular event rate in people with coronary disease.** *Circulation* 2008, **117:**163–168.
11. Ku NS, Kim HW, Oh HJ, Kim YC, Kim MH, Song JE, Oh DH, Ahn JY, Kim SB, Jeong SJ, Han SH, Kim CO, Song YG, Kim JM, Choi JY: **Red blood cell distribution width is an independent predictor of mortality in patients with gram-negative bacteremia.** *Shock* 2012, **38:**123–127.
12. Senol K, Saylam B, Kocaay F, Tez M: **Red cell distribution width as a predictor of mortality in acute pancreatitis.** *Am J Emerg Med* 2013. doi: 10.1016/j.ajem.2012.12.015. [Epub ahead of print].
13. Sadaka F, O'Brien J, Prakash S: **Red cell distribution width and outcome in patients with septic shock.** *J Intensive Care Med* 2012 [Epub ahead of print].
14. Andersson REB: **Meta-analysis of the clinical and laboratory diagnosis of appendicitis.** *Br J Surg* 2004, **91:**28–37.
15. Birchley D: **Patients with clinical acute appendicitis should have pre-operative full blood count and C-reactiveprotein assays.** *Ann R Coll Surg Engl* 2006, **88:**27–32.
16. Albayrak Y, Albayrak A, Albayrak F, Yildirim R, Aylu B, Uyanik A, Kabalar E, Güzel IC: **Mean platelet volume: a new predictor in confirming acute appendicitis diagnosis.** *Clin Appl Thromb Hemost* 2011, **17:**362–366.
17. Hallan S, Asberg A, Edna TH: **Additional value of biochemical tests in suspected acute appendicitis.** *Eur J Surg* 1997, **163:**5333–5338.
18. Ani C, Ovbiagele B: **Elevated red blood cell distribution width predicts mortality in persons with known stroke.** *J Neurol Sci* 2009, **277:**103–108.
19. Malandrino N, Wu WC, Taveira TH, Whitlatch HB, Smith RJ: **Association between red blood cell distribution width and macrovascular and microvascular complications in diabetes.** *Diabetologia* 2012, **55:**226–235.

20. Kim J, Kim K, Lee JH, Jo YH, Rhee JE, Kim TY, Kang KW, Kim YJ, Hwang SS, Jang HY: **Red blood cell distribution width as an independent predictor of all-cause mortality in out of hospital cardiac arrest.** *Resuscitation* 2012, **83:**1248–1252.
21. Spell DW, Jones DV Jr, Harper WF, David BJ: **The value of a complete blood count in predicting cancer of the colon.** *Cancer Detect Prev* 2004, **28:**37–42.
22. Patel KV, Ferrucci L, Ershler WB, Longo DL, Guralnik JM: **Red blood cell distribution width and the risk of death in middle-aged and older adults.** *Arch Intern Med* 2009, **169:**515–523.
23. Perlstein TS, Weuve J, Pfeffer MA, Beckman JA: **Red blood cell distribution width and mortality risk in a community-based prospective cohort.** *Arch Intern Med* 2009, **169:**588–594.
24. Lippi G, Targher G, Montagnana M, Salvagno GL, Zoppini G, Guidi GC: **Relation between red blood cell distribution width and inflammatory biomarkers in a large cohort of unselected outpatients.** *Arch Pathol Lab Med* 2009, **133:**628–632.

11

Emergency total thyroidectomy due to non traumatic disease: Experience of a surgical unit

Mario Testini[1], Francesco Logoluso[2], Germana Lissidini[1], Angela Gurrado[1*], Giuseppe Campobasso[4], Rocco Cortese[3], Giuseppe Massimiliano De Luca[1], Ilaria Fabiola Franco[1], Alessandro De Luca[1] and Giuseppe Piccinni[1]

Abstract

Background: Acute respiratory failure due to thyroid compression or invasion of the tracheal lumen is a surgical emergency requiring urgent management. The aim of this paper is to describe a series of six patients treated successfully in the emergency setting with total thyroidectomy due to ingravescent dyspnoea and asphyxia, as well as review related data reported in literature.

Methods: During 2005-2010, of 919 patients treated by total thyroidectomy at our Academic Hospital, 6 (0.7%; 4 females and 2 men, mean age: 68.7 years, range 42-81 years) were treated in emergency. All the emergency operations were performed for life-threatening respiratory distress. The clinical picture at admission, clinical features, type of surgery, outcomes and complications are described. Mean duration of surgery was 146 minutes (range: 53-260).

Results: In 3/6 (50%) a manubriotomy was necessary due to the extension of the mass into the upper mediastinum. In all cases total thyroidectomy was performed. In one case (16.7%) a parathyroid gland transplantation and in another one (16.7%) a tracheotomy was necessary due to a condition of tracheomalacia. Mean post-operative hospital stay was 6.5 days (range: 2-10 days). Histology revealed malignancy in 4/6 cases (66.7%), showing 3 primitive, and 1 secondary tumors. Morbidity consisted of 1 transient recurrent laryngeal palsy, 3 transient postoperative hypoparathyroidism, and 4 pleural effusions, treated by medical therapy in 3 and by drains in one. There was no mortality.

Conclusion: On the basis of our experience and of literature review, we strongly advocate elective surgery for patients with thyroid disease at the first signs of tracheal compression. When an acute airway distress appears, an emergency life-threatening total thyroidectomy is recommended in a high-volume centre.

Keywords: Thyroid surgery, Emergency Surgery, Thyroid emergency, Hemorrhage, Acute Air Obstruction

Background

Acute respiratory failure due to thyroid compression or invasion of the tracheal lumen is a surgical emergency requiring urgent management.

Total thyroidectomy is a routine elective operation, but exceptionally it has to be performed on an emergency basis especially when it is life-threatening due to airway obstruction [1-5].

Laryngo-tracheal compression may be caused by giant or cervico-mediastinal goiter, acute intra-thyroidal hemorrhage, anaplastic carcinoma, lymphoma, and metastases from breast, lung, gastro-enteric and renal cancer [6-12]. Bilateral recurrent laryngeal nerve infiltration by anaplastic cancer, lymphoma, metastasis can also result in vocal cord palsy with worsening dyspnoea [13].

Hemorrhage in cysts and adenoma of thyroid gland is a common asymptomatic event [6];

* Correspondence: angelagurrado@libero.it
[1]Department of Biomedical Sciences and Human Oncology, Unit of Endocrine, Digestive and Emergency Surgery, University Medical School of Bari "Aldo Moro", Bari, Italy
Full list of author information is available at the end of the article

On the contrary, massive hemorrhage, severe enough to result in acute airway distress is exceptional and more frequently secondary to neck trauma rather than a spontaneous complication of thyroid disease [14-16].

The aim of this paper is to describe a series of six patients treated successfully in the emergency setting with total thyroidectomy because of ingravescent dyspnoea and asphyxia, as well as review related data reported in literature.

Methods

During 2005-2010, of 919 patients treated by total thyroidectomy at our Academic Hospital, 6 (0.7%; 4 females and 2 men, mean age: 68.7 years, range 42-81 years) were treated in emergency. All the emergency operations were performed for life-threatening respiratory distress, and by the same surgeon (M.T.) with high level of thyroid surgical skill. The clinical picture at admission, clinical features, type of surgery, outcomes and complications are described below. Mean duration of surgery was 146 minutes (range: 53-260).

Case 1

An 81-year-old woman with dyspnoea, tachypnea, stridor, tachycardia, one week history of progressively increasing degree of breathlessness, and a 4-year history of anterior-lateral neck swelling came to our unit. Oxygen therapy was immediately set up, and an urgent CT scan of the neck (Figure 1) showed a huge multinodular goiter with retrosternal extension, producing left displacement of the trachea and its marked narrowing in laterolateral diameter. Because of rapidly worsening respiratory distress, an awake fiberoptic intubation using a small endotracheal tube, followed by induction of general anesthesia and emergency total thyroidectomy by manubriotomy were performed (Figure 2). Intraoperative surgical dissection helped by loupe magnification [17] revealed a mass adherent to the right common carotid artery and extending into the upper mediastinum. It also confirmed the marked left displacement of the trachea and permitted bilateral parathyroid gland and recurrent laryngeal nerve identification. Recovery showed a successfully treated atrial fibrillation and dysphonia due to a left vocal cord palsy confirmed by laryngoscopy. The patient was discharged 7 days after the operation. Microscopic examination revealed a Hürthle cell carcinoma. Transient recurrent laryngeal nerve palsy was successfully treated by logotherapy over a period of four months. The patient currently shows a five-year disease-free follow up.

Case 2

A 59-years-old woman with a large and mainly right-sided cervical mass (Figure 3) came to us with severe dyspnoea, stridor and visible use of accessory respiratory muscles, and cyanosis. Computed tomography scan was performed after an awake fiberoptic intubation followed by induction of general anesthesia, revealing a thyroid mass extending into the upper mediastinum, with displacement and compression of the right jugular vein

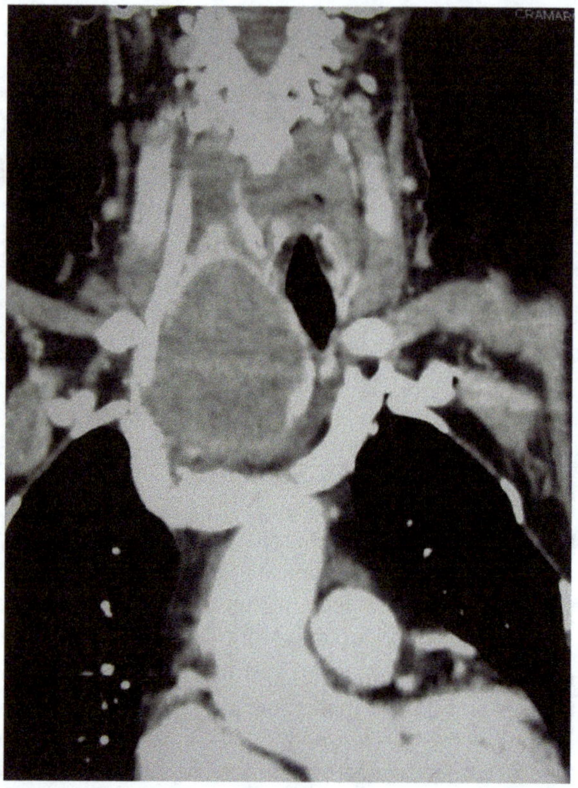

Figure 1 Contrast enhanced CT scan, coronal reconstructed image. The right lobe of the thyroid gland shows a voluminous mass compressing and dislocating trachea, and extending into the upper mediastinum.

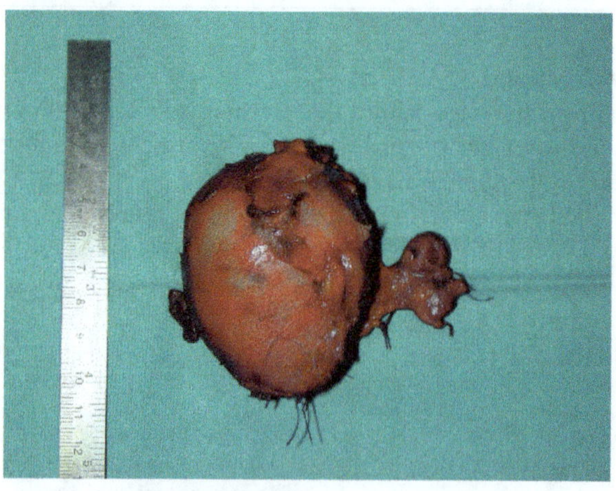

Figure 2 Total thryroidectomy.

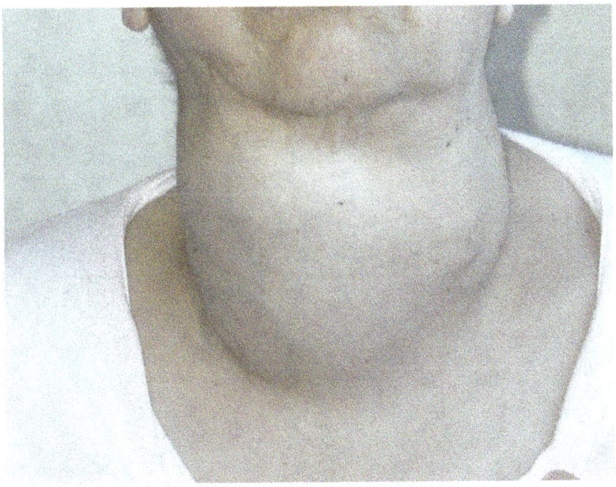

Figure 3 **Large and mainly right-sided cervical mass.**

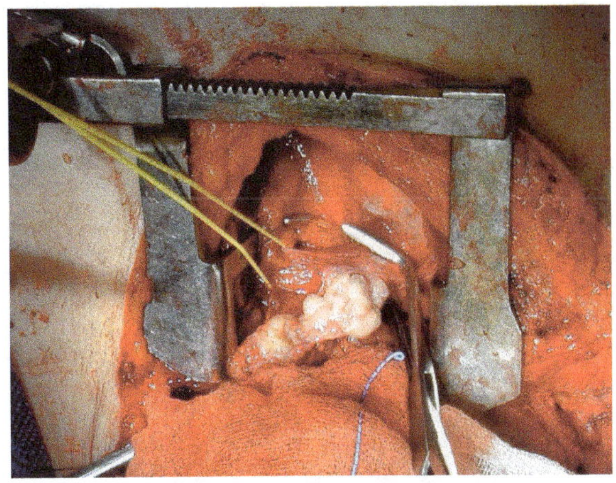

Figure 5 **The lower portion of this retrosternal goitre projected into the left innominate vein, with tumor floating into the lumen.**

and carotid artery on the lateral side and of the trachea on the medial one, with an apparent adherence to the superior vena cava and left innominate vein. Emergency surgery was performed. At operation, performed by sternal split, the lumen of the trachea seemed to be almost completely shut by the compression of the mass, and the lower portion of this retrosternal goitre projected into the left innominate vein, with tumor floating into the lumen (Figures 4, 5). Removal of the neoplastic thrombus through an incision in the vein was performed *en bloc* with the thyroid mass (Figure 6). Both tumor and thrombus were completely replaced by follicular carcinoma. Recovery was uneventful and the patient was discharged ten days after the operation. After four years, and after radioiodine therapy and chemotherapy, the patient is still in follow-up without recurrence or evidence of metastases.

Case 3

A 76-years old women was admitted in emergency with severe worsening respiratory distress due to a giant cervical goiter limiting cervical movements (Figure 7). Medical history revealed a developing mass over the past 50 years without toxic symptoms, increasing dysphagia and worsening ortopnea and paroximal dyspnoea. Physical examination revealed audible wheezing, inspiratory stridor, respiratory rate of 36 cycles/minute, with accessory respiratory muscles use, and tachycardia. Trachea was not reachable during palpation and carotid pulse was unpalpable on the right side and barely palpable on the left side. An urgent CT scan showed a thyroid mass extending from the submandibular and submental regions to the parapharyngeal space and superior mediastinum (Figure 8). A total thyroidectomy

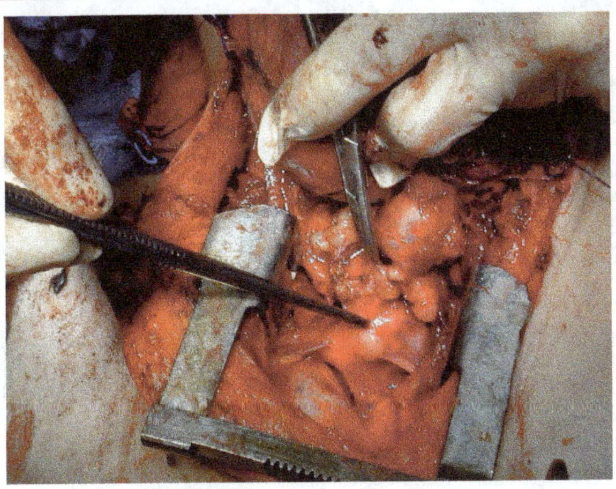

Figure 4 **At operation, performed by sternal split, the lumen of the trachea seemed to be almost completely shut by the compression of the mass.**

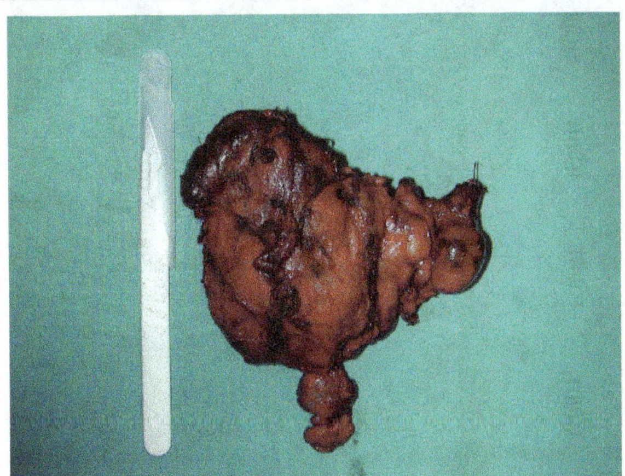

Figure 6 **Removal of the neoplastic thrombus through an incision in the vein was performed *en bloc* with the thyroid mass.**

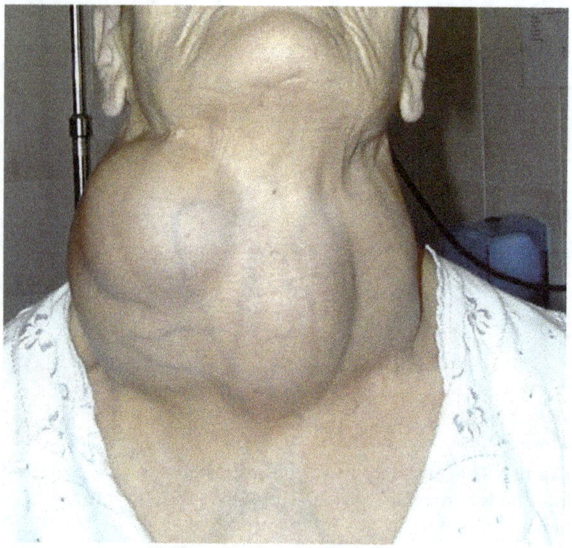

Figure 7 Giant cervical goiter.

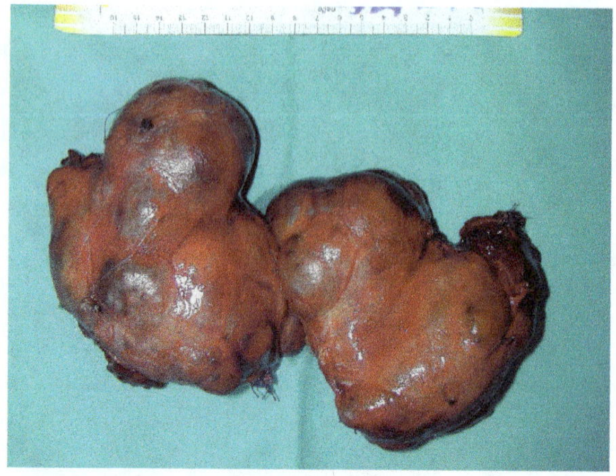

Figure 9 thyroid gland measuring 23 × 16 × 12 cm and weighing 950 g.

was performed in emergency under general anesthesia with a parathyroid gland autotrasplantation in the left sternocleidomastoid muscle according to our indications [18].

The recovery was uneventful and the patient was discharged on the third post-operative day. Pathologic examination revealed a thyroid gland measuring 23 × 16 × 12 cm and weighing 950 g (Figure 9), without histological signs of malignancy.

Case 4[12]

A 73-year-old man was admitted in emergency with a neck mass, sudden dyspnoea, stridor, dysphonia, and progressively worsening dysphagia. A history of multinodular goitre was noted in addition to a previous right radical nephrectomy for non-metastatic renal cell carcinoma 8 years before. The patient underwent fine-needle aspiration consistent with multinodular goitre 5 months before. Three days before admission the patient underwent a total-body CT scan showing a thyroid mass with substernal extension involving and completely obstructing the upper airways, the right vocal cord, with right jugular vein and carotid artery compression and displacement, in addition to diffuse lymphadenopathy (Figure 10). Physical examination revealed a large, painful, diffuse, and predominantly rightsided thyroid swelling. A

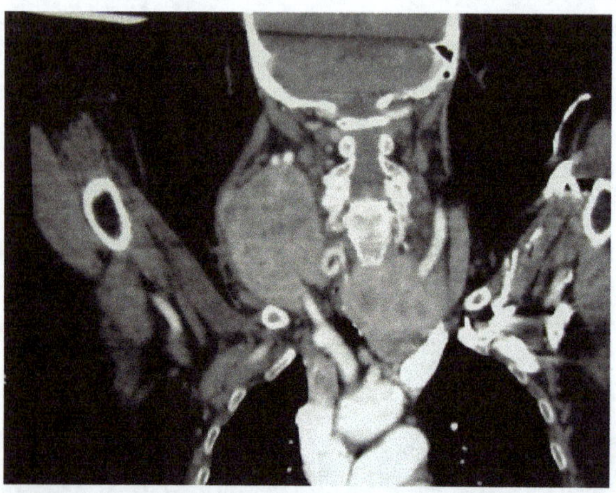

Figure 8 Contrast enhanced CT scan, coronal reconstructed image. A thyroid mass extending from the submandibular and submental regions to the parapharyngeal space and superior mediastinum is evident.

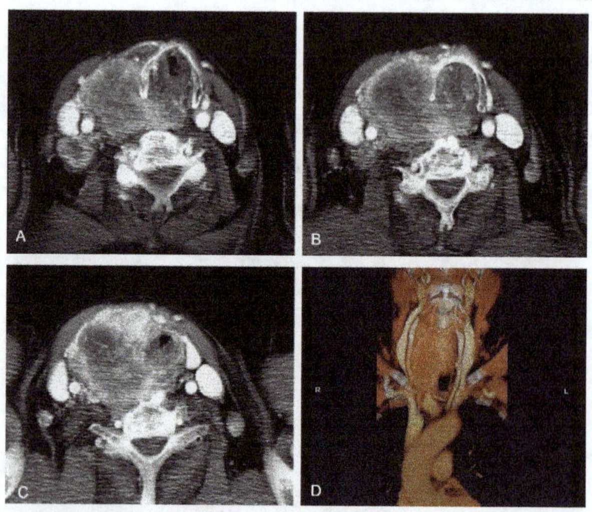

Figure 10 Contrast enhanced CT scan, axial images and coronal reconstructed image. Axial images sequences show the complete closure of the tracheal lumen. A thyroid mass with substernal extension, and with right jugular vein and carotid artery compression and displacement, in addition to diffuse lymphadenopathy are also evident.

flexible laryngoscopy revealed right vocal cord palsy and left cord paresis, with an almost total reduction of the laryngeal lumen. For these reasons, emergency endotracheal intubation was performed followed by total thyroidectomy with lymph node dissection (Figure 11). The operation was completed by a tracheotomy, considering the evident tracheomalacia (Figure 12). Histology revealed a poorly differentiated trabecular carcinoma, consisting of mainly clear cells with scanty oxyphil ones, with large nucleolated nuclei and frequent mitoses. Immunostains with alkaline phosphatase-anti-alkaline phosphatase showed strong and diffuse membrane positivity for CD10 antigen. These patterns were consistent with a renal cell primary carcinoma. The patient had an uneventful postoperative course and was discharged 10 days after the operation. Palliative chemotherapy was started, but the disease progressed and he died 7 months after surgery.

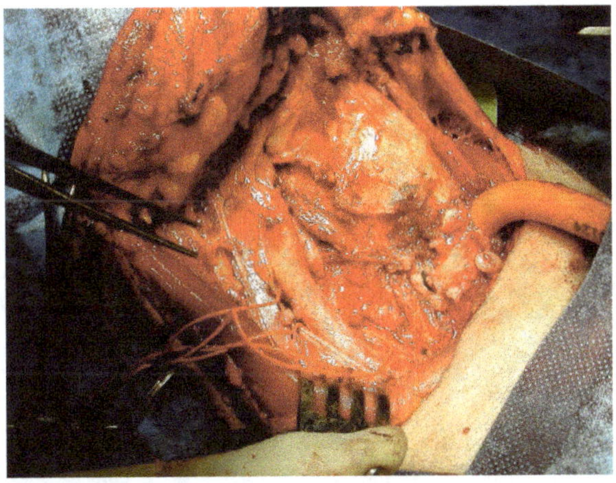

Figure 12 **Tracheostomy due to evident tracheomalacia.**

Case 5[19]

A 42-year-old woman with a previous history of no symptomatic multinodular goiter was evaluated for an emergency at our surgical department for acute, progressive dyspnea and intermittent inspiratory stridor, associated with a spontaneous and rapidly enlarging mass of the neck. Clinical examination revealed a large, firm, nonfluctuant thyroid swelling on the right side of the neck. Initial analyses of arterial blood gas, complete blood cell count, electrolyte levels, prothrombin and bleeding times, and thyroid function tests were normal. An urgent computerized tomography scan showed a hematoma within the right lobe of the thyroid, with substernal extension, and tracheal deviation with marked luminal narrowing (Figure 13). The rapid progression of respiratory distress meant performing endotracheal intubation by flexible laryngoscopy revealing normal vocal cord function and an emergency total thyroidectomy. During the operation, the thyroid gland revealed a huge, edematous, nonfluctuant, rubbery, firm swelling with easy bleeding on touch, but the capsule appeared to be intact without rupture (Figure 14). Microscopic examination revealed a colloid multinodular goiter with massive parenchymal hemorrhage. Recovery was uneventful, and the patient was discharged 2 days after the operation.

Case 6

An 81-year-old man with a forty-year history of substernal multinodular goiter was admitted in emergency with dysphonia and intermittent, sudden dyspnoea, and

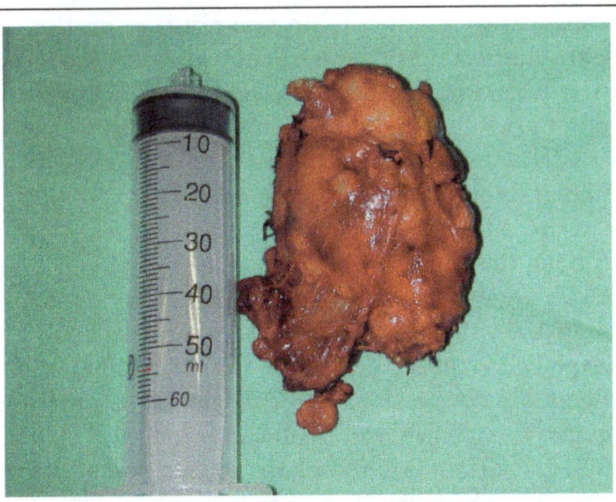

Figure 11 **Total thyroidectomy.**

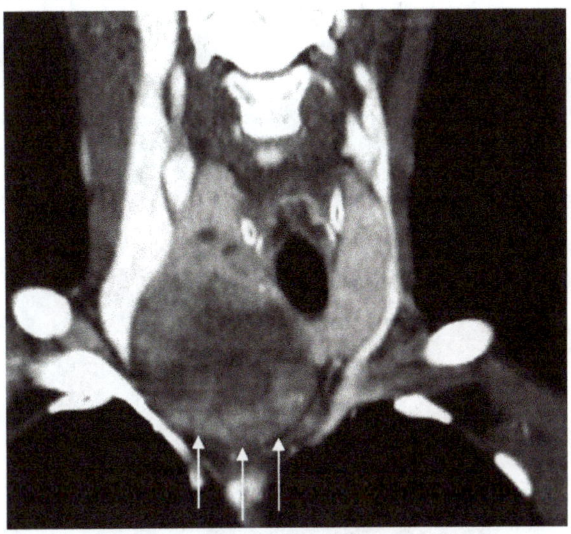

Figure 13 **Contrast enhanced CT scan with coronal reconstructed image: right lobe of the thyroid gland shows an inhomogeneous mass with focal areas of hemorrhage.** Compression and deviation of the trachea is also present.

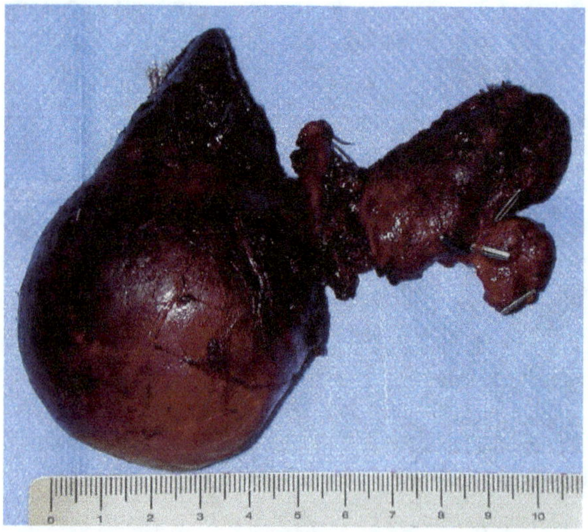

Figure 14 Thyroid gland revealing a huge, edematous, nonfluctuant, rubbery, firm swelling with easy bleeding on touch, but the capsule appeared to be intact without rupture.

stridor. A flexible laryngoscopy revealed right vocal cord palsy, with a nearly total reduction of the laryngeal lumen, and a CT scan confirmed the compression of the trachea by a cervicomediastinal goitre. An emergency endotracheal intubation was performed followed by total thyroidectomy by manubriotomy. The thyroid gland appeared wooden in consistency, strongly adherent to the trachea, and to the pre-thyroid muscles, without signs of infiltrations, caudally extending up to the left *Innominate* vein (Figure 15). The patient was discharged seven days after the operation without post-operative complications. Histology revealed a medullary carcinoma completely replacing the right lobe mass. A follow-up of four months showed a normal calcitonin haematic level.

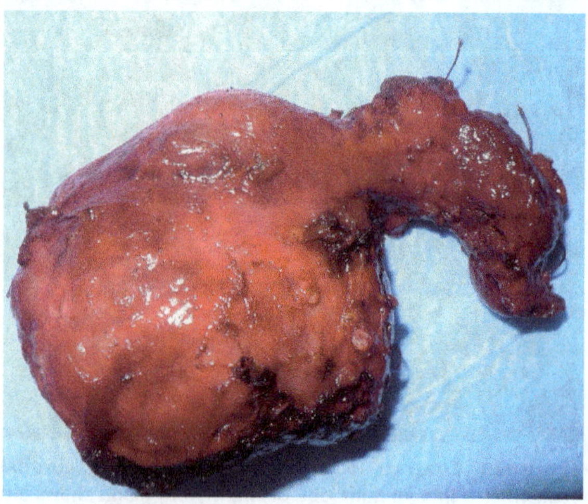

Figure 15 Total thyroidectomy for a medullary carcinoma completely replacing the right lobe mass.

Results

In 3/6 (50%) a manubriotomy was necessary due to the extension of the mass into the upper mediastinum. In all cases total thyroidectomy was performed by 3× loupe magnification [17] to aid dissection of parathyroid glands, and recurrent laryngeal nerves. In one case (16.7%) a parathyroid gland transplantation [18] and in another one (16.7%) a tracheotomy was necessary due to a condition of tracheomalacia. Mean post-operative hospital stay was 6.5 days (range: 2-10 days). Histology revealed malignancy in 4/6 cases (66.7%), showing 3 primitive, and 1 secondary tumors. Morbidity consisted of 1 transient recurrent laryngeal palsy, 3 transient post-operative hypoparathyroidism, and in 4 pleural effusions, treated by medical therapy in 3 cases and by drains in one. There was no mortality.

Discussion

In spite of *Hedenus* reporting successful thyroidectomies in six patients for goiters, which he described as "suffocating" [20] in 1821, nowadays airway obstruction due to goiter is exceptionally reported in literature [2-5,7,9,14] due to improved diagnostic methods and earlier treatment.

Although this dramatic occurrence seems to be more frequent in developing countries due to ignorance and lack of ready access to affordable medical services, in western countries the phenomenon of giant goiters is very uncommon though not completely absent [21,22]. A truly severe life-treating airway obstruction is, therefore, currently an extremely rare event [2,21,23,24], also because the tracheal lumen may be progressively compressed without causing symptoms up to 75% [2].

The causes of severe respiratory distress related to non traumatic thyroid disease show four different etiopathogeneses: rapidly progressive pressure on the tracheal lumen by spontaneous intrathyroideal hemorrhage, invasion of the tracheal lumen by primitive or secondary tumors, severe compression from benign or malignant masses and bilateral vocal cords palsy resulting from infiltration of recurrent nerves from thyroid malignancy.

Among the causes, spontaneous hemorrhage is often but not always [25] related to benign condition and is paradoxically the most insidious because it suddenly and unexpectedly appears in its full strength, sometimes in patients without previous history of thyroid disease; consequently diagnosis may be delayed. Indeed, literature [26-28] reports mortality related to this event of up to 27.8% [26]. The most likely explanation for hemorrhage in goiters is thought to be venous bleeding [19]. The adenomatous goiters are usually more fragile than normal thyroid because of the increased vascular flow and the lack of a true capsule; these aspects easily explain the great propensity for injury by blunt trauma [29], or iatrogenic bleeding resulting from fine-needle aspiration biopsy [30,31].

In the spontaneous thyroid hemorrhage, however, the mechanism is unclear. Johnson [32] and Terry [33] proposed that the inciting event for the hemorrhage was increased venous pressure resulting from the *Valsalva* maneuver. Therefore, most spontaneous cases are found to have an associated external event, such as various forms of light housework, coughing, straining at defecation, crying, which are, however, seemingly insignificant [6]. However, on appearance of a stable spontaneous hematoma of the thyroid gland without airway compromise, we believe that a conservative treatment could be safely performed; however, the increasing size of neck swelling or acute worsening of respiratory distress must be absolute, although rare indications point to early intubation and emergency surgery [19], as in the case reported in this series.

Anaplastic thyroid cancer is a rare tumor, ranging from 1-3% of all thyroid neoplasms, but is characterized by a very aggressive loco-regional disease, with mortality often related to respiratory failure from infiltration of the tracheal lumen [34]. Indeed, the main indication for surgery is just palliative decompression and debulking to prevent invasion of larynx, trachea, nerves and vessels of the neck, in the presence of a median survival of 4-5 months from the time of diagnosis [25].

Thyroid lymphoma [35], and leiomyosarcoma [36] are exceptionally described as causes of tracheal obstruction with respiratory distress treated by total or partial thyroidectomy.

On the other hand, well-differentiated thyroid carcinoma may, on occasion, cause airway obstruction [37]. The usual treatment of carcinoma invading the trachea is by "shaving" the tumor off the trachea, expecting to control residual neoplasm by postoperative radioactive iodine or external irradiations therapies [37,38]. However, the prognosis for well-differentiated carcinomas worsens when the neoplasm invades the trachea; indeed, the cause of death in nearly half of the fatal cases of papillary carcinomas is caused by obstruction of the trachea [37,39]. Moreover, the survival rate of patients treated by incomplete resection of the affected trachea is much worse than patients treated by complete resection [40,41]. For these reasons, with progress in tracheal surgical techniques, resection of portions of the trachea with primary anastomosis *en bloc* with thyroid is nowadays the treatment of choice [40-43]. Four cases (66.7%) in this reported series were well-differentiated carcinoma. In case 1, 2, and 6 (Hürthle cell, follicular, and medullary carcinomas, respectively), the airway obstruction was determined by the compression but not by the infiltration of trachea from the thyroid mass, and a comfortable cleavage plain between trachea and thyroid was evident at operation during dissection. For this reason a trachea resection was deemed unnecessary and the long-term disease-free follow up provides proof of the correctness of the surgical decision. In case 4 (thyroid metastasis from renal cancer), however, despite the invasion of the trachea, the staging of a metastatic disease contraindicated resection. Indeed, the patient died 7 months after the operation, due to the disease progress, but without local recurrence.

When the respiratory distress is caused by benign thyroid disease, usually the compression *ab estrinseco* of the trachea is determined by a giant cervical or cervico-mediastinal goiters. However, there being enough room to accommodate the gland, acute respiratory failure secondary to tracheal compression by goiter is extremely rare [2], affecting 0.6% of reported cases [44]. However, when the extension of the goiter is retroclavicular, it can cause airway obstruction that may progress to arrest respiration [2,45,46]. Nevertheless, in the presence of benign thyroid disease, chronic obstructive airways disease, substernal extension, and long-standing goiter are considered as risk factors for developing acute, life-threatening airway compromission [44].

It is clear that the appearance of an acute airway obstruction requires urgent management to ensure an adequate ventilation and oxygenation.

The first step in the management of this emergency is represented by the anesthesia. An awake fiberoptic intubation using a small endotracheal tube followed by induction of general anesthesia, as always performed in this reported series, seem to be the gold standard in the approach to this emergency. Indeed, a standard sequence of induction and intubation could be considered at risk of aspiration in an unfasted patient, and besides this, the possibility of unsuccessful intubation due to the compression by the goiter is very high. On the other hand, an inhalation induction followed by laringoscopy and orotracheal or blind nasal intubations, may be considered dangerous because of complete airway obstruction following loss of consciousness [47,48]. When assisted intubation cannot be achieved, local or regional anesthesia are described too [21].

The second step is the choice of surgical treatment to be performed. Indeed, surgery - emergency or early - is always indicated for severe airway obstruction caused by thyroid mass [23]. An emergency tracheostomy is hindered by the presence of the thyroid mass which prevents access to the trachea, obliterating all landmarks [21]. An isthmectomy to allow a tracheostomy, appears to be an incomplete treatment, referring to a second surgical procedure for removing the entire thyroid. Moreover, in the presence of diagnosis of proven or suspected malignancy, it would cause a further delay in cancer treatment and exposes the patient to the risk of tumor dissemination. However, even in the presence of a benign goiter, re-surgery would mean higher morbidity [49,50]. Finally, once an endotracheal intubation has been performed, tracheotomy is questionable. Since a total thyroidectomy is capable of resolving airway obstruction, tracheostomy would result in unnecessary discomfort for the patient, furthermore exposing then to the need of a second operation to close the stomy. In our experience tracheostomy was necessary in only one case (16.7%) due to the evidence of a marked tracheomalacia.

Then, total, near-total or sub-total thyroidectomy represents the treatment of choice of acute airway obstruction resulting from compression of thyroid mass.

On the basis of our experience and that in literature, in the presence of warning signs such as a developing mass in patients with history of thyroid disease, increasing and/or intermittent dyspnoea, stridor, sudden onset of neck swelling, we stress the importance of immediate hospitalization to perform a controlled approach to the progressively acute disease, avoiding treatment in emergency. But, when this event occurs, like in our reported series, the approach to this emergency operation should be performed in highly specialized high-volume centers combining multidisciplinary anesthesiological and surgical strategies. Indeed, when total thyroidectomy is performed for cervicomediastinal goiters, there is a higher risk of postoperative hypoparathyroidism, recurrent laryngeal nerve palsy and hemorrhage, as reported in literature [8,51-57] and in our experience too, [58] which sometimes requires sternal split, as in 50% of this series. However, in our experience, the use of loupe magnification and parathyroid autotransplantation during thyroid surgery showed a significant improvement of results, with faster and safer identification of the nerve, and decreasing permanent and transient hypoparathyroidism [17,18]. Some authors suggest the use of the recurrent nerve monitor, especially in the presence of a large retrosternal goiter [59,60].

Moreover, when the upper mediastinum is occupied by a goiter, the endocrine surgeon is not usually familiar with the course of the RNLs and their anatomical variability in this district, and the cardiothoracic surgeon is not familiar with endocrinosurgical challenges. Therefore, the emergency extracervical approach could require multidisciplinary collaboration [58].

In conclusion, on the basis of our experience and of the literature review, we strongly advocate elective surgery for patients with thyroid disease at the first signs of tracheal compression. When an acute airway distress appears, an emergency life-threatening total thyroidectomy is recommended in a high-volume centre.

Author details

[1]Department of Biomedical Sciences and Human Oncology, Unit of Endocrine, Digestive and Emergency Surgery, University Medical School of Bari "Aldo Moro", Bari, Italy. [2]Department of Emergency and Organ Transplantation, Unit of Endocrinology, University Medical School of Bari "Aldo Moro", Bari, Italy. [3]Department of Neurological and Psychiatric Sciences, Unit of Physical and Rehabilitation, University Medical School of Bari "Aldo Moro", Bari, Italy. [4]Unit of Otorhinolaryngology; "Di Venere Hospital", Bari, Italy.

References

1. Alagaratnam TT, Ong GB: **Carcinoma of the thyroid.** *Br J Surg* 1979, **66**:558-561.
2. Raftos JR, Ethell AT: **Goitre causing acute respiratory arrest.** *Aust New Zeal J Surg* 1996, **66**:331-332.
3. Kalawole IK, Rahman GA: **Emergency thyroidectomy in a patient with severe upper airway obstruction caused by goiter: case for regional anesthesia.** *J Natl Med Assoc* 2006, **98**:86-89.
4. Warren CP: **Acute respiratory failure and tracheal obstruction in the elderly with benign goiters.** *Can Med Assoc J* 1979, **121**:191-194.
5. Karbowitz SR, Edelman LB, Nath S, Owek JH, Rammohan G: **Spectrum of advanced upper airway obstruction due to goiters.** *Chest* 1985, **87**:18-21.
6. Armstrong WB, Funk GF, Rice DH: **Acute airway compromise secondary to traumatic thyroid hemorrhage.** *Arch Otolaryngol Head Neck Surg* 1994, **120**:427-430.
7. Shaha AR, Burnett C, Alfonso A, Jaffe BM: **Goiters and airway problems.** *Am J Surg* 1989, **158**:378-380.
8. McHenry CR, Piotrowski JJ: **Thyroidectomy in patients with marked thyroid enlargement: airway management, morbidity and outcome.** *Am Surg* 1994, **60**:586-591.
9. Myatt HM: **Acute airway obstruction due to primary thyroid lymphoma.** *Rev Laryngol Otol Rhinol (Bord)* 1996, **117**:237-239.
10. Poon D, Toh HC, Sim CS: **Two case reports of metastases from colon carcinoma to the thyroid.** *Ann Acad Med Singapore* 2004, **33**:100-102.
11. Haugen BR, Nawaz S, Cohn A, Shroyer K, Bunn PA Jr, Liechty DR, Ridgway EC: **Secondary malignancy of the thyroid gland: a case report and review of the literature.** *Thyroid* 1994, **4**:297-300.
12. Testini M, Lissidini G, Gurrado A, Lastilla G, Ianora A, Fiorella R: **Acute airway failure secondary to thyroid metastasis from renal carcinoma: Case Report.** *World J Surg Oncol* 2008, **6**:14-17.
13. Cornett WR, Sharma AK, Day TA, Richardson MS, Hoda RS, van Heerden JA, Fernandes JK: **Anaplastic thyroid carcinoma: an overview.** *Curr Oncol Rep* 2007, **9**:152-158.
14. Tsilchorozidou T, Vagropoulos I, Karagianidou C, Grigoriadis N: **Huge intrathyroidal hematoma causing airway obstruction: a multidisciplinary challange.** *Thiroid* 2006, **16**:795-799.
15. Weeks C, Moore FD Jr, Ferzoco SJ, Gates J: **Blunt trauma to the thyroid. A case report.** *Am Surg* 2005, **71**:518-521.
16. Paleri V, Marojou RS, Ali MS, Ruckley RW: **Spontaneous retro and parapharyngeal haematoma caused by intrathyroid bleed.** *J Laryngol Otol* 2002, **116**:854-858.
17. Testini M, Nacchiero M, Piccinni G, Portincasa P, Di Venere B, Lissidini G, Bonomo GM: **Total thyroidectomy is improved by loupe magnification.** *Microsurgery* 2004, **24**:39-42.
18. Testini M, Rosato L, Avenia N, Basile F, Portincasa P, Piccinni G, Lissidini G, Biondi A, Gurrado A, Nacchiero M: **The impact of single parathyroid gland autotransplantation during thyroid surgery on postoperative hypoparathyroidism: a multicenter study.** *Transplant Proc* 2007, **39**:225-230.
19. Testini M, Gurrado A, Lissidini G, Lardo D, Poli E, Piccinni G: **Energency surgery for acute respiratory failure secondary to spontaneous thyroid hemorrhage.** *Int Surg* 2008, **93**:158-162.
20. Farling PA: **Thyroid disease.** *Br J Anaesth* 2000, **85**:15-28.

21. Kolawole IK, Rahman GA: **Emergency thyroidectomy in a patient with severe upper airway obstruction caused by goiter: case for regional anesthesia.** *J Natl Med Assoc* 2006, **98**:86-89.
22. Olurin ED: **Surgical techniques in giant goiters.** *Br J Surg* 1971, **58**:739-746.
23. Gittoes NJ, Miller MR, Daykin J, Sheppard MC, Franklyn JA: **Upper airways obstruction in 153 consecutive patients presenting with thyroid enlargement.** *BMJ* 1996, **312**:484.
24. Chiriboga M, Oropello J, Padmanabhan K, Goldman JM: **Advanced upper airway obstruction caused by cervical goiter.** *Am J Med Sci* 1989, **297**:176-177.
25. Kumar S, Joshi MK: **Emergency total thyroidectomy for bleeding anaplastic thyroid carcinoma: a viable option for palliation.** *Indian J Palliat Care* 2011, **17**:67-69.
26. Schwoerer G: **Intrastrumose spontanbluntungen.** *Beir KlinChir (Tubingen)* 1924, **131**:362-372.
27. Simon P: **Sur un cas de mort rapide consecutive a une hemorrhagie primitive du corps thyroide.** *Rev Med (Nancy)* 1894, **26**:77-83.
28. Plummer WA, Brodens AC: **Acute capsulitis of cystic degenerated or partially degenerated adenoma of thyroid gland: clinical dinstinction from gross intra-adenomatous hemorrhage.** *Am J Surg* 1934, **23**:63-69.
29. Weeks C, Moore FD Jr, Ferzoco SJ, Gates J: **Blunt trauma to the thyroid: a case report.** *Am Surg* 2005, **71**:518-521.
30. Roh JL: **Intrathyroid haemorrhage acute upper airway obstruction after fine needle aspiration of the thyroid gland.** *Laryngoscope* 2006, **116**:154-156.
31. Noordzij JP, Goto MM: **Airway compromised caused by hematoma after thyroid fine-needle aspiration.** *A J Otholaryngol* 2005, **26**:3989-3999.
32. Johnson N: **The blood supply of the thyroid gland: II: the nodular gland.** *Aust N Z J Surg* 1954, **23**:241-252.
33. Terry WL: **Radium emanations in exophtalmic goiter: blood vessels of adenomas of thyroid.** *JAMA* 1922, **79**:1-3.
34. Blaivas M, Hom DB, Younger JG: **Thyroid gland hematoma after blunt cervical trauma.** *Am J Emerg Med* 1999, **17**:348-350.
35. Joshi A, Chan J, Bruch G, Jeannon JP, Mikhaeel NG, Fields PA, Simo R: **Thyroid lymphoma and airway obstruction - is there a rationale for surgical management?** *Int J Clin Pract* 2009, **63**:1647-1652.
36. Tsugawa K, Koyanagi N, Nakamnishi H, Wada H, Tanoue K, Hashizume M, Sugimachi K: **Leyomiosarcoma of the thyroid gland with rapid growth and tracheal obstruction: a partial thyroidectomy and tracheostomy using an ultrasonically activated scalpel can be safely performed with less bleeding.** *Eur J Med Res* 1999, **4**:483-487.
37. Yang CC, Lee CH, Wang LS, Huang BS, Hsu WH, Huang MH: **Resectional treatment for thyroid cancer with tracheal invasion.** *Arch Surg* 2000, **135**:704-707.
38. Grillo HC, Zannini P: **Resectional management of airway invasion by thyroid carcinoma.** *Ann Thorac Surg* 1986, **42**:287-298.
39. Ishihara T, Yamazaki S, Kobayashi K, Inoue H, Fukai S, Ito K, Mimura T: **Resection of the trachea infiltrated by thyroid carcinoma.** *Ann Surg* 1982, **195**:496-500.
40. Nakao K, Miyata M, Izukura M, Monden Y, Maeda M, Kawashima Y: **Radical operation for thyroid carcinoma invading the trachea.** *Arch Surg* 1984, **119**:1046-1049.
41. Pearson FG, Cooper JD, Nelems JM, Van Nostrand AW: **Primary tracheal anastomosis after resection of the cricoid cartilage with preservation of recurrent laryngeal nerves.** *J Thorac Cardiovasc Surg* 1975, **70**:806-816.
42. Ishihara T, Kikuchi K, Ikeda T, Inoue H, Fukai S, Ito K, Mimura T: **Resection of thyroid carcinoma infiltrating the trachea.** *Thorax* 1978, **33**:378-386.
43. Nomori H, Kobayashi K, Ishihara T, Torikata C, Hosada Y, Ozaki O, Ito K: **Thyroid carcinoma infiltrating the trachea: clinical, histologic, and morphometric analyses.** *J Surg Oncol* 1990, **44**:78-83.
44. Kadhim AL, Shehan P, Timon C: **Management of life-threatening airway obstruction caused by benign thyroid disease.** *L Laryngol Otol* 2006, **120**:1038-1041.
45. Georgiadis N, Katsas A, Leoutsakos B: **Substernal goiter.** *Int Surg* 1970, **54**:116-121.
46. Manfred B, Bruce JB, Donald AB: **The thyroid cork: obstruction of the thoracic inlet due to retroclavicular goiter.** *JAMA* 1974, **227**:189-191.
47. Buggy D, Shnittger T, Fox L: **Airway management after severe facial contracture.** *Br J Hosp Med* 1994, **52**:367.
48. Goh MH, Liu XY, Goh YS: **Anterior mediastinal masses: an anaesthetic challenge (case report).** *Anaesthesia* 1999, **54**:670-674.
49. Testini M, Nacchiero M, Portincasa P, Miniello S, Piccinni G, Di Venere B, Campanile L, Lissidini G, Bonomo GM: **Risk factors of morbidity in thyroid surgery: analysis of the last 5 years of experience in a general surgery unit.** *Int Surg* 2004, **89**:125-130.
50. Rosato L, Avenia N, Bernante P, De Palma M, Gulino G, Nasi PG, Pelizzo MR, Pezzullo L: **Complications of thyroid surgery: analysis of a multicentric study on 14,934 patients operated on in Italy over 5 years.** *World J Surg* 2004, **28**:271-276.
51. Shen WT, Kebebew E, Duh QY, Clark OH: **Predictors of airway complications after thyroidectomy for substernal goiters.** *Arch Surg* 2004, **138**:656-660.
52. Ozdemir A, Hasbahceci M, Hamaloglu E, Oznec A: **Surgical treatment of substernal goiter.** *Int Surg* 2000, **85**:194-197.
53. White ML, Doherty GM, Gauger PG: **Evidence-based surgical management of substernal goiter.** *World J Surg* 2008, **32**:1285-1300.
54. Sancho JJ, Kraimps JL, Sanchez-Blanco JM, Larrad A, Rodríguez JM, Gil P, Gibelin H, Pereira JA, Sitges-Serra A: **Increased mortality and morbidity associated with thyroidectomy for intrathoracic goiters reaching the carina tracheae.** *Arch Surg* 2006, **141**:82-85.
55. Zambudio AR, Rodriguez J, Riquelme J, Soria T, Canteras M, Parrilla P: **Prospective study of postoperative complications after total thyroidectomy for multinodular goiters by surgeons with experience in endocrine surgery.** *Ann Surg* 2004, **240**:18-25.
56. Bhattacharyya N, Fried MP: **Assessment of the morbidity and complications of total thyroidectomy.** *Arch Otolaryngol Head Neck Surg* 2002, **128**:389-392.
57. Arici C, Dertsiz L, Altunbas H, Demircan A, Emek K: **Operative management of substernal goiter: analysis of 52 patients.** *Int Surg* 2001, **86**:220-224.
58. Testini M, Gurrado A, Avenia N, Bellantone R, Biondi A, Brazzarola P, Calzolari F, Cavallaro G, De Toma G, Guida P, Lissidini G, Loizzi M, Lombardi CP, Piccinni G, Portincasa P, Rosato L, Sartori N, Zugni C, Basile F: **Does mediastinal extension of the goiter increase morbidity of total thyroidectomy? A multicenter study of 19,662 patients.** *Ann Surg Oncol* 2011, **18**:2251-2259.
59. Donnellan KA, Pitman KT, Cannon CR, Replogle WH, Simmons JD: **Intraoperative laryngeal nerve monitoring during thyroidectomy.** *Arch Otolaryngol Head Neck Surg* 2009, **135**:1196-1198.
60. Terris DJ, Anderson SK, Watts TL, Chin E: **Laryngeal nerve monitoring and minimally invasive thyroid surgery: complementary technologies.** *Arch Otolaryngol Head Neck Surg* 2007, **133**:1254-1257.

12

Safety and effectiveness of propranolol in severely burned patients

Ramiro Manzano-Nunez[1,2], Herney Andrés García-Perdomo[2], Paula Ferrada[3], Carlos Alberto Ordoñez Delgado[4], Diego Andrés Gomez[2] and Jorge Esteban Foianini[5*]

Abstract

Background: The objective of this systematic review was to determine the effectiveness and safety of propranolol compared to placebo or usual care for improving clinical relevant outcomes in severely burned patients (TBSA >20%).

Methods: Relevant articles from randomized controlled trials were identified by a literature search in MEDLINE, EMBASE, and CENTRAL. We included trials involving patients with a severe burn (>20% of total body surface area affected). Trials were eligible if they evaluated propranolol and compared to usual care or placebo. Two investigators independently assessed articles for inclusion and exclusion criteria and selected studies for the final analysis. We conducted a meta-analysis using a random-effects model.

Results: We included ten studies in our systematic review. These studies randomized a total of 1236 participants. There were no significant differences between propranolol and placebo with respect to mortality (RD −0.02 [95% CI −0.06 to 0.02]), sepsis (RD −0.03 [95% CI −0.09 to 0.04]), and the overall hospital stay (MD −0.37 [−4.52 to 3.78]). Propranolol-treated adults had a decrease in requirements of blood transfusions (MD −185.64 [95% CI −331.06 to −40.43]) and a decreased heart rate (MD −26.85 [95% CI −39.95 to −13.75]).

Conclusions: Our analysis indicates that there were no differences in mortality or sepsis in severely burned patients treated with propranolol compared with those who had usual care or placebo. However, the use of propranolol in these patients resulted in lower requirements of blood transfusion and lower values of heart rate. The evidence synthesized in this systematic review is limited to conclude that propranolol reduces the length of hospital stay among severely burned patients. Future trials should assess the impact of propranolol on clinically relevant outcomes such as mortality and adverse events.

Keywords: Propranolol, Burns, Pharmacology, Critical care, Adrenergic antagonist

Background

Burn injuries are among the most severe of all injuries [1] with approximately 90% of cases occurring in low- and middle-income countries [2]. Burns are a common cause of morbidity and mortality, and most occur in a domestic setting with children from birth through 4 years having the highest burden of the condition. Episodes occur commonly at home and principally due to scalds, hot objects, and fires [3, 4]. For adults, the incidence of burns is low until the 30s, with cases occurring at home, outdoors, and at workplaces in equal proportions [1]. The incidence of burns in low- and middle-income countries is 1.3 per 100,000 population whereas in high-income countries is approximately of 0.14 per 100,000 population with burn injuries ranking the top 15 leading causes of burden of disease globally [2, 5].

Burn injuries covering more than 20% of the total body surface area (TBSA) cause an inflammatory and subsequent hypermetabolic response that starts immediately post-burn and can persist for years [6, 7]. Hypermetabolic state has two aspects—the "ebb" and "flow" phases. The ebb phase, occurring within the first 48 h

* Correspondence: ruralcirugiatrauma@gmail.com; efoianini@hotmail.com
[5]Division of Surgery, Clinica Foianini, Av. Irala 468, Santa Cruz de la Sierra, Bolivia
Full list of author information is available at the end of the article

after injury, is associated with decreased cardiac output, oxygen consumption, and metabolic rate. The chronic "flow" phase is a critical phase that requires medical intervention to reduce the risk of fatal outcomes [8].

The release of cytokines and other pro-inflammatory mediators at the site of injury has a systemic effect once the burn reaches 20% of total body surface area. Injuries greater than this percentage invariably results in severe impairments of cardiovascular, respiratory, metabolic, and immunological functions derived from hypermetabolic changes [9]. The hypermetabolic response along with catecholamines and corticosteroids increase liver and cardiac work, impair muscle function, increase the risk of sepsis, and produce hormonal abnormalities that augment morbidity and mortality [6, 9–11].

Several interventions have been proposed to decrease the hypermetabolic response and to improve outcomes in the burned patient [12–16]. Propranolol through β-adrenergic receptor blockade has been proposed as an effective strategy for reducing post-burn catabolism and therefore to improve outcomes in burned patients. The objective of this systematic review was to determine the effectiveness and safety of propranolol compared to placebo or usual care for improving clinical relevant outcomes in severely burned patients (TBSA >20%).

Methods

This systematic review and meta-analysis was conducted according to the recommendations of the Cochrane Collaboration and following the PRISMA Statement. The PROSPERO registration number is CRD42016042230.

Inclusion criteria

We included only randomized controlled trials (RCTs) involving patients with a severe burn, defined as a burn with an affected area greater than 20% of the total body surface area (TBSA). Trials were eligible if they evaluated propranolol as the intervention of interest in adults or children and compared to usual care or placebo. We excluded trials where propranolol was compared to other pharmacologic interventions and trials evaluating the combination of propranolol with other interventions. Two investigators independently assessed articles for inclusion and exclusion criteria and selected studies for the final analysis, with divergences finally resolved by consensus.

Outcomes

We prespecified clinical relevant outcomes as our primary outcomes. Those included mortality, adverse events, need for transfusions/blood loss, the occurrence of infections/sepsis, and length of hospital stay. Secondary outcomes were heart rate, hypertriglyceridemia, and hyperglycemia. Only those trials providing sufficient information (i.e., measures of treatment effects and the associated precision) were included in our statistical analysis.

Search methods

Literature search strategy was built according to current recommendations (Additional file 1: Table S1) [17–19]. We searched MEDLINE, EMBASE, and CENTRAL from inception to 2016. We also hand-searched references from relevant narrative reviews and previous systematic reviews for more trials. Other sources were thesis databases, OpenGrey and Google Scholar. Authors were contacted to complement data by e-mail. No language restrictions were used.

Study selection and data collection

Two individuals independently assessed the titles and abstracts identified by the searches for potential eligibility, and the full-text articles were retrieved for those that appeared relevant. Two investigators independently assessed full-text articles for final eligibility. Disagreements were resolved by consensus or by a third, independent reviewer. The following information was independently extracted using a standardized form: study design, geographic location, authors names, title, objectives, inclusion and exclusion criteria, the number of patients included, losses to follow-up, the definition of interventions, definitions of outcomes, outcomes measures, funding, and status of data on clinical trials website.

Risk of bias

The internal validity of each trial included in this review was critically evaluated for bias according to the Cochrane Collaboration tool for assessing the risk of bias [20] which covers sequence generation, allocation concealment, blinding, incomplete data, selective reporting, and other biases. Two independent investigators made a judgment about the possible risk of bias from extracted information, rated as "high risk," "low risk," or "unclear risk". We computed a graphic representation of potential bias using RevMan 5.3.

Data analysis/synthesis of results

A meta-analysis was performed to assess the overall outcomes of propranolol compared to usual care or placebo. The statistical analysis was performed using Review Manager 5.3 (RevMan® 5.3). For dichotomous outcomes, we extracted data on the total number of participants, the number that experienced the outcomes, and the number analyzed. For continuous outcomes, we extracted end-value means with standard deviations (SD). Whenever possible, we used results from an intention-to-treat population.

Mean differences (MD) and risk differences were pooled using a random-effects model. The results were reported in forest plots of the estimated effects of the included studies with a 95% confidence interval (95% CI). Meta-analysis was considered since the included studies were similar in terms of participants, interventions, and outcomes (clinical homogeneity). Heterogeneity was evaluated using the I^2 test. For the interpretation, it was determined that the values of 25, 50, and 75% in the I^2 test corresponded to low, medium, and high levels of heterogeneity, respectively.

Results

We identified 164 records from our searches, of which 19 trials were eligible to be included in our systematic review. After applying inclusion and exclusion criteria, ten studies [21–30] were included in the systematic review, all of them in the qualitative synthesis and eight in quantitative synthesis (meta-analysis). Figure 1 shows the flowchart for the selection of randomized trials.

Characteristics of included studies

Included trials were published between 2001 and 2015. These trials randomized a total of 1236 participants with a sample size ranging from 25 to 406 (median, 76; interquartile range, 58.5–195.5). Five trials (50%) [22–25, 27] were single-center trials. Of the ten RCTs included, nine recruited participants from the USA and one trial recruited patients from Iran [27]. Losses to follow-up were reported in four trials [22–24, 29], and finally, an intention-to-treat analysis was performed in two trials [22, 24]. Main characteristics from included studies were summarized in Additional file 2: Appendix 1.

Six RCTs were done in adults and four were done in children [23–25, 29]. Regarding how the condition was defined, four RCTs [23, 25, 26, 28] included patients with burns greater than 40% of TBSA, five [21, 22, 24, 29, 30] included patients with burns greater than 30% of TBSA, and one trial [27] included patients with burns between 20 and 50% of TBSA. Interventions and comparators were very similar, with propranolol (at similar doses) and placebo or usual care being the intervention and comparator, respectively, in all trials. The similarity in interventions and comparators between trials could result in low clinical diversity at this point. Main characteristics of participants from individual RCTs are summarized in Table 1.

With respect to outcomes (see Additional file 1: Table S1), four trials [22, 24, 25, 27] presented mortality data, in three trials [21, 22, 27], the quantity of blood transfused was reported, three trials [23, 25, 27] measured occurrence of sepsis, five trials [22, 24, 25, 27, 29] reported length of hospital, eight trials [21–24, 26, 28–30] defined hemodynamic parameters such as heart rate, mean arterial pressure, cardiac output, and/or stroke volume as part of the outcomes measured. Three trials [21, 22, 27] presented data about wound healing in terms of the number of grafting procedures and the average time between grafting procedures, and only one trial [22] presented data about adverse effects of propranolol.

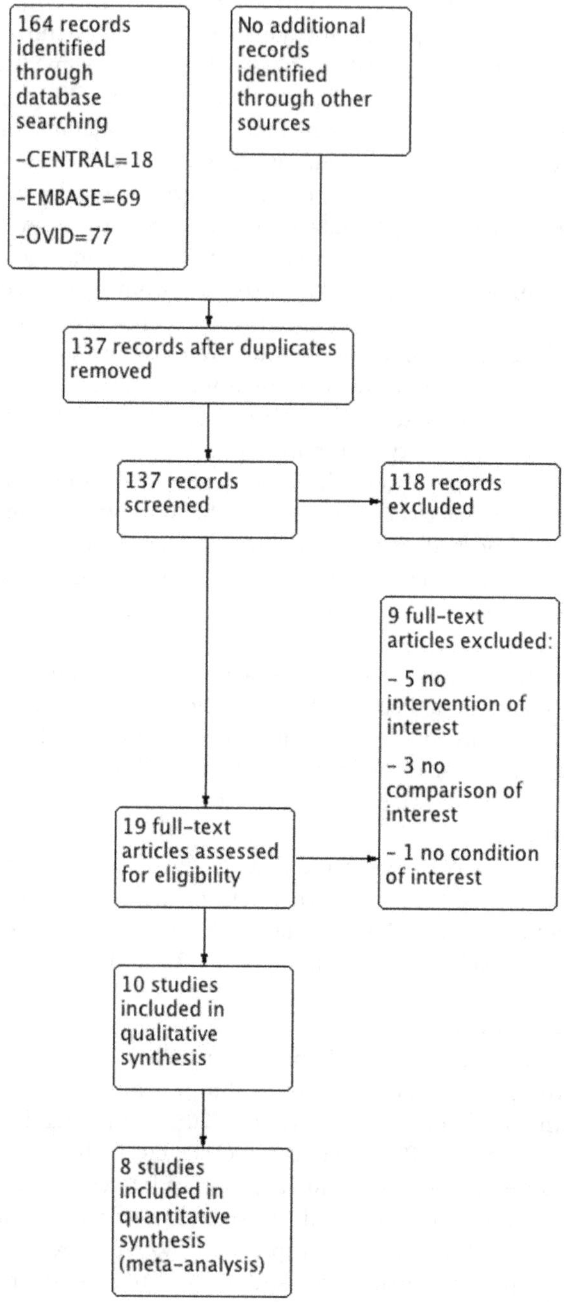

Fig. 1 Flowchart according to PRISMA guidelines

Risk of bias

Seven (70%) and ten trials (100%) were rated as unclear risk of bias for random sequence generation and allocation

Table 1 Characteristics of participants. Age is described as mean and standard deviation

No.	Study	Group	Total number of randomized patients	Age	TBSA (%) of patients to be included	Country	Socio-demographics
1	Williams 2011 [29]	Propranolol	125	7 (5)	Burns >30%	USA	Not described
		Standard care	215	8 (5)			
2	W Norbury 2007 [28]	Propranolol	33	Not described	Burns >40%	USA	Not described
		Standard care	33	Not described			
3	Wurzer 2015 [30]	Propranolol	43	Not described	Burns >30%	USA	Not described
		Standard care	39				
4	Ali 2014 [21]	Propranolol	21	Not described	Burns >30%	USA	Not described
		Standard care	21				
5	Komak 2012 [26]	Propranolol	29	Not described	Burns >40%	USA	Not described
		Standard care	35				
6	Ali 2015 [22]	Propranolol	35	41 (14)	Burns >30%	USA	Not described
		Standard care	34	38 (16)			
7	Herndon 2012 [24]	Propranolol	90	7 (5)	Burns >30%	USA	Majority of participants were Hispanic: 97% in the control group and 91% in the propranolol group
		Standard care	89	7 (5)			
8	Akbar Mohammadi 2009 [27]	Propranolol	37	27.21 (9.73)	Burns 20–50%	Iran	Not described
		Standard care	42	24.54 (12.06)			
9	Jeschke 2007 [25]	Propranolol	102	7.2 (0.6)	Burns >40%	USA	Not described
		Standard care	143	7.8 (0.4)			
10	Herndon 2001 [23]	Propranolol	12	6.6 (1.5)	Burns >40%	USA	Not described
		Standard care	12	7.8 (1.4)			

concealment, respectively; the remaining three trials (30%) from the random sequence generation domain were rated at low risk of bias. Only one trial (10%) reported masking of study participants, and the remaining nine trials (90%) were rated at unclear risk of bias for this domain. All trials were rated at unclear risk of bias in terms of blinding of outcome assessors. Three trials (30%) were rated as high risk of attrition bias because of losses to follow-up. High risk of selective reporting was found in eight trials (80%); thus, a dangerous quantity of reporting bias could have been introduced from those trials but it was difficult to estimate the likely magnitude and the likely direction of this bias. High risk of other biases was found in six trials (60%) due to small sample sizes. Five trials (50%) reported receiving funding for the research, and none was funded by pharmaceutical industry. Finally, none of the trials posted results in clinical trials website (https://clinicaltrials.gov/) and six trials reported receiving ethical approval. The overall risk of bias of the included RCTs is best represented in Figs. 2 and 3.

Outcomes

There were no significant differences between propranolol and placebo/usual care with respect to mortality (RD −0.02 [95% CI −0.06 to 0.02]), and also, no differences were found in the sub-group analysis when assessing this outcome in children (RD −0.02 [95% CI −0.06 to 0.02]) and adults (RD −0.05 [95% CI −0.17 to 0.07]) (Fig. 4). Similarly, no significant differences were found when assessing overall occurrence of sepsis (RD −0.03 [95% CI −0.09 to 0.04]) with no differences in children (RD −0.03 [95% CI −0.09 to 0.04]) and adults (RD −0.04 [95% CI −0.24 to 0.15]) (Fig. 5). When assessing the length of hospital stay, propranolol did not shorten the overall number of days of hospitalization when compared to usual care or placebo (MD −0.37 [−4.52 to 3.78]) but this was not sustained when assessing sub-groups. In the sub-group analysis, the use of propranolol was associated with a lower length of hospital stay in adults (MD −6.59 [95% CI −10.18 to −3.0]), a fact that did not occur in children (MD 2.30 [95% CI −3.36 to 7.96]).

With respect to blood transfused, propranolol was associated with a lower amount of transfused blood (measured in milliliters) in adults (MD −185.64 [95% CI −331.06 to −40.43]). Propranolol was associated with lower values of heart rate (beats per minute) when compared to usual care (MD −26.85 [95% CI −39.95 to −13.75]) and this was consistent in adults

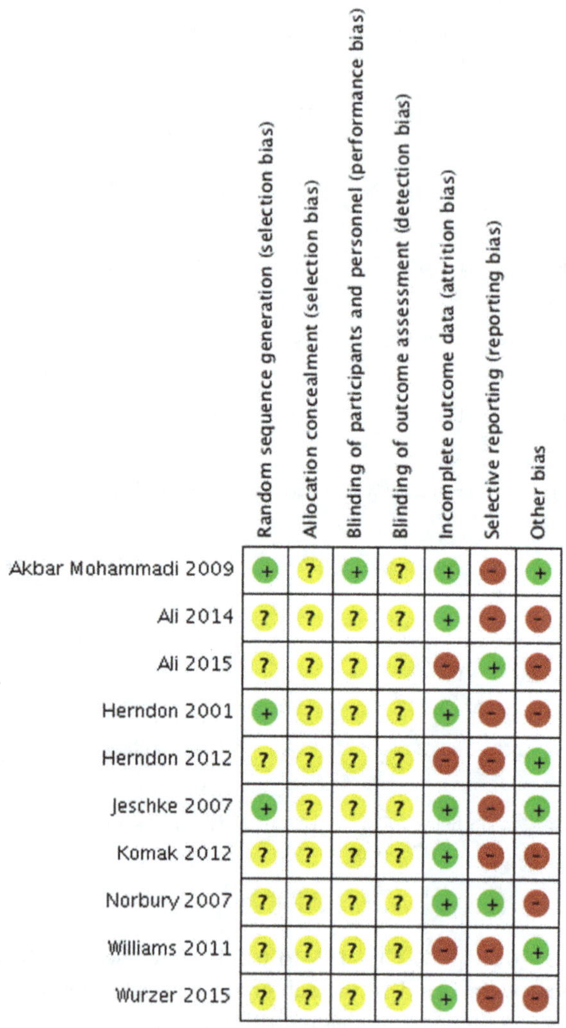

Fig. 2 Risk of bias from individual study

(MD −32.54 [95% CI −38.45 to −26.63]) and children (MD −19.0 [95% CI −31.12 to −6.88]).

Finally, it is important to mention that studies done in children did not report data about transfused blood. On the other hand, some of our primary outcomes are not reported and this is because primary research did not report data on hypertriglyceridemia and hyperglycemia.

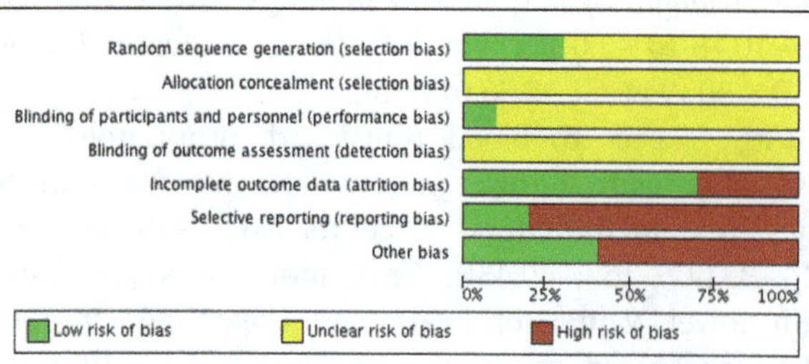

Fig. 3 Risk of bias across studies

Sensitivity analysis

Of the ten studies included in our systematic review, eight were rated as high risk for selective reporting; therefore, we decided to exclude those studies from our quantitative synthesis to evaluate the effect of this bias on results. We found that there were no differences in mortality (RD −0.12 [95% CI −0.32 to 0.07]) and quantity of blood transfused (MD −405 [95% CI −1343.48 to 533.48]) when comparing propranolol and usual care after excluding studies with high risk of selective reporting.

On the other hand, three of the ten studies were rated as high risk for attrition bias; thus, after excluding those studies from quantitative results, we found that propranolol was associated with a lower length of hospital stay in children (MD −2.0 [CI 95% −2.51 to −1.49]) and adults (MD −6.54 [95% CI −10.19 to −2.89]).

Discussion

The present study was designed to determine the effectiveness and safety of propranolol, compared to placebo or usual care, for improving clinical relevant outcomes in severely burned patients. In summary, no significant differences were found between propranolol and usual care in terms of mortality and sepsis occurrence. Propranolol-treated adults had a decrease in requirements of blood transfusion and a decreased heart rate. There was no difference in the overall length of hospital stay. However, the subgroup analysis showed decreased hospital stay in adults treated with propranolol. Furthermore, the sensitivity analysis revealed significantly decreased hospital stay in both adults and children treated with propranolol.

Severe burn injuries cause a hypermetabolic response driven by supraphysiologic elevations in stress hormones, catecholamines, and inflammatory mediators [6, 9, 11]. The hypermetabolic response is characterized by increased peripheral lipolysis, increased muscle wasting, elevated resting energy expenditure, and suppressed immune function. This response impedes recovery or leads to organ failure and death [9]. Therefore, the hypermetabolic response can be seen as an intermediate variable in the causal pathway between burns and relevant outcomes in burned patients; and thus, it is not irrational to think that the use of propranolol, by mitigating the deleterious effects of the hypermetabolic response, can result in improved outcomes among severely burned patients.

Burns impose a significant challenge and are associated with mortality rates between 1.4 and 18% with age groups and greater percentage total body surface area (TBSA) affected being associated with greater fatality rates [31–33]. It is estimated that 265,000 deaths every year are caused by burns, with the higher proportion of these fatalities occurring in low- and middle-income

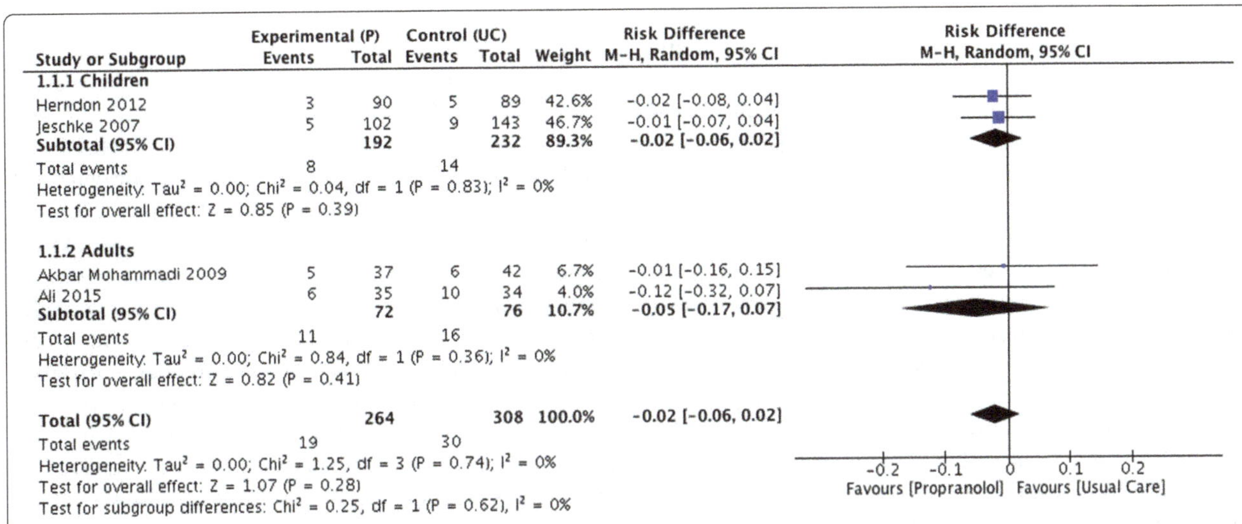

Fig. 4 Forrest plot for mortality (propranolol vs usual care)

countries [2, 34], places where burns are a leading cause of mortality and a public health problem; thus, interventions to reduce mortality in burned patients could be of great value. Our study found that the use of propranolol did not significantly reduce mortality in patients with severe burns, a result that is consistent with previous research [24].

Burns are associated with changes in the immune response. Severe burns induce a state of immunosuppression [35] that predisposes burn patients to infectious complications and sepsis [36]. In theory, the use of β-adrenergic blocking agents could improve immune status through the suppression of catecholamine-mediated hypermetabolism in critically ill patients. However, the potential immunological side effects of the β-adrenergic blockade are not well elucidated. Furthermore, research in animal models has found that the use of pharmacologic β-adrenergic blockade during sepsis is associated with disturbances in the immune system that predisposes to organ dysfunction and associated mortality [37, 38]. The current study found no significant differences between propranolol and placebo/usual care when measuring sepsis occurrence.

Overall, the use of propranolol in severely burned patients was not associated with a lower length of hospital stay. However, after performing subgroup and sensitivity analyses, the use of propranolol was associated with a lower length of hospital stay (LOS) in severely burned adults and children. This finding could be of great importance if we take into account that burn patient management requires significant financial resources, and LOS has a large impact on cost. It is not clear how propranolol could reduce the length of stay since many factors are related to this outcome. Such

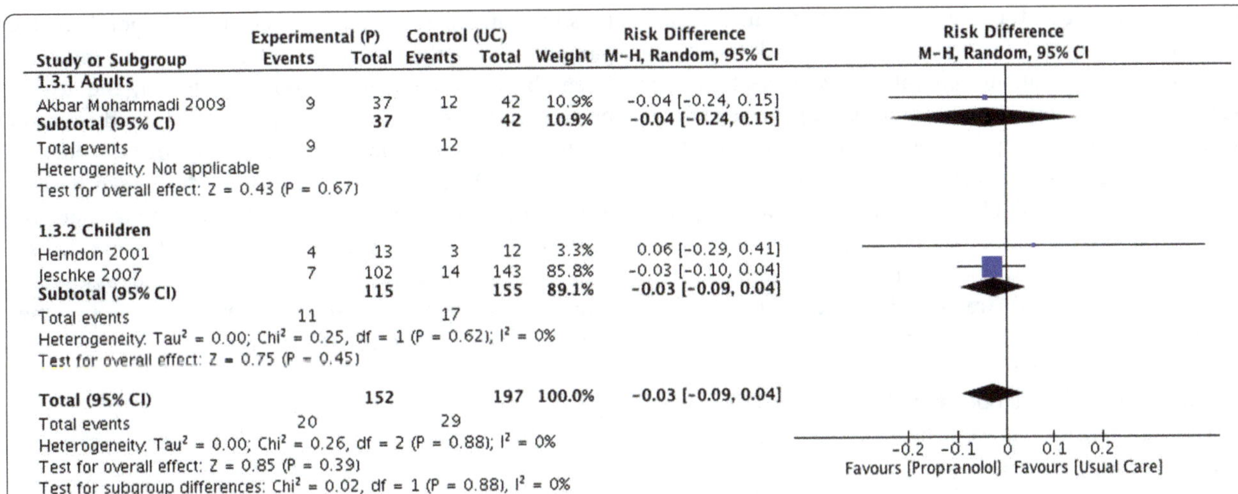

Fig. 5 Forrest plot for sepsis (propranolol vs usual care)

factors include the area and deepness of the burn, the sex and age of the patient, and the time until the initiation of the treatment [39, 40]. Although reductions of time spent in the hospital will reduce costs, and therefore are of great importance for managerial attention [41], our results provide limited evidence to conclude that propranolol decreases the length of hospital stay.

The sustained elevation of catecholamines after severe burn injuries may be detrimental to the myocardium. Severe burns may cause cardiac deficiency, myocardial hypoxia, and cardiac death [42]. In this setting, propranolol has been proposed as an intervention aimed to improve the hemodynamic state of severely burned patients. Our pooled analysis showed, as expected, that propranolol reduced heart rate in severely burned patients. This result seems to be consistent with other research which found that the administration of propranolol improves cardiac physiology and reduces cardiac stress among patients with severe burns [43, 44]. For example, Brown et al. [44] reported a 22% decrease in resting heart rate after 2 weeks of propranolol treatment in burned adults. Herndon et al. showed a 20% decrease in baseline heart rate with the use of propranolol in burned children [23]. Although the use of propranolol in severely burned patients can improve cardiac physiology, it is also associated with frequent episodes of hypotension and bradycardia [44].

Another important finding was that propranolol-treated adults had a decrease in requirements of blood transfusion. A possible explanation for this result might be that the use of propranolol in severe burns improves wound healing and therefore decreases the number of skin graft procedures [27]. In major burns, the blood loss from one debridement and grafting can be enormous. Such losses can result in cardiovascular derangements and even shock. Therefore, decreasing the number of skin graft procedures reduce the chance for major bleeding. Even if propranolol can decrease requirements of blood transfusion, it is important to keep in mind that several factors influence the decision to transfuse a burn patient and also several factors are associated with transfusions thresholds. A previous study explored the relationship between patient characteristics and number of transfusions. This study found that the number of PRBC and plasma transfusions was significantly influenced by TBSA burn, the presence of co-existing inhalation injury, and the type of anticoagulation used [45]. Palmieri and Greenhalgh [46] used a survey to identify burn center physician blood transfusions practices. They found that inhalation injury influenced the decision to transfuse blood and that the most frequent reasons for transfusions were hemorrhage, anemia, hypoxia, and cardiac disease.

A key component of evidence-based medicine is the knowledge about the balance of benefit to harm. Therefore, we must acknowledge that only one [22] of the trials reported adverse events of propranolol and that was one of the reasons why we rated eight trials as having a high risk for selective reporting. Adverse events reported in the trial by Ali et al. [22] included bradycardia, bradypnea, hypotension, and ischemia. Brown et al. [44] studied the safety of propranolol use in adult patients with burn injuries. In this study, the use of propranolol was associated with frequent episodes of hypotension and bradycardia. The authors concluded that despite the potential beneficial effects, burn care providers must recognize the potential iatrogenic hemodynamic effects of propranolol. Previous research on other conditions in children and adults have found that propranolol is associated with potentially life-threatening reactions such as pulmonary edema, shock, or complete heart block [47–49].

The most important limitation of this systematic review lies in the fact that only one study utilized mortality as a primary outcome [27]. From an orthodox view, evaluation of mortality in this study is preliminary as the remaining studies reporting mortality data are underpowered for this outcome. However, systematic reviews should include all outcomes that are likely to be meaningful to stakeholders even if those are not reported as primary endpoints in the primary research [20].

To develop a full picture of the effectiveness of propranolol on burns, additional studies will be needed that include clinical relevant outcomes, such as mortality as their primary outcomes. On the other hand, as only one trial reported data on adverse effects of propranolol, a further study with more focus on the safety of propranolol is therefore suggested.

Conclusions

Propranolol has been used as a therapy to reduce the deleterious effects of hypermetabolic response. Our analysis indicates that although lower in propranolol-treated patients, mortality and sepsis were not significantly different between compared groups. However, the use of propranolol in severely burned patients resulted in lower requirements of blood transfusion and lower values of heart rate. On the other hand, the evidence synthesized in this systematic review is limited to conclude that propranolol reduces the length of hospital stay among severely burned patients. Future trials should assess the impact of propranolol on clinically relevant outcomes such as mortality and adverse events.

Abbreviations

TBSA: Total body surface area

Acknowledgements

None.

Funding
No funding. This research received no specific grant from any funding agency in the public, commercial, or not-for-profit sectors.

Authors' contributions
RMN, HAG, PF, CAO, DAG, and EF contributed equally to this work. RMN and HAG designed the research. RMN, HAG, PF, CAO, DAG, and EF performed the research, analyzed the data, and wrote the paper. All authors read and approved the final manuscript.

Competing interests
The authors declare that they have no competing interests.

Author details
[1]Clinical Research Center, Fundación Valle del Lili, Cali, Colombia. [2]UROGIV Research Group, Universidad Del Valle, Cali, Colombia. [3]Surgical Critical Care, Virginia Commonwealth University, Richmond, VA, USA. [4]Division of Acute Care Surgery, Fundación Valle del Lili, Cali, Colombia. [5]Division of Surgery, Clinica Foianini, Av. Irala 468, Santa Cruz de la Sierra, Bolivia.

References

1. Forjuoh SN. Burns in low- and middle-income countries: a review of available literature on descriptive epidemiology, risk factors, treatment, and prevention. Burns. 2006;32:529–37. Available from: http://www.burnsjournal.com/article/S0305-4179(06)00120-3/abstract.
2. World Health Organization N. The global burden of disease: 2004 update. Update [Internet]. 2008;2010:146. Available from: http://www.who.int/healthinfo/global_burden_disease/2004_report_update/en/index.html.
3. Rossi LA, Braga ECF, Barruffini RCP, Carvalho EC. Childhood burn injuries: circumstances of occurrences and their prevention in Ribeirão Preto, Brazil. Burns. 1998;24:416–9. Available from: http://www.sciencedirect.com/science/article/pii/S0305417998000461.
4. Krishnamoorthy V, Ramaiah R, Bhananker SM. Pediatric burn injuries. Int J Crit Illn Inj Sci. India: Medknow Publications & Media Pvt Ltd; 2012;2:128–34. Available from: http://www.ncbi.nlm.nih.gov/pmc/articles/PMC3500004/.
5. Burton KR, Sharma VK, Harrop R, Lindsay R. A population-based study of the epidemiology of acute adult burn injuries in the Calgary Health Region and factors associated with mortality and hospital length of stay from 1995 to 2004. Burns. 2009;35:572–9. Available from: http://www.sciencedirect.com/science/article/pii/S0305417908003355.
6. Jeschke MG, Gauglitz GG, Kulp GA, Finnerty CC, Williams FN, Kraft R, et al. Long-term persistance of the pathophysiologic response to severe burn injury. PLoS One. 2011;6:e21245. Available from: http://journals.plos.org/plosone/article?id=10.1371/journal.pone.0021245.
7. Rojas Y, Finnerty CC, Radhakrishnan RS, Herndon DN. Burns: an update on current pharmacotherapy. Expert Opin Pharmacother. 2012;13:2485–94.
8. Cree MG, Aarsland A, Herndon DN, Wolfe RR. Role of fat metabolism in burn trauma-induced skeletal muscle insulin resistance. Crit Care Med. 2007;35:S476–83.
9. Atiyeh BS, Gunn SWA, Dibo SA. Metabolic implications of severe burn injuries and their management: a systematic review of the literature. World J Surg. 2008;32:1857–69. Available from: http://link.springer.com/article/10.1007/s00268-008-9587-8%E2%80%8b.
10. Gore DC, Chinkes DL, Hart DW, Wolf SE, Herndon DN, Sanford AP. Hyperglycaemia exacerbates muscle protein catabolism in burn injured patients. Crit Care Med. 2002;30:2438–42. Available from: https://www.ncbi.nlm.nih.gov/pubmed/12441751.
11. Williams FN, Herndon DN, Jeschke MG. The hypermetabolic response to burn injury and interventions to modify this response. Clin Plast Surg. 2009;36:583–96. Available from: http://www.ncbi.nlm.nih.gov/pmc/articles/PMC3776603/.
12. Ramirez RJ, Wolf SE, Barrow RE, Herndon DN. Growth hormone treatment in pediatric burns: a safe therapeutic approach. Ann Surg. 1998;228. Available from: http://journals.lww.com/annalsofsurgery/Fulltext/1998/10000/Growth_Hormone_Treatment_In_Pediatric_Burns__A.1.aspx
13. Hart DW, Wolf SE, Chinkes DL, Beauford RB, Mlcak RP, Heggers JP, et al. Effects of early excision and aggressive enteral feeding on hypermetabolism, catabolism, and sepsis after severe burn. J. Trauma Acute Care Surg. 2003;54. Available from: http://journals.lww.com/jtrauma/Fulltext/2003/04000/Effects_of_Early_Excision_and_Aggressive_Enteral.19.aspx
14. Celis MM, Suman OE, Huang TT, Yen P, Herndon DN. Effect of a supervised exercise and physiotherapy program on surgical interventions in children with thermal injury. J Burn Care Res. 2003;24. Available from: http://journals.lww.com/burncareresearch/Fulltext/2003/01000/Effect_of_a_Supervised_Exercise_and_Physiotherapy.14.aspx.
15. Wolf SE, Edelman LS, Kemalyan N, Donison L, Cross J, Underwood M, et al. Effects of oxandrolone on outcome measures in the severely burned: a multicentre prospective randomised double blind trial. J Burn Care Res. 2006;27:131–139. Available from: http://journals.lww.com/burncareresearch/pages/articleviewer.aspx?year=2006&issue=03000&article=00002&type=abstract.
16. Pierre EJ, Barrow RE, Hawkins HK, Nguyen TT, Sakurai Y, Desai M, et al. Effects of insulin on wound healing. J. Trauma Acute Care Surg. 1998;44. Available from: http://journals.lww.com/jtrauma/Fulltext/1998/02000/Effects_of_Insulin_on_Wound_Healing.19.aspx
17. Robinson KA. Development of a highly sensitive search strategy for the retrieval of reports of controlled trials using PubMed. Int J Epidemiol. 2002;31:150–3. Available from: http://ije.oxfordjournals.org/cgi/content/long/31/1/150.
18. Dickersin K, Scherer R, Lefebvre C. Identifying relevant studies for systematic reviews. BMJ. 1994;309:1286–91. Available from: http://www.pubmedcentral.nih.gov/articlerender.fcgi?artid=2541778&tool=pmcentrez&rendertype=abstract.
19. Glanville JM, Lefebvre C, Miles JN V, Camosso-Stefinovic J. How to identify randomized controlled trials in MEDLINE: ten years on. J Med Libr Assoc. 2006;94:130–6. Available from: http://www.pubmedcentral.nih.gov/articlerender.fcgi?artid=1435857&tool=pmcentrez&rendertype=abstract.
20. Higgins JP, Green S. Cochrane Handbook for Systematic Reviews of Interventions: Cochrane Book Series. Cochrane Handb. Syst. Rev. Interv. Cochrane B. Ser. John Wiley and Sons; 2008
21. Ali, A; Hasan, BS; Mamachen A, BS; Finnerty, CC; Herndon N. Treatment with propranolol limits blood loss during surgery in severely burned adults. J. Burn Care Res. 2014;35:S172
22. Ali A, Herndon DN, Mamachen A, Hasan S, Andersen CR, Grogans R-J, et al. Propranolol attenuates hemorrhage and accelerates wound healing in severely burned adults. Crit Care. 2015;19:217. Available from: http://www.pubmedcentral.nih.gov/articlerender.fcgi?artid=PMC4432824.
23. Herndon DN, Hart DW, Wolf SE, Chinkes DL, Wolfe RR. Reversal of catabolism by beta-blockade after severe burns. N Engl J Med. 2001;345:1223–1229. Available from: http://www.nejm.org/doi/full/10.1056/NEJMoa010342#t=article.
24. Herndon D, MD F, Rodriguez N, Diaz E, Hegde S, Jennings K, et al. Long-term propranolol use in severely burned pediatric patients: a randomized controlled study. Ann Surg. 2012;256:402–11. Available from: https://www.ncbi.nlm.nih.gov/pmc/articles/PMC3505887/.
25. Jeschke MG, Norbury WB, Finnerty CC, Branski LK, Herndon DN. Propranolol does not increase inflammation, sepsis, or infectious episodes in severely burned children. J Trauma. 2007;62:676–81. Available from: http://journals.lww.com/jtrauma/pages/articleviewer.aspx?year=2007&issue=03000&article=00020&type=abstract.
26. Komak S, Rodriguez NA, Branski LK, Diaz EC, Kinsky P, Finnerty CC, Herndon DN. The effect of propranolol on cardiovascular parameters measured by transpulmonary thermodilution in severely burned children. J Burn Care Res. 2012;33:S110.
27. Mohammadi AA, Bakhshaeekia A, Alibeigi P, Hasheminasab MJ, Tolide-ei HR, Tavakkolian AR, et al. Efficacy of propranolol in wound healing for hospitalized burn patients. J Burn Care Res. 2009;30:1013–7. Available from: http://journals.lww.com/burncareresearch/pages/articleviewer.aspx?year=2009&issue=11000&article=00013&type=abstract.
28. Norbury W. Propranolol attenuates factors affecting hypermetabolism in pediatric burn patients. Crit Care. 2007;11:P152.
29. Williams FN, Herndon DN, Kulp GA, Jeschke MG. Propranolol decreases cardiac work in a dose-dependent manner in severely burned children. Surgery. 2011;149:231–9. Available from: https://www.ncbi.nlm.nih.gov/pmc/articles/PMC3008513/.
30. Wurzer P, Clayton R, Branski L, Andersen C, Kamolz L, Woodson L, et al. 1111: Propranolol decreases cardiac stress in severely burned children. Crit Care Med. 2015;43. Available from: http://journals.lww.com/ccmjournal/Fulltext/2015/12001/1111___PROPRANOLOL_DECREASES_CARDIAC_STRESS_IN.1114.aspx

31. Brusselaers N, Monstrey S, Vogelaers D, Hoste E, Blot S. Severe burn injury in europe: a systematic review of the incidence, etiology, morbidity, and mortality. Crit Care. 2010;14:1–12. Available from: https://www.ncbi.nlm.nih.gov/pmc/articles/PMC3219295/.
32. Latenser BA, Miller SF, Bessey PQ, Browning SM, Caruso DM, Gomez M, et al. National Burn Repository 2006: a ten-year review. J Burn Care Res. 2007;28. Available from: https://www.ncbi.nlm.nih.gov/pubmed/17969244.
33. Bessey P, Caruso D, Casavant C, Edelman L, Jeng J, Kemalyan N, et al. National Burn Repository. Report of Data from 2001–2010. USA: American Burn Association; 2011.
34. Murray CJL, Lopez AD. The Global Burden of Disease a comprehensive assessment of mortality and disability from diseases, injuries, and risk factors in 1990 and projected to 2020 [Internet]. The Harvard School for Public Health; 1996. Available from: http://apps.who.int/iris/bitstream/10665/41864/1/0965546608_eng.pdf.
35. Heideman M, Bengtsson A. The immunologic response to thermal injury. World J Surg. 1992;16:53–6. Available from: http://link.springer.com/article/10.1007/BF02067115.
36. Greenhalgh DG, Saffle JR, Holmes JH, Gamelli RL, Palmieri TL, Horton JW, et al. American Burn Association consensus conference to define sepsis and infection in burns. J Burn Care Res. 2007;28:776–790. Available from: http://journals.lww.com/burncareresearch/pages/articleviewer.aspx?year=2007&issue=11000&article=00002&type=abstract.
37. Oberbeck R, Schmitz D, Wilsenack K, Schüler M, Pehle B, Schedlowski M, et al. Adrenergic modulation of survival and cellular immune functions during polymicrobial sepsis. Neuroimmunomodulation. 2004;11:214–23. Available from: http://www.karger.com/DOI/10.1159/000078439.
38. Schmitz D, Wilsenack K, Lendemanns S, Schedlowski M, Oberbeck R. Beta-adrenergic blockade during systemic inflammation: impact on cellular immune functions and survival in a murine model of sepsis. Resuscitation. 2016;72:286–94. Available from: http://www.resuscitationjournal.com/article/S0300-9572(06)00362-5/abstract.
39. Berry CC, Patterson TL, Wachtel TL, Frank HA. Behavioural factors in burn mortality and length of stay in hospital. Burns. 1984;10:409–14. Available from: http://www.sciencedirect.com/science/article/pii/0305417984900809.
40. Sánchez J, Perepérez S, Bastida J, Martínez M. Cost-utility analysis applied to the treatment of burn patients in a specialized center. Arch Surg. 2007;142:50–7. Available from: http://dx.doi.org/10.1001/archsurg.142.1.50.
41. Clarke A. Why are we trying to reduce length of stay? Evaluation of the costs and benefits of reducing time in hospital must start from the objectives that govern change. Qual Heal Care. 1996;5:172–9. Available from: http://www.ncbi.nlm.nih.gov/pmc/articles/PMC1055402/.
42. Williams FN, Herndon DN, Suman OE, Lee JO, Norbury WB, Branski LK, et al. Changes in cardiac physiology after severe burn injury. J Burn Care Res. 2011;32:269–74. Available from: http://www.ncbi.nlm.nih.gov/pmc/articles/PMC3391739/.
43. Finnerty CC, Herndon DN. Is propranolol of benefit in pediatric burn patients? Adv Surg. 2013 ;47:177–97. Available from: http://www.pubmedcentral.nih.gov/articlerender.fcgi?artid=3955897&tool=pmcentrez&rendertype=abstract. [cited 2016 May 27].
44. Brown DA, Gibbons J, Honari S, Klein MB, Pham TN, Gibran NS. Propranolol dosing practices in adult burn patients. J Burn Care Res. 2016;37:e218–26. Available from: https://www.ncbi.nlm.nih.gov/pubmed/25882517.
45. Lu RP, Lin F-C, Ortiz-Pujols SM, Adams SD, Whinna HC, Cairns BA, et al. Blood utilization in patients with burn injury and association with clinical outcomes. Transfusion. 2013;53:2212–21. Available from: http://www.ncbi.nlm.nih.gov/pmc/articles/PMC3620962/.
46. Palmieri TL, Greenhalgh DG. Blood transfusion in burns: what do we do? J Burn Care Rehabil. 2004;25:71–5. Available from: https://www.ncbi.nlm.nih.gov/pubmed/14726742.
47. Greenblatt DJ, Koch-Weser J. Adverse reactions to propranolol in hospitalized medical patients: a report from the Boston Collaborative Drug Surveillance Program. Am Heart J. 1973;86:478–84. Available from: http://www.sciencedirect.com/science/article/pii/0002870373901397.
48. Scheinman MM, Strauss HC, Evans GT, Ryan C, Massie B, Wallace A. Adverse effects of sympatholytic agents in patients with hypertension and sinus node dysfunction. Am J Med. 1978;64:1013–20. Available from: http://www.sciencedirect.com/science/article/pii/0002934378904576.
49. de Graaf M, Breur JMPJ, Raphaël MF, Vos M, Breugem CC, Pasmans SGMA. Adverse effects of propranolol when used in the treatment of hemangiomas: a case series of 28 infants. J Am Acad Dermatol. 2011;65:320–7. Available from: http://www.sciencedirect.com/science/article/pii/S0190962210007632.

13

WSES guidelines for emergency repair of complicated abdominal wall hernias

Massimo Sartelli[1*], Federico Coccolini[2], Gabrielle H van Ramshorst[3], Giampiero Campanelli[4], Vincenzo Mandalà[5], Luca Ansaloni[2], Ernest E Moore[6], Andrew Peitzman[7], George Velmahos[8], Fredrick Alan Moore[9], Ari Leppaniemi[10], Clay Cothren Burlew[6], Walter Biffl[6], Kaoru Koike[11], Yoram Kluger[12], Gustavo P Fraga[13], Carlos A Ordonez[14], Salomone Di Saverio[15], Ferdinando Agresta[16], Boris Sakakushev[17], Igor Gerych[18], Imtiaz Wani[19], Michael D Kelly[20], Carlos Augusto Gomes[21], Mario Paulo Faro Jr[22], Korhan Taviloglu[23], Zaza Demetrashvili[24], Jae Gil Lee[25], Nereo Vettoretto[26], Gianluca Guercioni[27], Cristian Tranà[1], Yunfeng Cui[28], Kenneth YY Kok[29], Wagih M Ghnnam[30], Ashraf El-Sayed Abbas[30], Norio Sato[11], Sanjay Marwah[31], Muthukumaran Rangarajan[32], Offir Ben-Ishay[12], Abdul Rashid K Adesunkanmi[33], Helmut Alfredo Segovia Lohse[34], Jakub Kenig[35], Stefano Mandalà[36], Andrea Patrizi[1], Rodolfo Scibé[1] and Fausto Catena[37]

Abstract

Emergency repair of complicated abdominal hernias is associated with poor prognosis and a high rate of post-operative complications.

A World Society of Emergency Surgery (WSES) Consensus Conference was held in Bergamo in July 2013, during the 2nd Congress of the World Society of Emergency Surgery with the goal of defining recommendations for emergency repair of abdominal wall hernias in adults. This document represents the executive summary of the consensus conference approved by a WSES expert panel.

Introduction

A large number of abdominal hernias require emergency surgery. However, these procedures are associated with poor prognoses and a higher rate of post-operative complications [1].

A World Society of Emergency Surgery (WSES) Consensus Conference was held in Bergamo on July 2013, during the 2nd Congress of the World Society of Emergency Surgery with the goal of defining recommendations for emergency repair of abdominal wall hernias in adults. This document represents the executive summary of the consensus conference approved by a WSES expert panel.

Abdominal hernias may be classified as groin hernias (femoral and inguinal) and ventral hernias (umbilical, epigastric, spigelian and incisional).

An incarcerated hernia may be defined as a hernia in which the contents have become irreducible due to a narrow opening in the abdominal wall or adhesions within the cavity. Intestinal obstruction can complicate an incarcerated hernia. In contrast, a strangulated hernia is one in which the blood supply to the contents of the hernia (eg omentum, bowel) s becomes compromised [2].

Strangulated hernias remain a significant challenge, as they are sometimes difficult to diagnose purely by physical examination yet require urgent surgical intervention. Early surgical intervention of a strangulated hernia with obstruction is crucial as delayed diagnosis can lead to bowel resection with longer recovery and its attendant complications. Strangulated hernias can have serious deleterious effects such as, bowel obstruction, bacterial translocation, and intestinal wall necrosis (potentially resulting in bowel perforation). It poses a significant risk to emergency hernia repair, as there is an increased incidence of surgical field contamination, leading to high rates of post-operative infection and probably recurrence.

Bacteria inherently colonize all surgical wounds, but only a fraction of these contaminates ultimately lead to infection. In most patients infection does not occur because innate host defences are able to eliminate microbes at the surgical

* Correspondence: m.sartelli@virgilio.it
[1]Department of Surgery, Macerata Hospital, Macerata, Italy
Full list of author information is available at the end of the article

site. However, there is some evidence that the implantation of foreign materials, such as prosthetic mesh, may lead to a decreased threshold for infection [3].

While many factors can influence surgical wound healing and post-operative infection, bacterial burden is the most significant risk factor. Wounds are classified according to the likelihood and degree of wound contamination at the time of operation. Classifications include: clean wounds, clean-contaminated wounds, contaminated wounds, and dirty or infected wounds [4].

The pathogens involved in an infection depend on the type of surgery. In an aseptic surgical procedure, *Staphylococcus aureus* is a common source of infection, either from the patient's own skin flora or surrounding environment. Surgeons can minimize the risk of infection and associated complications by routinely employing site-specific spectrum antibiotic prophylaxis.

In clean-contaminated, contaminated, and dirty surgical procedures, the polymicrobial aerobic and anaerobic flora closely resemble the normal endogenous microflora of the gastrointestinal (GI) tract and are the most frequently observed pathogens. The contaminating pathogens in GI surgery include gram-negative bacilli (e.g., *Escherichia coli*) and gram-positive microbes, such as enterococci and anaerobic organisms. A classification scheme has been demonstrated in multiple studies to predict the relative probability that a given wound will become infected [5,6].

Several studies show clear advantages of mesh use in elective cases, where infection should be uncommon. Mesh significantly reduces the rate of hernia recurrence yet is easy to use and has low complication rates. On the other hand, few studies have investigated the outcome of mesh use in an emergency setting, where there is often surgical field contamination due to bowel involvement [7,8].

The use of biological mesh has many advantages, including a decreased immune response mounted against the foreign body, as well as decreased incidence of fistulae formation, fibrosis, and erosions.

There is, however, a paucity of high quality evidence on the superiority of biological mesh and there remains a significant price premium with their use [9].

Recommendation guidelines are evaluated according to the Grading of Recommendations Assessment, Development, and Evaluation (GRADE), a hierarchical, evidence-based rubric [10,11] summarized in Table 1, which is a guideline used to assess the strength of recommendations.

Recommendations

Timing of intervention

Patients should undergo emergency hernia repair immediately when intestinal strangulation is suspected (grade 1C recommendation).

Systemic inflammatory response syndrome (SIRS) signs, contrast-enhanced CT findings as well as lactate, CPK and D-dimer levels are predictive of bowel strangulation (grade 1C recommendation).

Unfortunately, morbidity and mortality rates remain high for patients who undergo emergency repair of abdominal hernias. Early diagnosis of strangulated obstruction maybe difficult, and delayed diagnosis can lead to septic complications. However, in the case of suspected bowel strangulation the benefits outweigh the risks of surgery and patients should undergo immediate surgical intervention.

A recent study performed by Martínez-Serrano et al. prospectively analyzed morbidity and mortality rates following emergency hernia repair [12]. The study population included 244 patients with complicated abdominal wall hernias requiring surgical repair. In this study, the patients were treated according to standardized protocols with detailed actions to be taken during the pre-, intra-, and post-operative periods. Clinical outcomes were compared retroactively to that of 402 patients who had undergone similar procedures before the development and implementation of the protocols outlined in the study. Results showed higher rates of mortality in patients with acute complication as their first hernia-related symptom and whose treatment was delayed for more than 24 hours. Thus, the authors concluded that early detection of complicated abdominal hernias may be the best means of reducing the rate of mortality [12].

In 2007, Derici et al. published a retrospective study using univariate and multivariate analysis to investigate factors affecting morbidity and mortality rates in cases of incarcerated abdominal wall hernias [13]. Using univariate analysis, results showed that symptomatic periods lasting longer than 8 hours, the presence of comorbid disease, high American Society of Anesthesiology (ASA) scores, the use of general anesthesia, the presence of strangulation, and the presence of necrosis significantly affect morbidity rates. In contrast, advanced age, the presence of comorbid diseases, high ASA scores, the presence of strangulation, the presence of necrosis, and hernia repair with graft were found to significantly affect mortality rates by univariate analysis; the presence of necrosis, however, was the only factor that appeared to significantly affect mortality rates based on multivariate analysis [10].

A retrospective study was recently published evaluating the risk factors associated with bowel resection and treatment outcome in patients with incarcerated groin hernias [14].

The study analyzed 182 adult patients with incarcerated groin hernias who underwent emergency hernia repair in the 10-year period from January 1999 to June 2009. Of these patients, bowel resection was required in 15.4% of cases (28/182). A logistic regression model

Table 1 Grading of Recommendations Assessment, Development, and Evaluation (GRADE) from Guyatt and colleagues [10,11]

Grade of recommendation	Clarity of risk/benefit	Quality of supporting evidence	Implications
1A			
Strong recommendation, high-quality evidence	Benefits clearly outweigh risk and burdens, or vice versa	RCTs without important limitations or overwhelming evidence from observational studies	Strong recommendation, applies to most patients in most circumstances without reservation
1B			
Strong recommendation, moderate-quality evidence	Benefits clearly outweigh risk and burdens, or vice versa	RCTs with important limitations (inconsistent results, methodological flaws, indirect analyses or imprecise conclusions) or exceptionally strong evidence from observational studies	Strong recommendation, applies to most patients in most circumstances without reservation
1C			
Strong recommendation, low-quality or very low-quality evidence	Benefits clearly outweigh risk and burdens, or vice versa	Observational studies or case series	Strong recommendation but subject to change when higher quality evidence becomes available
2A			
Weak recommendation, high-quality evidence	Benefits closely balanced with risks and burden	RCTs without important limitations or overwhelming evidence from observational studies	Weak recommendation, best action may differ depending on the patient, treatment circumstances, or social values
2B			
Weak recommendation, moderate-quality evidence	Benefits closely balanced with risks and burden	RCTs with important limitations (inconsistent results, methodological flaws, indirect or imprecise) or exceptionally strong evidence from observational studies	Weak recommendation, best action may differ depending on the patient, treatment circumstances, or social values
2C			
Weak recommendation, Low-quality or very low-quality evidence	Uncertainty in the estimates of benefits, risks, and burden; benefits, risk, and burden may be closely balanced	Observational studies or case series	Very weak recommendation; alternative treatments may be equally reasonable and merit consideration

identified three independent risk factors for bowel resection: lack of health insurance (odds ratio [OR], 5, P = 0.005), obvious peritonitis (OR, 11.52, P = 0.019), and femoral hernia (OR, 8.31, P < 0.001) [14].

Many authors reported that early detection of progression from an incarcerated hernia to a strangulated hernia is difficult to achieve by either clinical or laboratory means, which presents a large challenge in early diagnosis [15-17]. Signs of SIRS including fever, tachycardia, and leukocytosis, as well as abdominal wall rigidity, are considered common indicators of strangulated obstruction. However, an investigation by Sarr et al. demonstrated that the combination of four classic signs of strangulation – continuous abdominal pain, fever, tachycardia, and leukocytosis – could not distinguish strangulated from simple obstructions [16]. Furthermore, Shatilla et al. reported a low incidence of these classical findings and stated that their presence indicated an advanced stage of strangulation, which would be of limited value for early diagnosis [16]. In 2006, Tsumura et al. published a retrospective study investigating SIRS as a predictor of strangulated small bowel obstruction. Multivariate analysis revealed that the presence of SIRS alongside abdominal muscle guarding was independently predictive of strangulated small bowel obstruction [18].

Among possible diagnostic tests, serum creatinine phosphokinase (CPK) appears to be a relatively reliable indicator of early intestinal strangulation [19,20]. Icoz et al. published a prospective study investigating the relevance of serum D-dimer measurement as a potential diagnostic indicator of strangulated intestinal hernia. The authors concluded that D-dimer assays should be performed on patients presenting with intestinal emergencies to better evaluate and predict ischemic events. Despite having low specificity, elevated D-dimer levels measured upon admission were found to correlate strongly with intestinal ischemia [21].

In 2012 an interesting retrospective study examining whether various laboratory parameters could predict viability of strangulation in patients with bowel obstruction was published. Forty patients diagnosed with bowel strangulation operated within 72 hours of the start of symptoms were included in the study. Lactate level was the only laboratory parameter significantly associated with viability ($P < 0.01$, Mann-Whitney test). Other laboratory data did not show statistically significant associations. The Authors concluded that arterial blood lactate level (2.0 mmol/L or greater) was a useful predictor of nonviable bowel strangulation [22].

Early diagnostic methods to detect bowel strangulation have advanced substantially following the development and refinement of radiological techniques, such as Computed Tomography (CT) scanning [23]. Jancelewicz et al. recently published a retrospective analysis demonstrating that CT findings of reduced wall enhancement were the most significant independent predictor of bowel strangulation, with 56% sensitivity and 94% specificity. By contrast, elevated white blood cell (WBC) count and guarding on physical examination were only moderately predictive. It should be noted, however, that an elevated WBC was the only variable found to be independently predictive of bowel strangulation in patients with small bowel obstruction [24].

Laparoscopic approach

Repair of incarcerated hernias – both ventral and groin – may be performed with a laparoscopic approach (grade 1C recommendation).

Recent prospective studies and recent guidelines [25-31] have focused on the laparoscopic approach to hernia repair in an elective setting.

By contrast, few studies have focused on the laparoscopic approach to hernia repair in an emergency setting. In 2004, Landau et al. published a retrospective study investigating the use of laparoscopy in the repair of incarcerated incisional and ventral hernias. The authors argued that laparoscopic repair was feasible and could be safely used to treat patients presenting with incarcerated incisional and ventral hernias [32].

Another retrospective study published in 2008 investigated the role of laparoscopy in the management of incarcerated (non-reducible) ventral hernias. The authors concluded that laparoscopic repair of ventral abdominal wall hernias could be safely performed with low subsequent complication rates, even in the event of an incarcerated hernia. Careful bowel reduction with adhesiolysis and mesh repair in an uncontaminated abdomen (without inadvertent enterotomy) using a 5-cm mesh overlap was an important factor predictive of successful clinical outcome [33].

In 2009, another retrospective study was published investigating laparoscopic techniques used to treat incisional hernias in an emergency setting. The results of this series also demonstrated the feasibility of laparoscopic surgery to treat incarcerated incisional hernias in an emergency setting [34].

Additionally, a systematic literature review performed in 2009 identified articles reporting on laparoscopic treatment, reduction, and repair of incarcerated or strangulated inguinal hernias from 1989 to 2008. It included seven articles on this topic, reporting on 328 cases treated with total extraperitoneal (TEP) or transabdominal preperitoneal (TAPP) repair. Laparoscopy can also be used to resect bowel, if necessary, or to repair an occult contralateral hernia, present in 11.2–50% of cases. The Authors concluded that the laparoscopic repair is a feasible procedure with acceptable results; however, its efficacy needs to be studied further, ideally with larger, multicenter randomized controlled trials [35]

In 2007 a series of patients with large irreducible groin hernias (omentoceles), treated by laparoscopy without conversions, was published. The Authors described a technique to facilitate complete removal of the the hernia contents. A laparoscopic transperitoneal repair for large irreducible scrotal hernias removing as much omentum as possible was performed. Then a small groin incision was made to excise the adherent omentum from the distal sac [36].

Hernioscopy is a mixed laparoscopic–open surgical technique for incarcerated inguinal hernias. Specifically, it is effective in evaluating the viability of the herniated loop, thus avoiding unnecessary laparotomy [37]. A prospective randomized study in 2009 aimed to evaluate the impact of hernia sac laparoscopy on the morbidity and mortality of cases with a spontaneous reduction of the strangulated hernia content before the assessment of its viability. Ninety-five patients were randomly assigned to 2 groups: group A (21 patients managed using hernia sac laparoscopy) and group B (20 patients managed without laparoscopy). The median hospital stay was 28 hours for group A and 34 hours for group B. Four patients of group B had major complications, whereas there was none observed in the group A. Two unnecessary laparotomies and 2 deaths occurred in group B. The authors concluded that hernia sac laparoscopy seems to be an accurate and safe method of preventing unnecessary laparotomy and in high-risk patients it contributes to decreased morbidity [38].

Emergency hernia repair in "clean surgical field"

The choice of technique repair is based on the contamination of the surgical field, the size of the hernia and the experience of the surgeon.

Prosthetic repair with synthetic mesh is recommended for patients with intestinal incarceration and no signs of intestinal strangulation or concurrent bowel resection (clean surgical field) (grade 1A recommendation).

The increased likelihood of surgical site infection may suggest additive risk for permanent synthetic mesh repair (grade 1C recommendation).

Primary suture repair as an elective hernia-related procedure can increase the risk of recurrence, thereby leading to subsequent follow-up surgery. This is the case in both ventral and inguinal abdominal wall hernias. Numerous studies have demonstrated the advantages of mesh use in clean, sterile cases; such advantages include ease of placement, low long-term complication rates, and reduction of recurrence for incisional hernias [39-42]. For patients with intestinal incarceration and no signs of intestinal strangulation or concurrent bowel resection, the surgical field is presumed clean and the infectious risk for synthetic mesh is low. The absence of intestinal wall ischemia renders patients less predisposed to bacterial translocation, and there is a low risk of need for concurrent bowel resection, which leads to contamination of the surgical field. However, this has not been proven for cases of acute irreducible hernias.

Researchers have published a variety of small-scale studies comparing mesh use to suture repair in the treatment of acute irreducible hernias [43-46]. In 2011, Nieuwenhuizen et al. published a retrospective study investigating the use of mesh in acute hernia-related procedures. A total of 203 patients were identified for the study: 76 inguinal, 52 umbilical, 39 incisional, 14 epigastric, 14 femoral, 5 trocar, and 3 spigelian hernias. For purposes of statistical analysis, epigastric, femoral, trocar, and spigelian hernia patients were pooled together due to their small individual group sizes. One patient was excluded from the analysis because the hernia was not ultimately corrected during surgery. In all, 99 hernias were repaired using mesh compared to 103 primary suture repairs. Additionally, univariate analysis demonstrated that female patients (P = 0.007), overweight patients (P = 0.016), patients with an umbilical hernia (P = 0.01), and patients who had undergone bowel resection (P = 0.015) featured significantly higher rates of wound infection. By contrast, the type of repair (i.e. primary suture vs. mesh), the use of antibiotic prophylaxis, ASA class, and patient age did not appear to share any statistically significant relationships with post-operative rates of surgical site infection. Based on logistic regression analysis, only bowel resection (P = 0.020) appeared to correlate significantly with post-operative surgical site infection [47].

An increased likelihood for surgical site infection may suggest additive risk for permanent synthetic mesh repair [48-50]. In a recent multicenter cohort study, patients who underwent incisional hernia repair during other concomitant intra-abdominal procedures experienced greater than 6-fold increases in the risk of subsequent mesh removal. Of the 1,071 mesh repairs retrospectively analyzed during the 4-year period from 1998 to 2002, 5.1% (55/1,071) underwent mesh removal at a median time of 7.3 months (interquartile range 1.4-22.2) following incisional hernia repair with permanent mesh prosthesis. Infection was the most common reason for mesh removal, accounting for 69% of cases. No statistically significant differences were observed based on the method of surgical repair. After adjusting for covariates, both same-site concomitant surgery (hazard ratio [HR] = 6.3) and post-operative surgical site infection (HR = 6.5) were associated with mesh removal [51].

Emergency hernia repair in "potentially contaminated surgical field"

For patients with intestinal strangulation and/or concurrent bowel resection (potentially contaminated surgical field), direct suture is recommended when the hernia defect in question is small. Synthetic mesh repair may be performed, but with caution. Biological meshes may be a valid option but merit detailed cost-benefit analysis (grade 2C recommendation).

Many studies discuss and advocate the use of prosthetic mesh in clean surgical fields. However, the use of prosthetic grafts in potentially-contaminated and contaminated settings is seldom described. Despite discrepancies in data and conflicting reports, prosthetic materials are not generally recommended for abdominal hernia repair in contaminated settings. Most studies on the subject do not focus on emergency repair, and as such, their results are of limited value. According to many researchers, the use of mesh is strongly discouraged in potentially contaminated surgical fields.

One study analyzed and compared post-operative outcome following ventral hernia repair using prosthetic mesh in clean-contaminated and contaminated wounds [52]. All patients of U.S. hospitals participating in the National Surgical Quality Improvement Program (NSQIP) who were admitted for mesh-mediated ventral hernia repair in the 5-year period from January 1, 2005, to April 4, 2010, were included in the study. Compared to clean cases, clean-contaminated cases featured a significantly greater likelihood of wound disruption, pneumonia, and sepsis as well as superficial, deep, and ventral surgical site infections (SSIs). Both clean-contaminated and contaminated mesh-mediated cases featured an increased risk of septic shock (5.82% and 26.74%, respectively) and ventilator use lasting longer than 48 hours (5.59% and 26.76%, respectively). Clean-contaminated cases of mesh-mediated ventral hernia repair also featured a significantly increased odds ratio for complications (2.52) [52].

In a recent study, Xourafas et al. examined the impact of mesh use on ventral hernia repairs with simultaneous bowel resections attributable to either cancer or bowel occlusion. Researchers found a significantly higher incidence of post-operative infection in patients with prosthetic mesh compared to those without mesh. According to multivariate regression analysis, prosthetic mesh use was the only significant risk factor irrespective of other variables such as drain use, defect size, or type of bowel resection [53]. By contrast, other researchers have asserted that prosthetic repair of abdominal hernias can be safely performed alongside simultaneous colonic operations. Such joint procedures, they argue, exhibit acceptable rates of infectious complications and recurrence, and consequently, they maintain that there is insufficient evidence to advocate the avoidance of prosthetic mesh in potentially contaminated fields, assuming that the appropriate technique is used [54,55].

In 2000 Mandalà et al. published a series of patients with incisional hernias treated with nonabsorbable prostheses and associated visceral surgery. The low incidence of suppurative complications, with neither removal of the patch nor recurrences in the short term, showed that nonabsorbable mesh repair in potentially contaminated fields was safe [56].

Studies by Vix et al., Birolini et al., and Geisler et al. report wound-related morbidity rates of 10.6%, 20%, and 7%, respectively, following mesh use in both clean-contaminated and contaminated procedures [57-59]. A different study by Campanelli et al. analyzed ten prosthetic hernia repairs in potentially contaminated fields and reported no major or minor complications after a 21-month follow-up period [60].

Recently a study by Carbonell et al. [61] investigated Open ventral hernia repairs performed with polypropylene mesh in the retro-rectus position in clean-contaminated and contaminated fields. The 30-day surgical site infection rate was 7.1% for clean-contaminated cases; for contaminated cases the 30-day surgical site infection rate was 19.0%.

It should be noted, however, that most of these studies did not focus on emergency repair of incarcerated hernias.

A study by Kelly et al. reported a 21% infection rate in a series of emergency and elective incisional hernia repairs [62]. A study by Davies et al. focused exclusively on a subset of hernia cases in which patients presented with an obstructed bowel and required emergency surgery. This study found high rates of infection in patients requiring emergency repair for all types of abdominal hernias [63]. A retrospective multivariate analysis by Nieuwenhuizen et al. revealed bowel resection to be a major factor associated with wound infection, but that other clinical ramifications of the procedure were relatively rare [47]. A recently published retrospective analysis of emergency repair of incarcerated incisional hernias with simultaneous bowel obstruction in potentially contaminated fields demonstrated that the use of permanent prosthetic mesh in these surgeries was associated with high rates of wound infection. No infections occurred in patients whose surgical wounds were left open to granulate [64].

In 2013 a prospective study to present a 7-year experience with the use of prosthetic mesh repair in the management of the acutely incarcerated and/or strangulated ventral hernias was published. The hernia was paraumbilical in 71 patients (89%), epigastric in 6 patients (8%) and incisional in 3 patients (4%). Eighteen patients (23%) had recurrent hernias. Resection-anastomosis of non-viable small intestine was performed in 18 patients (23%) and was not regarded as a contraindication for prosthetic repair [65].

Biological mesh prosthetics are most commonly used in infected fields involving large, complex abdominal wall hernia repairs. The use of biological mesh, which becomes vascularized and remodelled into autologous tissue after implantation, may offer a low-morbidity alternative to prosthetic mesh products in these complex settings, with good results also in immunocompromised patients [66]. The use of biological materials in clinical practice has led to innovative methods of treating abdominal wall defects in contaminated surgical fields.

Many retrospective studies have explored the promising role of biological mesh in contaminated fields, but most of these investigations did not focus on emergency repair of incarcerated hernias [67-87].

Although biologic mesh in these situations is safe, long-term durability has still not been demonstrated [88]. A study by Catena et al. published in 2007 focused on complicated incisional hernia repair using mesh prosthetics made of porcine dermal collagen (PDC). Incisional hernioplasty using PDC grafts was found to be a safe and efficient approach to difficult cases complicated by potential contamination [82].

A recent literature review by Coccolini et al. covered the use of biological meshes for abdominal reconstruction in emergency and elective setting in transplanted patients, and reported a complication rate of 9.4% [85].

By incorporating biological mesh, surgeons hope to provide a collagen-based extracellular matrix scaffold by which host fibroblasts can induce angiogenesis and deposit new collagen. The non-synthetic material of biological mesh makes it less susceptible to infection, and several biological grafts are available in the current market. Their classification is based on the species of origin (allogenic or xenogenic), the type of collagen matrix utilized (dermis, pericardium, or intestinal submucosa), the decellularization process, the presence or absence of cross-linkage, temperature-related storage requirements, and the use of rehydration [86].

On the basis of either the presence or not of the cross-linking, biological prosthesis are divided into two subgroups: the partially remodeling (cross-linked) and the completely remodeling ones (not cross-linked). Thanks to the presence of additional linkages the partially remodeling ones resist better and for a longer period to mechanical stress [66].

Coccolini et al. recently published the results of the first 193 patients of the Italian Register of Biological Prosthesis (IRBP) [87]. This prospective multi-centre study, suggests the usefulness, versatility and ease of using biological prosthesis in many different situations, including clean or contaminated surgical fields. Despite the lack of a cohesive body of evidence, published studies on biological mesh suggest that cross-linked mesh prosthetics have the lowest failure rate in potentially contaminated and outright infected fields. This trend should be investigated further by means of large, prospective, randomized studies [89].

Recently a critical review of biologic mesh use in ventral hernia repairs under contaminated field was published. All literature reviews found in medline database supported biologic mesh use, especially in the setting of contaminated fields, but the primary literature included in these reviews consisted entirely of case series and case reports with low levels of evidence [90]. To better guide surgeons, prospective, randomized trials should be undertaken to evaluate the short- and long-term outcomes associated with biological meshes under the various surgical wound classifications [91].

Emergency hernia repair in "contaminated-dirty surgical field"

For stable patients with strangulated obstruction and peritonitis by bowel perforation (contaminated-dirty surgical field) direct tissue suture is recommended when the hernia defect is small; in the events that direct tissue suture is not possible, biological mesh repair may be suggested (grade 2C recommendation). The choice between a cross-linked or a non cross-linked biological mesh should be evaluated depending on the defect size and degree of contamination (grade 2C recommendation).

If biological mesh is not available, both polyglactin mesh repair and open management with delayed repair may be a viable alternative (grade 2C recommendation).

For unstable patients (those experiencing severe sepsis or septic shock), open management is recommended to prevent abdominal compartment syndrome; intra-abdominal pressure may be measured intra-operatively (grade 2C recommendation).

Following stabilization of the patient, surgeons should attempt early, definitive closure of the abdomen. Primary fascial closure may be possible when there is minimal risk of excessive tension or recurrence of intra-abdominal hypertension (IAH) (grade 2C recommendation).

In the event that early, definitive fascial closure is not possible, surgeons must resort to progressive closure performed incrementally each time the patient returns for a subsequent procedure. Cross-linked biological meshes may be considered an option in abdominal wall reconstruction (grade 2C recommendation).

In cases of bacterial peritonitis, patients must undergo contaminated surgical intervention, which means that the surgical field is infected and the risk of surgical site infection is very high. As mentioned earlier, the use of biological materials in clinical practice has led to innovative methods of treating abdominal wall defects in contaminated surgical fields, although there is still insufficient level of high-quality evidence on their value, and there is still a very huge price difference between the synthetic and biological meshes (9).

Some authors investigated the use of absorbable prosthetic materials [86]. However, the use of absorbable prosthesis exposes the patient to an inevitable hernia recurrence. These meshes, once implanted, initiate an inflammatory reaction that, through a hydrolytic reaction, removes and digests the implanted prosthetic material completely. In this case, the high risk of hernia recurrence is explained by the complete dissolution of the prosthetic support [92].

Patients with strangulated obstruction and peritonitis caused by bowel perforation are often considered critically ill due to septic complications; further, they may experience high intra-operative intra-abdominal pressure, which can lead to abdominal compartment syndrome. Although intra-abdominal hypertension has been known to cause physiological perturbation since the early 19th century, its clinical implications have only recently been recognized in patients sustaining intra-abdominal trauma. Such hypertension may be the underlying cause of increased pulmonary pressures, reduced cardiac output, splanchnic hypoperfusion, and oliguria. In summary, this clinical condition is known as abdominal compartment syndrome. Abdominal compartment syndrome results from shock and resuscitation yielding ischemic reperfusion-related injury. Cellular damage results from ischemia, subsequent cellular membrane dysfunction, and intra- and extra-cellular edema. This capillary leak results in massive edema of local tissues, most notably those of the intestines. Prophylactic treatment to avoid abdominal compartment syndrome involves refraining from abdominal closure when fascial approximation becomes problematic due to excessive tension [93].

Intestinal strangulation can lead to increased intra-abdominal pressure, and ultimately, to abdominal compartment syndrome. A study published by Beltran et al. examined 81 consecutive unselected patients presenting with complicated hernias and intestinal obstruction. The researchers measured intra-abdominal pressure using the intra-vesicular pressure method, and these serial measurements of intra-abdominal pressure were used to assess the clinical severity of strangulated hernias. Intra-abdominal pressure measurement may be used as a predictor of intestinal strangulation for patients presenting with acute abdominal compartment syndrome secondary to complicated herniation [94].

Following stabilization of the patient, the primary objective is early and definitive closure of the abdomen to minimize complications. For many patients, primary fascial closure may be possible within a few days of the initial operation. In other patients, early definitive fascial closure may not be possible. In these cases, surgeons must resort to progressive closure, in which the abdomen is incrementally closed each time the patient undergoes a subsequent surgery.

Many methods of fascial closure have been described in the medical literature [95-100].

In 2012 a retrospective analysis evaluating the use of vacuum-assisted closure and mesh-mediated fascial traction (VACM) as temporary abdominal closure was published. The study compared 50 patients treated with (VACM) and 54 using non-traction techniques (control group).

VACM resulted in a higher fascial closure rate and lower planned hernia rate than methods that did not provide fascial traction [100].

Occasionally abdominal closure is only partially achieved, resulting in large, debilitating hernias of the abdominal wall that will eventually require complex surgical repair. In these cases, delayed repair or use of biological meshes may be suggested. Bridging meshes will often result in bulging or recurrences [101]. The Italian Biological Prosthesis Working Group (IBPWG) proposed a decisional algorithm in using biological meshes to restore abdominal wall defects [60].

Another option if definitive fascial closure is not possible could be skin only closure and subsequent management of the eventration with deferred abdominal closure with synthetic meshes after hospital discharge (grade 1C recommendation).

Damage control surgery has been widely used in trauma patients and its use is rapidly expanding in the setting of Acute Care Surgery. Damage control surgery can be used in patients with strangulated obstruction and peritonitis caused by bowel perforation. Skin only closure could be an alternative for patients with failure of definitive fascia closure, reducing the risk of complications of open abdomen and abdominal compartmental syndrome [102]. Patients could be deferred for definitive abdominal closure with mesh after hospital discharge.

The component separation technique may be useful for the repair of large midline abdominal wall hernias (grade 1B recommendation).

This technique for reconstructing abdominal wall defects without the use of prosthetic material was descibed in 1990, by Ramirez et al. [103].

The technique is based on enlargement of the abdominal wall surface by translation of the muscular layers without severing the innervation and blood supply of the muscles [104].

Reherniation rates in the literature vary between 0% and 8.6%. In these series, several modifications are used, including application of prosthetic material [105-109].

In a prospective randomized trial comparing CST with bridging the defect with prosthetic material, CST was found to be superior to the insertion of prosthetic material, although a similar reherniation rate was found after a follow-up of 24 months [110].

When other means of reconstruction have already been used or are insufficient also a microvascular tensor fasciae latae (TFL) flap is a feasible option for reconstruction of exceptionally large abdominal wall defects. It can also be combined with other methods of reconstruction.

Vascularized flaps provide healthy autologous tissue coverage without implantation of foreign material at the closure site. A close collaboration between plastic and abdominal surgeons is important for this reconstruction [111].

Antimicrobial prophylaxis

For patients with intestinal incarceration with no evidence of ischaemia and no bowel resection, short term prophylaxis is recommended.

For patients with intestinal strangulation and/or concurrent bowel resection, 48-hour antimicrobial prophylaxis is recommended. Antimicrobial therapy is recommended for patients with peritonitis (grade 2C recommendation).

In aseptic hernia repair, *Staphylococcus aureus* from the exogenous environment or the patient's skin flora is typically the source of infection. In patients with intestinal strangulation, the surgical field may be contaminated by bacterial translocation [7,8] from intestinal villi of incarcerated ischemic bowel loops as well as by concomitant bowel resections. In patients with peritonitis both antimicrobial therapy and surgery is always recommended.

Competing interests

The authors declare that they have no competing interests.

Authors' contributions
MS wrote the manuscript. All authors reviewed and approved the final manuscript.

Author details
[1]Department of Surgery, Macerata Hospital, Macerata, Italy. [2]General Surgery Department, Papa Giovanni XXIII hospital, Bergamo, Italy. [3]Department of Surgery, Red Cross Hospital Beverwijk, Erasmus University Medical Center, Rotterdam, Netherlands. [4]Department of Surgical Science, Istituto clinic Sant'Ambrogio, Milan, Italy. [5]Department of Surgery, Buccheri La Ferla Hospital, Palermo, Italy. [6]Department of Surgery, Denver Health Medical Center, Denver, CO, USA. [7]Department of Surgery, University of Pittsburgh School of Medicine, Pittsburgh, USA. [8]Harvard Medical School, Division of Trauma, Emergency Surgery and Surgical Critical Care Massachusetts General Hospital, Boston, MA, USA. [9]Department of Surgery, University of Florida, Gainesville, Florida, USA. [10]Department of Abdominal Surgery, University Hospital Meilahti, Helsinki, Finland. [11]Department of Primary Care & Emergency Medicine, Kyoto University Graduate School of Medicine, Kyoto, Japan. [12]Department of General Surgery, Rambam Health Care Campus, Haifa, Israel. [13]Division of Trauma Surgery, Hospital de Clinicas -, School of Medical Sciences, University of Campinas, Campinas, Brazil. [14]Department of Surgery, Fundacion Valle del Lili, Universidad del Valle, Cali, Colombia. [15]Department of Surgery, Maggiore Hospital, Bologna, Italy. [16]Department of Surgery, Adria Civil Hospital, Adria, RO, Italy. [17]First Clinic of General Surgery, University Hospital /UMBAL/ St George Plovdiv, Plovdiv, Bulgaria. [18]Department of Surgery 1, Lviv Regional Hospital, Danylo Halytsky Lviv National Medical University, Lviv, Ukraine. [19]Department of Surgery, Sheri-Kashmir Institute of Medical Sciences, Srinagar, India. [20]Griffith Base Hospital, Griffith, NSW, Australia. [21]Faculdade de Ciências Médicas e da Saúde de Juiz de Fora (SUPREMA), Federal University of Juiz de Fora (UFJF), Juiz de Fora, MG, Brazil. [22]Department of General Surgery, Trauma and Emergency Surgery Division, ABC Medical School, Santo André, SP, Brazil. [23]Department of General Surgery, Istanbul Doctor's Center, Istanbul, Turkey. [24]Department of Surgery, Tbilisi State Medical University, Tbilisi, Georgia. [25]Department of Surgery, Yonsei University College of Medicine, Seoul, Korea. [26]Laparoscopic Surgical Unit, M. Mellini Hospital, Chiari, BS, Italy. [27]Department of Surgery, Mazzoni Hospital, Ascoli Piceno, Italy. [28]Department of Surgery, Tianjin Nankai Hospital, Nankai Clinical School of Medicine, Tianjin Medical University, Tianjin, China. [29]Department of Surgery, Ripas Hospital, Bandar Seri Begawan, Brunei. [30]Department of Surgery Mansoura, Faculty of Medicine, Mansoura University, Mansoura, Egypt. [31]Department of Surgery, Pt BDS Post-graduate Institute of Medical Sciences, Rohtak, India. [32]Department of Laparoscopic Surgery, GEM Hospital & Research Center, Coimbatore, India. [33]Department of Surgery, College of Health Sciences, Obafemi Awolowo University Hospital, Ile-Ife, Nigeria. [34]II Cátedra de Clínica Quirúrgica, Hospital de Clínicas, Facultad de Ciencias Médicas, Universidad Nacional de Asuncion, San Lorenzo, Paraguay. [35]3rd Department of General Surgery, Jagiellonian University Collegium Medium, Krakow, Poland. [36]Department of Surgery, G. Giglio Hospital Cefalù, Palermo, Italy. [37]Emergency Surgery, Maggiore Parma Hospital, Parma, Italy.

References

1. Helgstrand F, Rosenberg J, Kehlet H, Bisgaard T: **Outcomes after emergency versus elective ventral hernia repair: a prospective nationwide study.** *World J Surg* 2013, **37**(10):2273–2279.
2. Miserez M, Alexandre JH, Campanelli G, Corcione F, Cuccurullo D, Pascual MH, Hoeferlin A, Kingsnorth AN, Mandala V, Palot JP, Schumpelick V, Simmermacher RK, Stoppa R, Flament JB: **The European hernia society groin hernia classification: simple and easy to remember.** *Hernia* 2007, **11**(2):113–116.
3. Horan TC, Gaynes RP, Martone WJ, Jarvis WR, Emori TG: **CDC definitions of nosocomial surgical site infections, 1992: a modification of CDC definitions of surgical wound infections.** *Am J Infect Control* 1992, **20**:271–274.
4. Falagas ME, Kasiakou SK: **Mesh-related infections after hernia repair surgery.** *Clin Microbiol Infect* 2005, **11**(1):3–8.
5. Cruse PJE, Foord R: **The epidemiology of wound infection. A ten-year prospective study of 62,939 wounds.** *Surg Clin North Am* 1980, **60**:27–40.
6. Olson M, O'Connor MO, Schwartz ML: **A 5-year prospective study of 20,193 wounds at the Minneapolis VA Medical Center.** *Ann Surg* 1984, **199**:253–259.
7. Samel S, Keesse M, Kleczka M, Lanig S, Gretz N, Hafner M, Sturm J, Post S: **Microscopy of bacterial translocation during small bowel obstruction and ischemia in vivo: a new animal model.** *BMC Surg* 2002, **2**(1):6.
8. Akcay MN, Capan MY, Gundogdu C, Polat M, Oren D: **Bacterial translocation in experimental intestinal obstruction.** *J Int Med Res* 1996, **24**(1):17–26.
9. Montgomery A: **The battle between biological and synthetic meshes in ventral hernia repair.** *Hernia* 2013, **17**(1):3–11.
10. Guyatt G, Gutterman D, Baumann MH, Addrizzo-Harris D, Hylek EM, Phillips B, Raskob G, Lewis SZ, Schunemann H: **Grading strength of recommendations and quality of evidence in clinical guidelines: report from an American college of chest physicians task force.** *Chest* 2006, **129**:174–181.
11. Brozek JL, Akl EA, Jaeschke R, Lang DM, Bossuyt P, Glasziou P, Helfand M, Ueffing E, Alonso-Coello P, Meerpohl J, Phillips B, Horvath AR, Bousquet J, Guyatt GH, Schunemann HJ: **Grading quality of evidence and strength of recommendations in clinical practice guidelines: part 2 of 3. The GRADE approach to grading quality of evidence about diagnostic tests and strategies.** *Allergy* 2009, **64**:1109–1116.
12. Martínez-Serrano MA, Pereira JA, Sancho J, Argudo N, López-Cano M, Grande L: **Specific improvement measures to reduce complications and mortality after urgent surgery in complicated abdominal wall hernia.** *Hernia* 2012, **16**(2):171–177.
13. Derici H, Unalp HR, Bozdag AD, Nazli O, Tansug T, Kamer E: **Factors affecting morbidity and mortality in incarcerated abdominal wall hernias.** *Hernia* 2007, **11**(4):341–346.
14. Ge BJ, Huang Q, Liu LM, Bian HP, Fan YZ: **Risk factors for bowel resection and outcome in patients with incarcerated groin hernias.** *Hernia* 2010 Jun, **14**(3):259–264.
15. Sarr MG, Bulkley GB, Zuidoma GD: **Preoperative recognition of intestinal strangulation obstruction. Prospective evaluation of diagnostic capability.** *Am J Surg* 1983, **145**:176–182.
16. Shatlla AH, Chamberlain BE, Webb WR: **Current status of diagnosis and management of strangulation obstruction of the small bowel.** *Am J Sur* 1978, **132**:299–303.
17. Bizer LS, Liebling RW, Delany HM, Gliedman ML: **Small bowel obstruction. The role of nonoperative treatment in simple intestinal obstruction and predictive criteria for strangulation obstruction.** *Surgery* 1981, **89**:407–413.
18. Tsumura H, Ichikawa T, Hiyama E, Murakami Y, Sueda T: **Systemic inflammatory response syndrome (SIRS) as a predictor of strangulated small bowel obstruction.** *Hepatogastroenterology* 2004, **51**(59):1393–1396.
19. Graeber GM, O'Neil JF, Wolf RE, Wukich DK, Caffery PJ, Harman JW: **Elevated levels of peritoneal serum creatine phosphokinase with strangulated small bowel obstruction.** *Arch Surg* 1983, **118**:837–840.
20. Davies MG, Hagen PO: **Systemic inflammatory response syndrome.** *Br J Surg* 1997, **84**:920–935.
21. Icoz G, Makay O, Sozbilen M, Gurcu B, Caliskan C, Firat O, Kurt Z, Ersin S: **Is D-dimer a predictor of strangulated intestinal hernia?** *World J Surg* 2006 Dec, **30**(12):2165–2169.
22. Tanaka K, Hanyu N, Iida T, Watanabe A, Kawano S, Usuba T, Iino T, Mizuno R: **Lactate levels in the detection of preoperative bowel strangulation.** *Am Surg* 2012 Jan, **78**(1):86–88.
23. Balthazar EJ: **CT of small-bowel obstruction.** *AJR* 1994, **162**:255–261.
24. Jancelewicz T, Vu LT, Shawo AE, Yeh B, Gasper WJ, Harris HW: **Predicting strangulated small bowel obstruction: an old problem revisited.** *J Gastrointest Surg* 2009, **13**(1):93–99.
25. Pring CM, Tran V, O'Rourke N, Martin IJ: **Laparoscopic versus open ventral hernia repair: a randomized controlled trial.** *ANZ J Surg* 2008, **78**(10):903–906.
26. Ballem N, Parikh R, Berber E, Siperstein A: **Laparoscopic versus open ventral hernia repairs: 5 year recurrence rates.** *Surg Endosc* 2008, **22**(9):1935–1940.
27. Olmi S, Scaini A, Cesana GC, Erba L, Croce E: **Laparoscopic versus open incisional hernia repair: an open randomized controlled study.** *Surg Endosc* 2007, **21**(4):555–559.
28. Lomanto D, Iyer SG, Shabbir A, Cheah WK: **Laparoscopic versus open ventral hernia mesh repair: a prospective study.** *Surg Endosc* 2006, **20**(7):1030–1035.
29. Cuccurullo D, Piccoli M, Agresta F, Magnone S, Corcione F, Stancanelli V, Melotti G: **Laparoscopic ventral incisional hernia repair: evidence-based**

guidelines of the first Italian consensus conference. *Hernia* 2013: [Epub ahead of print].
30. Bittner R, Arregui ME, Bisgaard T, Dudai M, Ferzli GS, Fitzgibbons RJ, Fortelny RH, Klinge U, Kockerling F, Kuhry E, Kukleta J, Lomanto D, Misra MC, Montgomery A, Morales-Conde S, Reinpold W, Rosenberg J, Sauerland S, Schug-Pass C, Singh K, Timoney M, Weyhe D, Chowbey P: **Guidelines for laparoscopic (TAPP) and endoscopic (TEP) treatment of inguinal hernia [International Endohernia Society (IEHS)].** *Surg Endosc* 2011, **25**(9):2773–2843.
31. Cavazzola LT, Rosen MJ: **Laparoscopic versus open inguinal hernia repair.** *Surg Clin North Am* 2013, **93**(5):1269–1279.
32. Landau O, Kyzer S: **Emergent laparoscopic repair of incarcerated incisional and ventral hernia.** *Surg Endosc* 2004, **18**(9):1374–1376. Epub 2004 May 28.
33. Shah RH, Sharma A, Khullar R, Soni V, Baijal M, Chowbey PK: **Laparoscopic repair of incarcerated ventral abdominal wall hernias.** *Hernia* 2008, **12**(5):457–463.
34. Olmi S, Cesana G, Erba L, Croce E: **Emergency laparoscopic treatment of acute incarcerated incisional hernia.** *Hernia* 2009, **13**(6):605–608.
35. Deeba S, Purkayastha S, Paraskevas P, Athanasiou T, Darzi A, Zacharakis E: **Laparoscopic approach to incarcerated and strangulated inguinal hernias.** *JSLS* 2009, **13**(3):327–331.
36. Palanivelu C, Rangarajan M, John SJ: **Modified technique of laparoscopic intraperitoneal hernioplasty for irreducible scrotal hernias (omentoceles): how to remove the hernial contents.** *World J Surg* 2007, **31**(9):1889–1891. discussion 1892-3.
37. Agresta F, Ansaloni L, Baiocchi GL, Bergamini C, Campanile FC, Carlucci M, Cocorullo G, Corradi A, Franzato B, Lupo M, Mandalà V, Mirabella A, Pernazza G, Piccoli M, Staudacher C, Vettoretto N, Zago M, Lettieri E, Levati A, Pietrini D, Scaglione M, De Masi S, De Placido G, Francucci M, Rasi M, Fingerhut A, Uranüs S, Garattini S: **Laparoscopic approach to acute abdomen from the consensus development conference of the Società Italiana di Chirurgia Endoscopica e nuove tecnologie (SICE), Associazione Chirurghi Ospedalieri Italiani (ACOI), Società Italiana di Chirurgia (SIC), Società Italiana di Chirurgia d'Urgenza e del Trauma (SICUT), Società Italiana di Chirurgia nell'Ospedalità Privata (SICOP), and the European Association for Endoscopic Surgery (EAES).** *Surg Endosc* 2012, **26**:2134–2164.
38. Sgourakis G, Radtke A, Sotiropoulos GC, Dedemadi G, Karaliotas C, Fouzas I, Karaliotas C: **Assessment of strangulated content of the spontaneously reduced inguinal hernia via hernia sac laparoscopy: preliminary results of a prospective randomized study.** *Surg Laparosc Endosc Percutan Tech* 2009, **19**(2):133–137.
39. Burger JW, Luijendijk RW, Hop WC, Halm JA, Verdaasdonk EG, Jeekel J: **Long-term follow-up of a randomized controlled trial of suture versus mesh repair of incisional hernia.** *Ann Surg* 2004, **240**(4):578–583.
40. Luijendijk RW, Hop WC, van den Tol MP: **A comparison of suture repair with mesh repair for incisional hernia.** *N Engl J Med* 2000, **343:**392.
41. Korenkov M, Sauerland S, Arndt M, Bograd L, Neugebauer EA: **Troidl H Randomized clinical trial of suture repair, polypropylene mesh or autodermal hernioplasty for incisional hernia.** *Br J Surg* 2002, **89**(1):50–56.
42. Sanjay P, Reid TD, Davies EL: **Retrospective comparison of mesh and sutured repair for adult umbilical hernias.** *Hernia* 2005, **9:**248.
43. Abdel-Baki NA, Bessa SS, Abdel-Razek AH: **Comparison of prosthetic mesh repair and tissue repair in the emergency management of incarcerated para-umbilical hernia: a prospective randomized study.** *Hernia* 2007, **11**(2):163–167.
44. Lohsiriwat V, Sridermma W, Akaraviputh T, Boonnuch W, Chinsawangwatthanakol V, Methasate A, Lert-akyamanee N, Lohsiriwat D: **Surgical outcomes of Lichtenstein tension-free hernioplasty for acutely incarcerated inguinal hernia.** *Surg Today* 2007, **37**(3):212–214.
45. Wysocki A, Kulawik J, Poźniczek M, Strzałka M: **Is the Lichtenstein operation of strangulated groin hernia a safe procedure?** *World J Surg* 2006, **30**(11):2065–2070.
46. Wysocki A, Poźniczek M, Krzywoń J, Bolt L: **Use of polypropylene prostheses for strangulated inguinal and incisional hernias.** *Hernia* 2001, **5**(2):105–106. doi:10.1007/s100290100013.
47. Nieuwenhuizen J, van Ramshorst GH, ten Brinke JG, de Wit T, van der Harst E, Hop WC, Jeekel J, Lange JF: **The use of mesh in acute hernia: frequency and outcome in 99 cases.** *Hernia* 2011 Jun, **15**(3):297–300.
48. Dunne JR, Malone DL, Tracy JK, Napolitano LM: **Abdominal wall hernias: risk factors for infection and resource utilization.** *J Surg Res* 2003, **111**(1):78–84.
49. Finan KR, Vick CC, Kiefe CI, Neumayer L, Hawn MT: **Predictors of wound infection in ventral hernia repair.** *Am J Surg* 2005, **190**(5):676–681.
50. Petersen S, Henke G, Freitag M, Faulhaber A, Ludwig K: **Deep prosthesis infection in incisional hernia repair: predictive factors and clinical outcome.** *Eur J Surg* 2001, **167**(6):453–457.
51. Hawn MT, Gray SH, Snyder CW, Graham LA, Finan KR, Vick CC: **Predictors of mesh explantation after incisional hernia repair.** *Am J Surg* 2011, **202**(1):28–33.
52. Choi JJ, Palaniappa NC, Dallas KB, Rudich TB, Colon MJ, Divino CM: **Use of mesh during ventral hernia repair in clean-contaminated and contaminated cases: outcomes of 33,832 cases.** *Ann Surg* 2012, **255**(1):176–180.
53. Xourafas D, Lipsitz S, Negro P: **Impact of mesh use on morbidity following ventral hernia repair with a simultaneous bowel resection.** *Arch Surg* 2010, **145**(8):739–744.
54. Machairas A, Liakakos T, Patapis P, Petropoulos C, Tsapralis D, Misiakos EP: **Prosthetic repair of incisional hernia combined with elective bowel operation.** *Surgeon* 2008, **6:**274–277.
55. Atila K, Guler S, Inal A, Sokmen S, Karademir S, Bora S: **Prosthetic repair of acutely incarcerated groin hernias: a prospective clinical observational cohort study.** *Langenbecks Arch Surg* 2010, **395**(5):563–568. doi:10.1007/s00423-008-0414-3. Epub 2008 Aug 29.
56. Mandalà V, Bilardo G, Darca F, Di Marco F, Luzza A, Lupo M, Mirabella A: **Some considerations on the use of heterologous prostheses in incisional hernias at risk of infection.** *Hernia* 2000, **4:**268–271.
57. Vix J, Meyer C, Rohr S, Bourtoul C: **The treatment of incisional and abdominal hernia with a prosthesis in potentially infected tissues–a series of 47 cases.** *Hernia* 1997, **1:**157–161.
58. Birolini C, Utiyama EM, Rodrigues AJ Jr, Birolini D: **Elective colonic operation and prosthetic repair of incisional hernia: does contamination contraindicate abdominal wall prosthesis use?** *J Am Coll Surg* 2000, **191:**366–372.
59. Geisler DJ, Reilly JC, Vaughan SG, Glennon EJ, Kondylis PD: **Safety and outcome of use of nonabsorbable mesh for repair of fascial defects in the presence of open bowel.** *Dis Colon Rectum* 2003, **46:**1118–1123.
60. Campanelli G, Nicolosi FM, Pettinari D, Avesani EC: **Prosthetic repair, intestinal resection, and potentially contaminated areas: safe and feasible?** *Hernia* 2004, **8:**190–192.
61. Carbonell AM, Criss CN, Cobb WS, Novitsky YW, Rosen MJ: **Outcomes of synthetic mesh in contaminated ventral hernia repairs.** *J Am Coll Surg* 2013:. doi:10.1016/j.jamcollsurg.2013.07.382. [Epub ahead of print].
62. Kelly ME, Behrman SW: **The safety and efficacy of prosthetic hernia repair in clean-contaminated and contaminated wounds.** *Am Surg* 2002, **68:**524–528. discussion 528-529.
63. Davies M, Davies C, Morris-Stiff G, Shute K: **Emergency presentation of abdominal hernias: outcome and reasons for delay in treatment – a prospective study.** *Ann R Coll Surg Engl* 2007, **89:**47–50.
64. Zafar H, Zaidi M, Qadir I, Memon AA: **Emergency incisional hernia repair: a difficult problem waiting for a solution.** *Ann Surg Innov Res* 2012, **6**(1):1.
65. Bessa SS, Abdel-Razek AH: **Results of prosthetic mesh repair in the emergency management of the acutely incarcerated and/or strangulated ventral hernias: a seven years study.** *Hernia* 2013, **17**(1):59–65.
66. Coccolini F, Agresta F, Bassi A, Catena F, Crovella F, Ferrara R, Gossetti F, *et al*: **Italian Biological Prosthesis Work-Group (IBPWG): proposal for a decisional model in using biological prosthesis.** *World J Emerg Surg* 2012, **7**(1):34.
67. Saettele TM, Bachman SL, Costello CR, Grant SA, Cleveland DS, Loy TS, Kolder DG, Ramshaw BJ: **Use of porcine dermal collagen as a prosthetic mesh in a contaminated field for ventral hernia repair: a case report.** *Hernia* 2007, **11:**279–285.
68. Smart N, Immanuel A, Mercer-Jones M: **Laparoscopic repair of a Littre's hernia with porcine dermal collagen implant [Permacol].** *Hernia* 2007, **11:**373–376.
69. Liyanage SH, Purohit GS, Frye JN, Giordano P: **Anterior abdominal wall reconstruction with a Permacol implant.** *J Plast Reconstr Aesthet Surg* 2006, **59:**553–555.
70. Gupta A, Zahriya K, Mullens PL, Salmassi S, Keshishian A: **Ventral herniorrhaphy: experience with two different biosynthetic mesh materials, Surgisis and Alloderm.** *Hernia* 2006, **10:**419.
71. Albo D, Awad SS, Berger DH, Bellows CF: **Decellularized human cadaveric dermis provides a safe alternative for primary inguinal hernia repair in**

contaminated surgical fields. *Am J Surg* 2006, **192:**e12–e17. doi:10.1016/j.amjsurg.2006.08.029.

72. Schuster R, Singh J, Safadi BY, Wren SM: **The use of acellular dermal matrix for contaminated abdominal wall defects: wound status predicts success.** *Am J Surg* 2006, **192:**594–597.
73. Alaedeen DI, Lipman J, Medalie D, Rosen MJ: **The single-staged approach to the surgical management of abdominal wall hernias in contaminated fields.** *Hernia* 2007, **11:**41–45.
74. Kim H, Bruen K, Vargo D: **Acellular dermal matrix in the management of high-risk abdominal wall defects.** *Am J Surg* 2006, **192:**705–709. doi:10.1016/j.amjsurg.2006.09.003.
75. Diaz JJ Jr, Guy J, Berkes MB, Guillamondegui O, Miller RS: **Acellular dermal allograft for ventral hernia repair in the compromised surgical field.** *Am Surg* 2006, **72:**1181–1188.
76. Patton JH Jr, Berry S, Kralovich KA: **Use of human acellular dermal matrix in complex and contaminated abdominal wall reconstructions.** *Am J Surg* 2007, **193:**360–363.
77. Bellows CF, Albo D, Berger DH, Awad SS: **Abdominal wall repair using human acellular dermis.** *Am J Surg* 2007, **194:**192–198.
78. Jin J, Rosen MJ, Blatnik J, McGee MF, Williams CP, Marks J, Ponsky J: **Use of acellular dermal matrix for complicated ventral hernia repair: does technique affect outcomes?** *J Am Coll Surg* 2007, **205:**654–660.
79. Franklin ME, Gonzalez JJ, Michaelson RP, Glass JL, Chock DA: **Preliminary experience with new bioactive prosthetic material repair of hernias in infected fields.** *Hernia* 2002, **6:**171–174.
80. Franklin ME, Gonzalez JJ, Glass JL: **Use of porcine small intestinal submucosa as a prosthetic device for laparoscopic repair of hernias in contaminated fields: 2-year follow-up.** *Hernia* 2004, **8:**186–189.
81. Helton WS, Fisichella PM, Berger R, Horgan S, Espat NJ, Abcarian H: **Short-term outcomes with small intestinal submucosa for ventral abdominal hernia.** *Arch Surg* 2005, **140:**549–562.
82. Catena F, Ansaloni L, Gazzotti F, Gagliardi S, Di Saverio S, D'Alessandro L, Pinna AD: **Use of porcine dermal collagen graft [Permacol] for hernia repair in contaminated fields.** *Hernia* 2007, **11:**57–60.
83. Treviño JM, Franklin ME Jr, Berghoff KR, Glass JL, Jaramillo EJ: **Preliminary results of a two-layered prosthetic repair for recurrent inguinal and ventral hernias combining open and laparoscopic techniques.** *Hernia* 2006, **10:**253–257.
84. Shaikh FM, Giri SK, Durrani S, Waldron D, Grace PA: **Experience with porcine acellular dermal collagen implant in one-stage tension-free reconstruction of acute and chronic abdominal wall defects.** *World J Surg* 2007, **31**(10):1966–1972. discussion 1973-4.
85. Coccolini F, Catena F, Bertuzzo VR, Ercolani G, Pinna A, Ansaloni L: **Abdominal wall defect repair with biological prosthesis in transplanted patients: single center retrospective analysis and review of the literature.** *Updates Surg* 2013. in press.
86. Cavallaro A, Lo Menzo E, Di Vita M, Zanghì A, Cavallaro V, Veroux PF, Cappellani A: **Use of biological meshes for abdominal wall reconstruction in highly contaminated fields.** *World J Gastroenterol* 2010, **16**(15):1928–1933.
87. Coccolini F, Poiasina E, Bertoli P, Gossetti F, Agresta F, Dassatti MR, Riccio P, Cavalli M, Agrusti S, Cucchi M, Negro P, Campanelli G, Ansaloni L, Catena F: **The italian register of biological prosthesis (IRBP).** *Eur Surg Res* 2013, **50:**262–272.
88. Smart NJ, Marshall M, Daniels IR: **Biological meshes: a review of their use in abdominal wall hernia repairs.** *Surgeon* 2012, **10**(3):159–171.
89. Rosen MJ, Krpata DM, Ermlich B, Blatnik JA: **A 5-year clinical experience with single-staged repairs of infected and contaminated abdominal wall defects utilizing biologic mesh.** *Ann Surg* 2013, **257**(6):991–996.
90. Primus FE, Harris HW: **A critical review of biologic mesh use in ventral hernia repairs under contaminated conditions.** *Hernia* 2013, **17**(1):21–30.
91. Harth KC, Krpata DM, Chawla A, Blatnik JA, Halaweish I, Rosen MJ: **Biologic mesh use practice patterns in abdominal wall reconstruction: a lack of consensus among surgeons.** *Hernia* 2013, **17**(1):13–20.
92. Dayton MT, Buchele BA, Shirazi SS, Hunt LB: **Use of an absorbable mesh to repair contaminated abdominal-wall defects.** *Arch Surg* 1986, **121:**954–960.
93. Jernigan TW, Fabian TC, Croce MA, Moore N, Pritchard FE, Minard G, Bee TK: **Staged management of giant abdominal wall defects: acute and long-term results.** *Ann Surg* 2003, **238**(3):349–355. discussion 355-7.
94. Beltrán MA, Villar RA, Cruces KS: **Abdominal compartment syndrome in patients with strangulated hernia.** *Hernia* 2008, **12**(6):613–620.
95. Tsuei BJ, Skinner JC, Bernard AC, *et al*: **The open peritoneal cavity: etiology correlates with the likelihood of fascial closure.** *Am Surg* 2004, **70:**652–656.
96. Reimer MW, Yelle JD, Reitsma B, *et al*: **Management of open abdominal wounds with a dynamic fascial closure system.** *Can J Surg* 2008, **51:**209–214.
97. Urbaniak RM, Khuthaila DK, Khalil AJ, *et al*: **Closure of massive abdominal wall defects: a case report using the abdominal reapproximation anchor (ABRA) system.** *Ann Plast Surg* 2006, **57:**573–577.
98. Rasilainen SK, Mentula PJ, Leppäniemi AK: **Vacuum and mesh-mediated fascial traction for primary closure of the open abdomen in critically ill surgical patients.** *Br J Surg* 2012, **99**(12):1725–1732.
99. Leppäniemi A, Tukiainen E: **Planned hernia repair and late abdominal wall reconstruction.** *World J Surg* 2012, **36**(3):511–515.
100. Kissane NA, Itani KM: **A decade of ventral incisional hernia repairs with biologic acellular dermal matrix: what have we learned?** *Plast Reconstr Surg* 2012, **130**(5 Suppl 2):194S–202S.
101. Boele Van Hensbroek P, Wind J, Dijkgraaf MG, *et al*: **Temporary closure of the open abdomen: a systematic review on delayed primary fascial closure in patients with an open abdomen.** *World J Surg* 2009, **33:**199–207.
102. Ramirez OM, Ruas E, Lee Dellon A: **"Components separation" method for closure of abdominal wall defects: an anatomic and clinical study.** *Plast Reconstr Surg* 1990, **86:**519–526.
103. De Vries Reilingh TS, van Goor H, Rosman C, Bemelmans MH, de Jong D, van Nieuwenhoven EJ, *et al*: **"Components separation technique" for the repair of large abdominal wall hernias.** *J Am Coll Surg* 2003, **196:**32–37.
104. DiBello JN, Moore JH: **Sliding myofascial flap of the rectus abdominis muscle for the closure of recurrent ventral hernias.** *Plast Reconstr Surg* 1996, **98:**464–469.
105. Girotto JA, Ko MJ, Redett R, *et al*: **Closure of chronic abdominal wall defects: a long-term evaluation of the component separation method.** *Ann Plast Surg* 1999, **42:**385–395.
106. Shestak KC, Edington HJD, Johnson RR: **The separation of anatomic components technique for the reconstruction of massive midline abdominal wall defects: anatomy, surgical technique, application and limitations revisited.** *Plast Reconstr Surg* 2000, **105:**731–738.
107. Lowe JB, Garza JR, Bowman JL, *et al*: **Endoscopically assisted separation for closure of abdominal wall defects.** *Plast Reconstr Surg* 2000, **105:**720–729.
108. Cohen M, Morales R, Fildes J, *et al*: **Staged reconstruction after gunshot wounds to the abdomen.** *Plast Reconstr Surg* 2001, **108:**83–92.
109. de Vries Reilingh TS, van Goor H, Charbon JA, Rosman C, Hesselink EJ, van der Wilt GJ, Bleichrodt RP: **Repair of giant midline abdominal wall hernias: "components separation technique" versus prosthetic repair: interim analysis of a randomized controlled trial.** *World J Surg* 2007, **31**(4):756–763.
110. Tukiainen E, Leppäniemi A: **Reconstruction of extensive abdominal wall defects with microvascular tensor fasciae latae flap.** *Br J Surg* 2011, **98**(6):880–884.

14

Off-pump suture repair of left ventricular rupture utilizing TachoComb® sheet

Hiroki Yamaguchi*, Tatsuya Nakao, Noriyuki Tokunaga, Hiromasa Nakamura and Masami Takagaki

Abstract

A 70-year-old woman was admitted to our institution with acute myocardial infarction. Coronary angiography demonstrated total occlusion of the left anterior descending artery, which was successfully revascularized. Four days later, the patient suddenly went into shock. The subsequent emergency operation revealed a blowout rupture of the left ventricular free wall. Several TachoComb® (CSL Behring, Tokyo, Japan) sheets were applied to control bleeding and avoid the need for a cardiopulmonary bypass. Horizontal mattress sutures were used in combination with a pair of Teflon felt strips for reinforcement. The combination of TachoComb® sheets and sutures is a novel hybrid method and an effective life-saving procedure for the treatment of left ventricular blowout ruptures. This approach avoids the need for a cardiopulmonary bypass. Sutureless repairs with TachoComb® sheet achieve rapid hemostasis without the need for cardiopulmonary bypass. This stabilizes patient hemodynamics immediately and preserves the fragile myocardium. This allows emergency room physicians to open the chest and apply the TachoComb® sheet to stabilize the patient before the cardiac surgeons arrive at the operating room. This technique will be very useful in emergency situations.

Keywords: Myocardial infarction, Left ventricular rupture, Off-pump surgery, Emergency room

Background

Left ventricular (LV) free wall rupture is a serious complication of acute myocardial infarction that may result in acute cardiac tamponade and sudden death. Among the various surgical procedures available for its treatment, sutureless repair using layered sheets of collagen fleece with fibrinogen-based impregnation (TachoComb®, CSL Behring, Tokyo, Japan) has proved the most effective [1-3]. Unlike prepare-to-use fibrin sealants, which require the coating of fibrin glue onto fleece or patching immediately before or during surgery, TachoComb® is a ready-to-use fixed combination that is activated by moisture upon application, providing adherence to the resection surface. Hemostasis is generally achieved after 3–5 min of compression [4]. However, this technique alone is associated with a potential risk for future complications such as pseudoaneurysm formation and rerupture [5,6]. We therefore developed a novel hybrid method for the treatment of blowout ruptures of the LV free wall that combines TachoComb® sheets with suture repair, avoiding cardiopulmonary bypass (CPB). Because this procedure can be performed without CPB, it is easily applicable even in an emergency room.

Case presentation

A 70-year-old woman was admitted to our hospital with a 3-day-old acute myocardial infarction. Although the patient reported adherence to the prescribed medication regimen, she developed heart failure with hypotension and oliguria the next day. Coronary angiography performed under intra-aortic balloon pumping demonstrated total occlusion of the proximal left anterior descending artery (LAD). Subsequent percutaneous coronary intervention achieved successful revascularization of LAD. The patient recovered steadily and gradually. However, four days later, her condition deteriorated suddenly and she went into shock. Her echocardiography results revealed cardiac tamponade with substantial pericardial effusion. Pericardiocentesis was

* Correspondence: r-shibata@sth-medical.co.jp
Department of Cardiovascular Surgery, New Tokyo Hospital, 1271 Wanagaya, Matsudo, Chiba 270-2232, Japan

performed, resulting in massive continuous drainage, and she was referred to us for emergency surgery.

The patient was markedly cyanotic and in cardiogenic shock with systolic blood pressure of 70 mm Hg. A large dose of dopamine had been administered. She was intubated immediately, and the results of blood gas analysis showed marked metabolic acidosis with a pH of 7.251 and a base excess of −13.2 mmol/l. Emergency surgery was undertaken via a median sternotomy. Upon opening the pericardium, a blowout rupture of the LV free wall was found. A large volume of fresh blood was expelled rapidly from the tear at the LV base, between LAD and its diagonal branch. We were unable to measure the size of the tear, because we had to cover the area quickly with TachoComb® sheets to achieve hemostasis. The LV apex was dyskinetic. A total of three TachoComb® sheets (5 × 5 cm each) were applied to the bleeding point and the surrounding area of fragile necrotic tissue. The major source of bleeding was controlled, but a small amount of blood continued to flow out the lower part of the sheet (Figure 1). Four 3–0 polypropylene (SH) horizontal mattress sutures were then used to secure a pair of Teflon felt strips over the TachoComb® sheets. The sutures were placed approximately 1 cm from the perforated myocardial region. Extreme care was taken to avoid LAD and its diagonal branch. After complete hemostasis was achieved, an additional TachoComb® sheet and fibrin glue were applied (Figure 2). The entire LV repair was performed without CPB. The patient was transferred to the intensive care unit with dramatically improved hemodynamics. The postoperative course was uneventful, and she walked out of the hospital on day 35. The patient was followed up until 3 months, when she died because of cerebral bleeding.

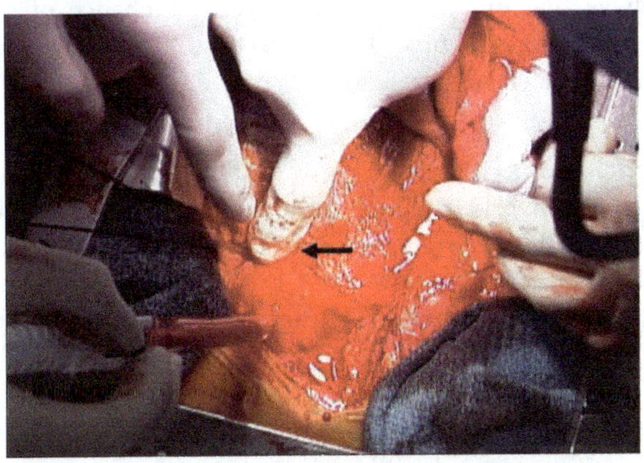

Figure 1 Operative view of the ruptured left ventricle. The major source of bleeding was a blowout rupture between the left anterior descending artery and its diagonal branch, which was controlled by manual compression (black arrow).

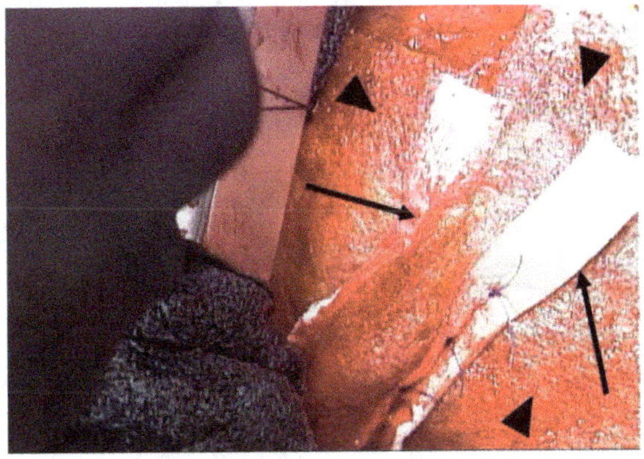

Figure 2 Intraoperative view after repair. TachoComb® sheets applied to the ventricle (black arrowheads) followed by Teflon felt strip sutures (black arrows).

Discussion and literature review

LV free wall rupture is the third-most serious complication and the second-most common cause of death after myocardial infarction [1,7]. The patient reported herein was in an extremely serious condition on referral, and the emergency surgery performed at our institution was necessary to save her life. The new hybrid method described here was designed to control the bleeding as quickly as possible without increasing the risks for future complications such as pseudoaneurysms and reruptures [5,6].

Various procedures and strategies have been developed to treat LV free wall ruptures (Table 1). The choice among them is made on the basis of three main considerations: (1) type of rupture, (2) with or without CPB, and (3) suture closure or sutureless repair. Blowout ruptures are often treated by infarctectomy combined with suture closure and/or patch repair, usually with CPB [7-10]. Oozing/sealed ruptures are often treated by sutureless repair without CPB [1-3,10]. Recent myocardial infarction decreases the heart's tolerance to subsequent global ischemia even when protected by hypothermic cardioplegia. Therefore, it is preferable to repair a ruptured LV free wall without CPB. Although the suture closure technique is a classic standard procedure, it is difficult to suture fragile myocardium because of the risk of mechanical tearing [1,2,11]. Many surgeons have recently reported that sutureless repair using TachoComb® sheets can efficiently achieve hemostasis [3,5,6,11]. However, this strategy is not usually suitable for blowout ruptures, where the myocardial tear is often large and bleeding is copious [1-3]. Although Nishizaki et al. [11] reported successful sutureless repairs with use of the TachoComb® sheet for a blowout rupture from a 1-cm tear, the risks of such an approach are possible future complications such as pseudoaneurysm and rerupture [5,6].

The advantages of sutureless repairs with TachoComb® sheets include rapid hemostasis without the need for

Table 1 Reference review for surgical repair of the left ventricular free wall rupture

Reference	Year	Article type	No. of pts.	Rupture type	Surgical procedures	CPB
Stiegel et al. [9]	1987	Case report	1	Blow-out	Suture closure and patch repair	Yes
Sutherland et al. [8]	1996	Case report/Review	1	Blow-out	Suture closure	Yes
Reardon et al. [7]	1997	Case report	1	Blow-out	Infarctectomy and patch repair	Yes
Iemura et al. [1]	2001	Original article	17	Oozing (n=14), Blow-out (n=3)	Infarctectomy and patch repair (n=1), Direct closure (n=4), Patch repair (n=4), Sutureless patch repair (n=7), Endventricular patch closure (VSP) (n=1)	Yes (n=12) No (n=5)
Lachapelle et al. [2]	2002	Original article	6	Oozing (n=3), Blow-out (n=3)	Sutureless patch repair (n=6)	Yes (n=4) No (n=2)
Fukushima et al. [5]	2003	Case report	1	Oozing	Sutureless repair with TachoComb	No
Nishizaki et al. [11]	2004	Case report	1	Blow-out	Sutureless repair with TachoComb	No
Muto et al. [3]	2005	Case report	1	Oozing	Sutureless repair with TachoComb	No
Kimura et al. [6]	2005	Case report	1	Blow-out	Sutureless repair with TachoComb	No
Sakaguchi et al. [10]	2008	Original article	32	Unknown (n=28), Blow-out(n=4)	Sutureless repair with autologous pericardial patch and gelatinresorcin formaldehyde glue +− additional sutures	Yes (n=6) No (n=26)
Pocar et al. [13]	2012	Original article	3	Unknown	Sutureless repair with TachoSil combined with pericardial patch and fibrin glue	Yes
Raffa et al. [14]	2013	Original article	6	Oozing (n=4), Blow-out (n=2)	Sutureless repair with TachoSil	Yes (n=3) No (n=3)

No. of pts. Number of patients, *CPB* Cardiopulmonary bypass, *VSP* Ventricular septal perforation.

CPB, which allows for the immediate stabilization of patient hemodynamics and preservation of the fragile myocardium [2,3,5,6]. Furthermore, even physicians in an emergency room can open the chest and apply a TachoComb® sheet to stabilize the patient before the cardiac surgeons arrive at the operating room. We therefore developed a new hybrid method that combines use of the TachoComb® sheet with suture closure to utilize the advantages of both procedures. Because of the risk of mechanical tearing, we do not recommend the use of this technique for tears >1 cm. However, the procedure can be performed safely without CPB, which represents a substantial advantage in emergency situations.

Although TachoComb® has frequently been used for the treatment of both venous and arterial bleeding, anaphylactic reactions have been reported after the repeated use of hemostatic agents such as TachoComb® that contain aprotinin. Because aprotinin is also associated with risks of renal failure, a new product, TachoSil® (Nycomed, Zurich, Switzerland), which lacks aprotinin and contains human rather than bovine thrombin, has been developed. TachoSil® is known to be equally hemostatic to TachoComb® [12]. Several cases of LV rupture have been treated successfully utilizing TachoSil® (Table 1) [13,14].

Our report has some limitations. First, the report here describes a single case. Further investigation including postoperative follow-up in a large number of patients will be necessary to support our hypothesis. Second, our technique does not address LV aneurysms, which could lead to heart failure and/or thromboembolisms. TachoComb® sheets covering the LV surface could complicate a concomitant or subsequent coronary artery bypass graft. Indeed, Iemura et al. [1] maintain that if subsequent coronary artery bypass grafting is needed, identification and exposure of the coronary artery will be difficult because of the widely and deeply piled collagen hemostats. However, the main goal of surgery for LV rupture is to save the patient's life by relieving the cardiac tamponade and to close the rupture [2,3]. We believe that our method maximizes the chance of patient survival and provides a novel option for emergency room physicians.

Conclusions

A novel hybrid method that combines TachoComb® sheets with reinforcing sutures was effective in quickly achieving hemostasis without the need for CPB. This represents a substantial advantage in the context of emergency medicine.

Competing interests

We declare that we have no competing interests.

Authors' contributions

HY performed the surgery, supervised the patient's care, drafted the manuscript, and approved the version submitted for publication. TN, NT, and

HN assisted with patient care and have been involved in drafting the manuscript. MT has been involved in drafting and revising the manuscript. All authors read and approved the final manuscript.

Acknowledgements
The authors would like to thank Enago (www.enago.com) for the English language review.

References

1. Iemura J, Oku H, Otaki M, Kitayama H, Inoue T, Kaneda T: **Surgical strategy for left ventricular free wall rupture after acute myocardial infarction.** *Ann Thorac Surg* 2001, **71:**201–204.
2. Lachapelle K, de Varennes B, Ergina PL, Cecere R: **Sutureless patch technique for postinfarction left ventricular rupture.** *Ann Thorac Surg* 2002, **74:**96–101.
3. Muto A, Nishibe T, Kondo Y, Sato M, Yamashita M, Ando M: **Sutureless repair with TachoComb sheets for oozing type postinfarction cardiac rupture.** *Ann Thorac Surg* 2005, **79:**2143–2145.
4. Maisano F, Kjaergard HK, Bauernschmitt R, Pavie A, Rabago G, Laskar M, Marstein JP, Falk V: **TachoSil surgical patch versus conventional haemostatic fleece material for control of bleeding in cardiovascular surgery: a randomised controlled trial.** *Eur J Cardiothorac Surg* 2009, **36:**708–714.
5. Fukushima S, Kobayashi J, Tagusari O, Sasako Y: **A huge pseudoaneurysm of the left ventricle after simple gluing of an oozing-type postinfarction rupture.** *Interact Cardiovasc Thorac Surg* 2003, **2:**94–96.
6. Kimura N, Kawahito K, Murata S, Yamaguchi A, Adachi H, Ino T: **Pitfalls of sutureless repair of a blow-out type left ventricular free wall rupture.** *Jpn J Thorac Cardiovasc Surg* 2005, **53:**382–385.
7. Reardon MJ, Carr CL, Diamond A, Letsou GV, Safi HJ, Espada R, Baldwin JC: **Ischemic left ventricular free wall rupture: prediction, diagnosis, and treatment.** *Ann Thorac Surg* 1997, **64:**1509–1613.
8. Sutherland FW, Guell FJ, Pathi VL, Naik SK: **Postinfarction ventricular free wall rupture: strategies for diagnosis and treatment.** *Ann Thorac Surg* 1996, **61:**1281–1285.
9. Stiegel M, Zimmern SH, Robicsek F: **Left ventricular rupture following coronary occlusion treated by streptokinase infusion: successful surgical repair.** *Ann Thorac Surg* 1987, **44:**413–415.
10. Sakaguchi G, Komiya T, Tamura N, Kobayashi T: **Surgical treatment for postinfarction left ventricular free wall rupture.** *Ann Thorac Surg* 2008, **85:**1344–1347.
11. Nishizaki K, Seki T, Fujii A, Nishida Y, Funabiki M, Morikawa Y: **Sutureless patch repair for small blowout rupture of the left ventricle after myocardial infarction.** *Jpn J Thorac Cardiovasc Surg* 2004, **52:**268–271.
12. Agger P, Langhoff J, Smerup MH, Hasenkam JM: **Comparison between TachoComb® and TachoSil® for surgical hemostasis in arterial bleeding: an animal experimental study.** *J Trauma* 2010, **68**(4):838–842.
13. Pocar M, Passolunghi D, Bregasi A, Donatelli F: **TachoSil® for postinfarction ventricular free wall rupture.** *Interact Cardiovasc Thorac Surg* 2012, **14:**866–867.
14. Raffa GM, Tarelli G, Patrini D, Settepani F: **Sutureless repair for postinfarction cardiac rupture: a simple approach with a tissue-adhering patch.** *J Thorac Cardiovasc Surg* 2013, **145**(2):598–599.

Hepato-pancreato-biliary emergencies for the acute care surgeon: etiology, diagnosis and treatment

Jean M Butte[1], Morad Hameed[2] and Chad G Ball[1*]

Abstract

Hepatopancreatobiliary (HPB) emergencies include an ample range of conditions with overlapping clinical presentations and diverse therapeutic options. The most common etiologies are related to cholelithiasis (acute cholecystitis, pancreatitis, and cholangitis) and non-traumatic injuries (common bile duct or duodenal). Although the true incidence of HPB emergencies is difficult to determine due to selection and reporting biases, a population-based report showed a decline in the global incidence of all severe complications of cholelithiasis, primarily based on a reduction in acute cholecystitis. Even though patients may present with overlapping symptoms, treatment options can be varied. The treatment of these conditions continues to evolve and patients may require endoscopic, surgical, and/or percutaneous techniques. Thus, it is essential that a multidisciplinary team of HPB surgeons, interventional gastroenterologists and radiologists are available on an as needed basis to the Acute Care Surgeon. This focused manuscript is a contemporary review of the literature surrounding HPB emergencies in the context of the acute care surgeon. The main aim of this review is to offer an update of the diagnosis and management of HPB issues in the acute care setting to improve the care of patients with potential HPB emergencies.

Keywords: Emergency surgery, Hepatopancreatobiliary, Acute care surgeon, Pancreatitis, Acute cholecystitis, Acute cholangitis, Surgery, Initial treatment

Introduction

Hepatopancreatobiliary (HPB) emergencies for the Acute Care Surgeon (ACS) include a wide range of diseases with variable clinical presentations and diverse therapeutic options. Fortunately most acute presentations can be classified as consequences of either inflammatory (gallstones, pancreatitis, cholangitis) or injury (common bile duct, duodenum) etiologies [1-3].

It is estimated that 1% to 4% of asymptomatic or mildly symptomatic patients will develop an acute complication of cholelithiasis [4]. These include cholecystitis, cholangitis and pancreatitis. Acute cholecystitis is the most frequent of these diseases [1,5]. Unfortunately determining the true incidence of HPB emergencies remains difficult due to selection and reporting biases. A recent population-based study showed a decline in the global incidence of all severe complications of cholelithiasis [6]. This was primarily based on a reduction in acute cholecystitis due to the wide spread adoption of laparoscopic cholecystectomy. Conversely, the incidence of acute biliary pancreatitis and cholangitis has increased during the same interval [6,7].

Although many of these HPB emergencies present with overlapping symptoms, treatment options can be diverse [8]. They may require endoscopic, surgical, and/or percutaneous techniques. As a result, it is essential that a multidisciplinary team of HPB surgeons, interventional gastroenterologists and radiologists are available on an as needed basis to the Acute Care Surgeon. Similarly, those patients who are not able to receive complete or gold standard therapy should be referred elsewhere without delay.

The aim of this review is to update the management of patients diagnosed with non-trauma HPB emergencies in the context of the ACS service.

* Correspondence: ball.chad@gmail.com
[1]Department of Surgery, Foothills Medical Center, University of Calgary, Calgary, AB, Canada
Full list of author information is available at the end of the article

General assessment

Similar to trauma, the initial evaluation of patients presenting with a HPB emergency should include simultaneous diagnosis and therapy. This concurrent rapid assessment and treatment is particularly important for patients who present with sepsis. A detailed clinical history of the acute event, including a focused past medical history (i.e. history of gallstones, pancreatitis, duodenal ulcer/NSAID use, and/or cancer) and complete physical examination are crucial. These details may suggest the likely diagnosis, determine the severity of the acute event, and guide both immediate and subsequent treatments. It is important to note that most patients present with an inflammatory and/or septic complication of a previously known disease, as opposed to a completely de novo etiology. Thus, patients presenting with acute cholecystitis or another complication of gallstones typically have a known history of symptomatic cholelithiasis. By contrast, patients suffering from pancreatic diseases generally develop symptoms after an acute new event.

The first step in caring for these patients requires a direct assessment of the severity of the acute event itself. Septic shock and acute bleeding represent the most common causes of hemodynamic compromise and must be addressed immediately. These methodologies include intravenous fluid resuscitation, early initiation of antimicrobial therapy, and blood product transfusion as needed. It is important to highlight that these patients often present with nausea and vomiting, dehydration, acute kidney injury, electrolyte imbalances, anemia, and/or coagulation abnormalities. A recent systematic review of 78 trials showed that resuscitation with colloids does not reduce the risk of death, nor improve survival [9]. It is also more expensive than resuscitation with crystalloids [9]. Another prospective randomized trial showed that patients with severe sepsis undergoing resuscitation with Ringer's solution had a decreased 90-day mortality and renal-replacement therapy rate when they were compared with patients who received Hydroxyethyl starch 130/0.42 [10]. Thus, it is recommended that patients with HPB emergencies undergo active and early resuscitation with crystalloids [9].

Numerous scoring models have been created to determine the severity of the acute HPB event [11]. These include, but are not limited to, the acute and physiology and chronic health evaluation (APACHE) III and IV, the simplified acute physiology score (SAPS) 3, and the mortality probability model (MPM) III. These scores were recently compared in 2596 patients with the aim of determining their value in predicting mortality [12]. The discriminatory performances of APACHE III and IV were similar, but also superior to both SAPS 3 and MPM III scores. Despite superior calibration and discrimination amongst surgical patients in particular, the APACHE III or IV assessments are not overly simple to determine in the initial resuscitation phase. It is also clearly important to obtain focused liver and pancreatic function, as well as liver enzyme tests during the evaluation to guide resuscitation and narrow the differential diagnosis.

Once effectively resuscitated, patients should undergo diagnostic imaging tests to rapidly determine the etiology and guide further treatment. The type of study required will depend on patient status and clinical suspicion. These may include bedside and/or formal abdominal ultrasound (US), hepatobiliary scintigraphy (HIDA), computed tomography (CT), endoscopic retrograde cholangiography (ERCP), magnetic resonance (MR) cholangiography and/or endoscopic ultrasound (EUS).

Biliary inflammatory diseases

Acute calculous cholecystitis (AC)

Acute inflammation of the gallbladder is a frequent complication of cholelithiasis, and affects up to 20% of patients with recurrent symptomatic gallstones [4]. Despite the history that most patients provide (previous episodes of transient colic pain in their right upper quadrant), acute presentations to a health care facility are typically longer and associated with additional symptoms (nausea or vomiting after ingesting high fat foods). Obstruction of the cystic duct by a gallstone or sludge produces dilation of the gallbladder and increases its internal pressure [8]. Subsequent biliary stasis and the proliferation of microorganisms is typical. If the obstruction persists, venous outflow decreases, with dilatation of capillaries and lymphatics resulting in gallbladder wall edema and thickening [4]. Eventually the gallbladder develops areas of hemorrhage and necrosis due to vascular occlusion. Imaging and exploration may reveal both fluid and air within the gallbladder wall. If the ischemia and necrosis is located within the posterior wall (i.e. apposed to the liver), a pericholecystic abscess eroding into the liver commonly occurs. It is also important to note that specific complications such as perforation, biliary peritonitis, pericholecystic abscess and biliary fistula (between the gallbladder and duodenum, colon, or stomach) may alter the clinical presentation and increase morbidity and mortality of the disease. Bouveret's syndrome, gastric outlet obstruction, biliary ileus and gallstone-related small bowel obstruction are uncommon complications that should be identified.

The initial assessment of these patients includes 2 dominant objectives: [1] confirming the diagnosis and [2] establishing its severity. Despite a wide array of options (US, HIDA, CT, MR), the revised Tokyo consensus guidelines represent the best parameters for directing diagnosis and treatment [5,13]. Based on diagnostic sensitivities of 90% to 95%, abdominal US remains the initial modality of choice [4]. Because it can be performed by the ACS within the emergency department itself, it is also cost saving and rapid. Identification of gallbladder wall thickening (>5 mm), an obstructing gallstone in the gallbladder neck, pericholecystic fluid, US Murphy's sign and/or dilation and thickening of the common bile duct (CBD) are important signs that contribute to defining the diagnosis. Unfortunately CT imaging is far less specific and frequent in confirming this diagnosis. After confirmation however, the disease should be classified according its severity (grade I = mild, II = moderate, III = severe). While grade II refers to the presence of systemic signs of inflammation, grade III cholecystitis includes dysfunction of at least one organ/system [13] (Table 1).

The treatment of patients with AC should include general medical therapy (nil per mouth (NPO), intravenous fluids, antibiotics and analgesia) followed by urgent cholecystectomy. The 2 dominant surgical issues include the type (open vs. laparoscopic) and timing (early vs. delayed) of the procedure. Two small prospective randomized trials compared open with laparoscopic surgery for acute cholecystitis. The first study showed that open cholecystectomy had a significantly higher number of postoperative complications, as well as a longer postoperative hospital stay (6 vs. 4 days). No mortality or bile duct injuries were observed in this study [14]. A more recent trial included 70 patients and did not show any significant difference in the rate of postoperative complications [15]. The laparoscopic group had a significantly longer median operating time (90 vs. 80 minutes) and shorter median postoperative stay. The timing of cholecystectomy has also been evaluated in prospective randomized trials. Numerous small studies have observed that patients undergoing early cholecystectomy have a shorter hospital stay, without any other significant differences [16-22]. A recent meta-analysis that included 451 patients from 5 trials comparing early (less than 7 days from the onset of symptoms) with delayed (more than six weeks after the index admission) cholecystectomy revealed no statistically significant difference between the groups with regard to bile duct injuries (BDI) or conversion to open surgery [23]. The hospital stay was 3 days shorter in the early group however. Importantly, 40 (17.5%) patients in the delayed group required an emergency cholecystectomy during their waiting period for non-resolving or recurrent AC. It is also evident from large population based studies that the rate of BDI increases with higher grades of cholecystitis [4]. The most recent prospective multicenter trial comparing the optimal timing for cholecystectomy (early, during the first 24 hours vs. delayed) in patients with acute cholecystitis confirmed that early cholecystectomy was associated with significantly lower morbidity (11.8 vs. 34.4%). Although conversion to open surgery, nor mortality differed between groups, the mean length of hospital stay (5.4 vs. 10 days) and hospital costs were significantly lower in the group treated with early cholecystectomy [24]. Taken together, these results suggest that early laparoscopic surgery should be considered the treatment of choice.

Table 1 "Severity assessment criteria for acute cholecystitis"

Grade	Definition
I (mild)	Acute cholecystitis does not meet the criteria of "Grade III" or "Grade II"
	It can also be defined as acute cholecystitis in a healthy patient with no organ dysfunction and mild inflammatory changes in the gallbladder, making cholecystectomy a safe and low-risk operative procedure.
II (moderate)	Acute cholecystitis is associated with any one of the following conditions:
	1. Elevated white blood cell count (>18,000/mm3)
	2. Palpable tender mass in the right upper abdominal quadrant
	3. Duration of complaints > 72 hours
	4. Marked local inflammation (gangrenous cholecystitis, pericholecystic abscess, hepatic abscess, biliary peritonitis, emphysematous cholecystitis).
III (severe)	"Grade III" (severe) acute cholecystitis is associated with dysfunction of any one of the following organs/systems
	1. Cardiovascular dysfunction defined as hypotension requiring treatment with dopamine ≥ 5 µg/kg per min, or any dose of norepinephrine
	2. Neurological dysfunction defined as decreased level of consciousness
	3. Respiratory dysfunction defined as a PaO2/FiO2 ratio < 300
	4. Renal dysfunction defined as oliguria, creatinine > 2.0 mg/dl
	5. Hepatic dysfunction defined as PT-INR > 1.5
	6. Hematological dysfunction defined as platelet count < 100,000/mm3

From "Yokoe M, et al. [1] (with permission).

In summary, patients with grade I or II acute cholecystitis should undergo early laparoscopic cholecystectomy, with awareness of the extent of the gallbladder's inflammation (i.e. defining biliary anatomy to prevent BDI). More specifically, the ACS surgeon must be particularly wary of the inflamed gallbladder that is contracted into the liver bed because the anatomy in this scenario represents the most common etiology for BDI. Patients with grade III acute cholecystitis should undergo cholecystectomy once organ dysfunction is reversed [25]. In the setting of persistent organ failure or poor surgical candidacy, antimicrobial therapy and concurrent percutaneous cholecystostomy should be performed [26].

The role for antibiotic prophylaxis prior to elective laparoscopic cholecystectomy has been studied in prospective randomized trials. Unfortunately the evidence remains insufficient to either support or refute their use in an attempt to reduce surgical site and global infections. This question has not been evaluated for patients undergoing urgent cholecystectomy for acute cholecystitis in any trials however. As a result, consensus guidelines recommend that antibiotic therapy should be started if infection is suspected on the basis of clinical, laboratory, and/or radiographic findings [27]. Treatment should include coverage for the Enterobacteriaceae family (i.e. second generation cephalosporin, or a combination of a quinolone and metronidazole) [4]. Treatment of enterococci is debated. Elderly patients and those with diabetes mellitus or immunosuppressive disorders should receive antibiotics even when infection has not been confirmed. Obtaining aerobic and anaerobic cultures from the bile during surgery is also recommended to guide treatment in complex cases [4].

The role of *routine* intraoperative cholangiography has been evaluated in patients undergoing elective cholecystectomy [28]. Eight randomized trials (1715 patients) were analyzed in a recent systematic review without showing any clear evidence to support its routine use [29]. When this is combined with the fact that there are no randomized studies in patients undergoing cholecystectomy for acute cholecystitis, intraoperative cholangiography should be performed selectively in the setting of concerning pre- and/or intra-operative findings.

AC in specific scenarios (jaundice, acalculous acute cholecystitis, pregnancy)

The presence of jaundice should be evaluated with caution because it reflects a wide spectrum of potentially benign and malignant conditions. These include, but are not limited to, CBD obstruction from external compression (cholangiocarcinoma, periampullary cancers, gallbladder cancer), choledocholithiasis, and liver failure (e.g. secondary to sepsis). Although US continues to be the diagnostic gold standard for detecting choledocholithiasis (especially within the distal CBD), MR cholangiography (MRC) may also be useful to define the etiology [30]. The dominant goals in the treatment of patients with choledocholithiasis are three-fold: [1] treat concurrent sepsis, [2] evacuate the CBD, and [3] prevent future recurrences. Although the order of the latter 2 goals is debated on the basis of length of stay, safety and economics, it is clear that ERCP and laparoscopic cholecystectomy represent the 2 dominant therapies [31,32]. Laparoscopic CBD exploration (transcystic or transductal) is also a viable option and has the added benefit of being performed as a single procedure [33,34].

Acalculous cholecystitis is an uncommon and serious presentation observed in 5% to 10% of patients with biliary emergencies [35]. It is typically associated with critical illness, immunosuppressive conditions, uncommon pathogens (anaerobes), and/or sepsis [35]. On a global basis, patients with acquired immunodeficiency syndrome (AIDS) continue to represent the most common immunosuppressive cases and are younger, present with elevations in their alkaline phosphatase and serum bilirubin, and may have cytomegalovirus and cryptosporidium associated infections [36]. Other rare causes of acalculous cholecystitis are chemical cholecystitis after hepatic artery infusion, antibiotic-related cholecystitis, and parasites (ascaris). Since patients with acalculous cholecystitis often present with organ dysfunction and are poor surgical candidates, medical treatment is often the therapy of choice, with surgery performed in selected cases (i.e. if cholecystostomy is ineffective) [35].

Pregnant patients carry a higher risk of developing both gallstones and acute cholecystitis than non-pregnant patients [37,38]. Complications of gallstones remain the second most common cause of surgery during pregnancy [39]. Despite this epidemiology, surgery should be avoided during the first (i.e. abortion) and third (i.e. premature delivery) trimesters if possible. Most symptomatic patients treated with nonoperative therapy present with recurrence of their symptoms however. Of this cohort, approximately 30% eventually require surgery during their pregnancy [40].

Acute cholangitis

Acute cholangitis is defined as acute inflammation and infection of the biliary tree. This is most commonly a consequence of biliary obstruction followed by bacterial overgrowth within bile [41]. The dominant cause of acute cholangitis is choledocholithiasis, followed by benign biliary stenosis and cancer. Interestingly, a recent report that included 794 patients did not show a significant difference between the incidence of gallstones (50.6%) and malignancies (49.4%) as the main source of obstruction [8,42]. This likely reflects an aging populous. Regardless of the cause or site, obstruction of the biliary tree (most commonly of the common bile duct), leads to an increase in the number of microorganisms followed by a rise in the intraductal pressure of the bile duct. This increases ductal permeability and facilitates translocation of bacteria and their products into the vascular system. This process is highly dependent upon contamination of normally aseptic bile. It is also supported by data that reports 16% of patients undergoing a non-biliary operation, 72% with acute cholangitis, 44% with chronic cholangitis, 50% with acute biliary obstruction, and 90% of patients with choledocholithiasis and jaundice have positive biliary cultures [8].

Patients with cholangitis may present with a wide variety of symptoms from nonspecific findings to severe infection and fatal septic shock. Morbidity and mortality are minimized only via early diagnosis and treatment. Given that Charcot's triad (jaundice, fever and right upper quadrant peritonitis) has a high specificity (>90%), but is observed in only 18.5% of patients, a high level of suspicion for the diagnosis is essential [3].

This reality is reinforced by the Tokyo guidelines that summarize the diagnosis must include at least [1] signs of systemic inflammation (i.e. fever), [2] cholestasis, and [3] specific findings on imaging [3,5] (Table 2). Current recommendations also grade the severity of cholangitis (I (mild = diagnosis of exclusion), II (moderate = systemic inflammation without organ dysfunction), or III (severe = concurrent dysfunction of at least 1 organ system)). Despite this grading system, most patients (54%) present with grade I disease (only 11% develop grade III).

The treatment of acute cholangitis has shown dramatic improvement over the past decade with a current mortality of less than 30% (i.e. sepsis leading to multiorgan failure) [3]. Patients should receive general medical therapy including NPO, intravenous fluids, antibiotics, and analgesia [27]. In addition to critical care, various techniques for biliary decompression are also mandated [43]. Approaches include endoscopic, percutaneous and/or operative approaches based on the etiology of the cholangitis and patient physiology [44,45]. Medical treatment may be sufficient in selected cases of grade I, but biliary drainage should be considered for all non-responders [46]. This scenario often incorporates postoperative patients. Patients with grade II disease require early endoscopic, percutaneous or emergent operative (T-tube) biliary drainage. These drainage procedures may be definitive for patients with gallstone-associated cholangitis [46]. Although it remains controversial if patients with cancer should undergo a definitive resection concurrent to their emergent decompression procedure, this is generally not recommended due to a lack of complete staging, higher postoperative complications, and known hospital volume-outcome relationships. Patients with cancer should be stabilized, undergo emergency drainage, and be referred for definitive treatment to a high volume HPB center. In the most critically ill patients, a

Table 2 "Severity assessment criteria for acute cholangitis"

Grade	Definition
I (mild)	Acute cholangitis does not meet the criteria of "Grade II or III", representing acute cholangitis at initial diagnosis. Notes
	Patients should have early diagnosis, biliary drainage and/or treatment for etiology, and antimicrobial administration.
	It is recommended that patients with acute cholangitis who do not respond to the initial medical treatment (general supportive care and antimicrobial therapy) undergo early biliary drainage or treatment for etiology.
II (moderate)	Acute cholangitis associated with any two of the following conditions:
	1. Abnormal white blood cell count (>12,000/mm^3, < 4,000/mm^3)
	2. High fever (≥39°C)
	3. Age (≥75 years old)
	4. Hyperbilirubinemia (total bilirubin ≥ 5 mg/dL)
	5. Hypoalbuminemia (< STD × 0.7)
III (severe)	Acute cholangitis associated with the onset of dysfunction in at least one of any of the following organs/systems:
	1. Cardiovascular dysfunction defined as hypotension requiring treatment with dopamine ≥ 5 μg/kg per min, or any dose of norepinephrine
	2. Neurological dysfunction defined as decreased level of consciousness
	3. Respiratory dysfunction defined as a PaO2/FiO2 ratio < 300
	4. Renal dysfunction defined as oliguria, creatinine > 2.0 mg/dl
	5. Hepatic dysfunction defined as PT-INR > 1.5
	6. Hematological dysfunction defined as platelet count < 100,000/mm3

STD lower limit of normal value.
Kiriyama S, et al. [5] (with permission).

multidisciplinary team of endoscopists, intensive care physicians and sometimes HPB surgeons should participate with the ACS in the management of these patients. The type of biliary drainage selected by the surgeon is particularly important. Patients with hilar cholangiocarcinoma most often benefit from a percutaneous technique (percutaneous transhepatic catheter (PTC) as opposed to endoscopic). ERCP-based attempts at drainage of hilar cholangiocarcinoma are notorious for failing to achieve adequate drainage within the proximal liver and subsequently often develop significant cholangitis due to instrumentation of the biliary system during this attempt. These patients *must* also receive high fidelity cholangiographic information either prior to (MRCP), or concurrent to the insertion of the PTC (i.e. via the PTC itself) to define resectability and reconstruction options. Patients with any periampullary malignancy should undergo ERCP-based stenting as the initial choice.

Patients with grade III cholangitis require admission to the intensive care unit for physiologic support, in addition to general medical treatment [46]. Urgent endoscopic, percutaneous or surgical biliary drainage must also be performed. Considering that these patients are often physiologically unstable, the most rapid and least invasive procedure should be selected (operative intervention should be the last resort given the high associated mortality). Once the cholangitis has resolved, definitive treatment of the etiology (i.e. laparoscopic cholecystectomy for cholelithiasis, resection for cancer) is indicated.

Severe acute pancreatitis (SAP)

Acute pancreatitis is a common disease that affects approximately 200,000 people per year in the United States [47]. It was classically defined by the Atlanta guidelines in 1992 as "an acute inflammatory process of the pancreas with variable involvement of regional or distant organ/systems and high levels of pancreatic enzyme in blood and/or urine" [48]. Although the differential diagnosis for causes of pancreatitis is broad, choledocholithiasis remains the most common [49]. SAP is observed in approximately 20% of patients, and depends on the presence of organ failure and local complications (necrosis, pseudocyst, and walled off pancreatic necrosis). The dominant definition of SAP includes subsets of patients with organ failure, necrotizing pancreatitis without organ failure, and infected pancreatic necrosis with organ failure [2,50]. Given that this definition considers groups with vastly different prognoses, it has been recently revised by a group of experts [50]. It is now based on local and systemic determinants of severity. The *local determinants* include pancreatic and/or peripancreatic necrosis (P-PN). These 2 entities have been included together and represent all non-viable tissue (solid or semisolid) that does not have a radiologically defined wall. Thus, pancreatic necrosis is defined as any area of non-enhancement on contrast-enhanced CT and peripancreatic necrosis includes every heterogeneous peripancreatic collection on CT until proven otherwise. P-PN may be considered infected when gas bubbles are observed on CT scan, or when a culture obtained by percutaneous or surgical techniques is positive [50]. It should be noted that the routine use of broad-spectrum prophylactic antibiotics has altered the bacteriology of secondary pancreatic infection in severe acute pancreatitis, from predominantly gram-negative to gram-positive bacteria without changing the rate of beta-lactam resistance or fungal super-infection [51]. *Systemic determinants* refer to distant organ failure, which is defined for 3 systems on the basis of the worst measurement in a 24-hour period or when the creatinine is ≥ 2 mg/dl, PaO_2/FiO_2 is ≤ 300, or inotropic agents are required. *Transient failure* is defined as failure of the same organ/system for less than 48 hours, while *persistent failure* implies more than 48 hours. Based on this new consensus grading, acute pancreatitis is described as [1] *mild* (P-PN and organ failure are absent), [2] *moderate* (sterile P-PN and/or transient organ failure), [3] *severe* (either infected P-PN or persistent organ failure), or [4] *critical* (infected P-PN with persistent organ failure) [50].

Despite guideline recommendations, every patient should receive personalized treatment based on the severity of their disease and the direction of a multidisciplinary team. The surgical treatment of patients with SAP has evolved dramatically and includes open, laparoscopic, radiologic, and endoscopic techniques of debridement and drainage [52,53]. These approaches may be used alone, or in combination [54]. Despite this long list of potential techniques to remove necrotic tissue, the more dominant issue for the ACS surgeon is one of timing. It is clear that early debridement increases blood loss, morbidity, the number of operative interventions, and mortality across all groups of patients with SAP [55]. More specifically, almost every patient should be physiologically supported without major intervention until the 28-day mark. Patients with SAP follow a predictable pattern of early SIRS and potentially multi-organ failure as a result. This interval observation is often misinterpreted as sepsis requiring treatment with antimicrobial therapy. Within the first 7 to 10 days, very few of these patients have infected necrosis (and therefore require antibiotics). The most common exceptions to this rule of delayed (28-day) intervention remains patients with concurrent ischemia of the bowel or gallbladder [56]. As a result, it is ischemia of these 2 organs that must be ruled out if a critically ill patient decompensates, as opposed to focusing on the status of the pancreas itself (infected or not).

Once the patient is stabilized and the pancreatic necrosum is mature, operative therapies may include both minimally invasive (laparoscopic cystgastrostomies and debridements, utilization of percutaneous drains as access guides for rigid scope debridement, step-up procedures, endoscopic transmural debridements) and open (transperitoneal, retroperitoneal-flank) approaches [47,57-59]. The best choice amongst these options is based on patient anatomy and the specific location(s) of the necrosum.

The recent publication popularity in percutaneous techniques as treatment for pancreatic necrosis deserves specific mention. CT-guided drainage followed by repeated irrigation procedures in the context of ever increasingly larger drains placed by involved and committed radiologists may improve the clinical course in up to 75% of patients. It has also been shown to resolve the necrotic collection in 45% of cases. This technique is incredibly labor intensive however, and therefore not available in most centers.

In addition to the role of surgery, significant literature exists with reference to the role of prophylactic antibiotics, early ERCP decompression in persistent biliary pancreatitis [60,61], type of nutrition [62], role of octreotide, and probiotic prophylaxis. The use of prophylactic antibiotics has been evaluated in numerous underpowered prospective randomized trials and meta-analyses [63-66]. These 7 RCTs are best summarized by stating that there is no good evidence to support the routine use of prophylactic antibiotics in patients with SAP [67,68]. Furthermore, the general recommendation is to stop all antibiotics if they have been previously started in this scenario.

The optimal type of nutrition (enteral vs. parenteral) has also been evaluated in multiple prospective randomized trials. A systematic review that included 348 patients from 8 trials showed that enteral nutrition decreased the risk of death (OR 0.50, 95% CI 0.28 to 0.91), multiple organ failure (OR 0.55, 95% CI 0.37 to 0.81), systemic infection (OR 0.39, 95% CI 0.23 to 0.65), operative interventions (OR 0.44, 95% CI 0.29 to 0.67), local septic complications (OR 0.74, 95% CI 0.40 to 1.35) and length of hospital stay (reduced by 2.4 days) [69]. More importantly, in patients with SAP, enteral nutrition decreased the risk of death (RR = 0.18, 95% CI 0.06 to 0.58) and multiple organ failure (RR = 0.46, 95% CI 0.16 to 1.29), suggesting that patients should receive enteral over parenteral nutrition [69]. In many patients, regardless of the extent of necrosis on CT, oral ingestion of a regular diet is well tolerated. If this fails, progression to nasogastric followed by nasojejunal tube feeding as needed is recommended.

The role of early ERCP in the context of choledocholithiasis has also been evaluated in prospective studies [61,70-74]. Amongst 153 patients in a multicenter prospective study, patients were divided into 2 groups (with and without signs of cholestasis) [75]. Although ERCP was associated with fewer complications than the observation group (25% vs. 54%, p = 0.02) in patients with signs of cholestasis, mortality was not significantly lower (6% vs. 15%, p = 0.2). Additionally, ERCP neither reduced complications (45% vs. 41%, p = 0.8) nor mortality (14% vs. 17%, P = 0.7) in patients without cholestasis, suggesting that ERCP should be indicated only in selected patients with *persistent* cholestasis [61,74].

Finally, trials evaluating probiotic use reported that prophylaxis did not reduce the risk of infectious complications, but actually increased the risk of mortality in patients with predicted SAP [76]. Similarly, another trial of 302 patients with moderate to SAP who received either octreotide or placebo had similar rates of mortality, complications, duration of pain, surgical interventions, and length of hospital stay. This finding suggests that octreotide should not be used in SAP [77].

Non-traumatic injuries

Iatrogenic bile duct injuries (BDI)

BDIs can be physically and psychologically challenging errors for both the injurious surgeon, as well as their colleague asked to repair the injury [78]. Although a detailed description of BDIs and their reconstructions is beyond the scope of this review, it is important to consider this diagnosis, as the ACS surgeon is often called as the initial consultant by a surgeon in need. Based on large population studies, the rate of BDIs approaches 0.4% using laparoscopic techniques and 0.1% with open approaches [79]. Most BDIs are not recognized intraoperatively and instead patients return to the hospital with complaints of nausea, vomiting, abdominal discomfort and potentially obstructive biliary symptoms [80]. The ACS surgeon must hold diagnoses of a BDI and/or biloma high in their differential diagnosis when assessing these postoperative patients. Intraoperative diagnoses of BDIs should be suspected in cases of extensive inflammation, severely contracted gallbladders, unexpected bleeding that requires multiple clips for control, abnormal anatomy, bile within the operative field, or difficultly in defining the triangle of Calot, sulcus of Rouvier, median umbilical fissure, hepatic artery and critical view of safety [81]. If an injury is suspected, but not clearly evident, an intraoperative cholangiogram should be performed to evaluate the biliary tree as a first assessment [82]. Given the tremendous frequency of general surgeons to misinterpret intraoperative cholangiograms however, more than one surgeon with experience and/or a radiologist is ideal. If doubt persists, consultation with an HPB surgeon experienced in BDI reconstruction prior to conversion to an open procedure is highly recommended. The status of the right hepatic artery (90%) in addition to the proximity of the injury and the quality/loss of ductal tissue will define recommendations from the referral surgeon [83]. If the surgical team does not have the expertise to repair the bile duct, 2 closed suction drains should be placed within the gallbladder fossa to manage a potential bile leak, followed by immediate referral and/or transfer. Intentional occlusion (clip or tie) of a transected common bile duct during the index operation is not helpful due to a lack of subsequent proximal dilation, as well as necrosis of the duct leading to a more proximal injury.

Delayed presentation of a BDI should be suspected by the ACS in patients who present with nausea, vomiting, fever and persistent abdominal pain that does not decrease with regular analgesics. Liver function tests may be abnormally elevated not only due to obstruction, but also because of a biloma. Patients should be studied immediately with an abdominal US and/or CT to define the presence of collections or abnormal free fluid. It is important to note that the absence of fluid does not exclude the occurrence of a BDI. Any fluid collection should be drained with a percutaneous approach. The biliary tree, and specifically the level of injury, may then be defined with an MRC and/or ERCP [84,85]. In scenarios where the posterior sector has been isolated or there has been a complete common ductal transection, retrograde drain cholangiograms and percutaneous transhepatic cholangiograms (and catheters) are required respectively [86].

It should be noted that in all BDI patients, the cause of sepsis may be multifold: [1] intraabdominal collections/biloma (usually related to the gallbladder bed), [2] biliperitoneum, [3] cholangitis (when the bile duct has been completely transected and clipped), and [4] liver necrosis/failure when the BDI is associated with a vascular injury [87]. Since the specific cause of sepsis is usually unknown at the time of presentation, all critically ill patients should receive immediate fluid resuscitation and antibiotics. A CT scan should be obtained to assess the etiology of sepsis. Blood and intraabdominal cultures are mandatory to guide the therapy.

Duodenal perforation following ERCP

ERCP is a diagnostic and therapeutic procedure that is employed in a wide range of benign and malignant diseases. It has been described that approximately 10% to 15% of patients sustain procedural complications. Although pancreatitis remains the most common, duodenal perforations occur in approximately 1% of patients [88-90]. Unfortunately the mortality associated with these perforations is as high as 20% depending on the series [88]. Treatment depends entirely on patient clinical presentation, location of the perforation, and the initial indication for the ERCP [91,92]. Injuries are classified as type I (created in the lateral wall of duodenum or jejunum during the ERCP scope's "long view") or type II (small perforations of the ampulla of Vater including the periampullary tissues) [93]. Unlike BDIs during laparoscopic cholecystectomy, most cases (74%) of ERCP perforations are detected during the ERCP itself [94]. The majority of type I injuries (81%) require surgical management (duodenal wall repair and periduodenal drainage with occasional Roux-en-Y duodenojejunostomy), whereas most type II (97%) injuries are treated conservatively (antibiotic therapy and drainage of retroperitoneal collections). It should be noted however that failure of medical management (including percutaneous drainage) is typical in scenarios of significant retroperitoneal fluid [95]. In contrast, patients with significant retroperitoneal air and very little fluid often recover well with nonoperative therapies (antibiotics, NPO).

In conclusion, HPB emergencies for the ACS surgeon are broad in nature and presentation. Although the appropriate treatments can be complex and require multimodality care, they are each approached similarly in the acute phase. This initial assessment involves both diagnosis, as well as treatment with resuscitation, antimicrobial therapy and multidisciplinary input. By approaching HPB emergencies in this manner, the ACS surgeon will be well equipped to deal with all patients.

Competing interests
The authors declare that they have no competing interests.

Authors' contributions
Each author contributed with the conception of the manuscript, participated in the analysis and interpretation of the data, drafting the manuscript, and approved the last version after reading it carefully. JMB, Literature search, study design, data analysis and interpretation, writing, critical revision. SMH, Study design, data interpretation, writing, critical revision. CGB, Literature search, study design, data analysis and interpretation, writing, critical revision.

Author details
[1]Department of Surgery, Foothills Medical Center, University of Calgary, Calgary, AB, Canada. [2]University of British Columbia, Vancouver, BC, Canada.

References

1. Yokoe M, Takada T, Strasberg SM, Solomkin JS, Mayumi T, Gomi H, et al. New diagnostic criteria and severity assessment of acute cholecystitis in revised Tokyo Guidelines. J Hepatobiliary Pancreat Sci. 2012;19(5):578–85.
2. Bollen TL, van Santvoort HC, Besselink MG, van Leeuwen MS, Horvath KD, Freeny PC, et al. The Atlanta Classification of acute pancreatitis revisited. Br J Surg. 2008;95(1):6–21.
3. Kiriyama S, Takada T, Strasberg SM, Solomkin JS, Mayumi T, Pitt HA, et al. New diagnostic criteria and severity assessment of acute cholangitis in revised Tokyo Guidelines. J Hepatobiliary Pancreat Sci. 2012;19(5):548–56.
4. Strasberg SM. Clinical practice. Acute calculous cholecystitis. N Engl J Med. 2008;358(26):2804–11.
5. Kiriyama S, Takada T, Strasberg SM, Solomkin JS, Mayumi T, Pitt HA, et al. TG13 guidelines for diagnosis and severity grading of acute cholangitis (with videos). J Hepatobiliary Pancreat Sci. 2013;20(1):24–34.
6. Urbach DR, Stukel TA. Rate of elective cholecystectomy and the incidence of severe gallstone disease. CMAJ. 2005;172(8):1015–9.

7. Yadav D, Lowenfels AB. Trends in the epidemiology of the first attack of acute pancreatitis: a systematic review. Pancreas. 2006;33(4):323–30.
8. Kimura Y, Takada T, Kawarada Y, Nimura Y, Hirata K, Sekimoto M, et al. Definitions, pathophysiology, and epidemiology of acute cholangitis and cholecystitis: Tokyo Guidelines. J Hepato-Biliary-Pancreat Surg. 2007;14(1):15–26.
9. Perel P, Roberts I, Ker K. Colloids versus crystalloids for fluid resuscitation in critically ill patients. Cochrane Database Syst Rev. 2013;2:CD000567.
10. Perner A, Haase N, Guttormsen AB, Tenhunen J, Klemenzson G, Aneman A, et al. Hydroxyethyl starch 130/0.42 versus Ringer's acetate in severe sepsis. N Engl J Med. 2012;367(2):124–34.
11. Nassar Jr AP, Mocelin AO, Nunes AL, Giannini FP, Brauer L, Andrade FM, et al. Caution when using prognostic models: a prospective comparison of 3 recent prognostic models. J Crit Care. 2012;27(4):423 e1–7.
12. Keegan MT, Gajic O, Afessa B. Comparison of APACHE III, APACHE IV, SAPS 3, and MPM0III and influence of resuscitation status on model performance. Chest. 2012;142(4):851–8.
13. Yamashita Y, Takada T, Kawarada Y, Nimura Y, Hirota M, Miura F, et al. Surgical treatment of patients with acute cholecystitis: Tokyo Guidelines. J Hepato-Biliary-Pancreat Surg. 2007;14(1):91–7.
14. Kiviluoto T, Siren J, Luukkonen P, Kivilaakso E. Randomised trial of laparoscopic versus open cholecystectomy for acute and gangrenous cholecystitis. Lancet. 1998;351(9099):321–5.
15. Johansson M, Thune A, Nelvin L, Stiernstam M, Westman B, Lundell L. Randomized clinical trial of open versus laparoscopic cholecystectomy in the treatment of acute cholecystitis. Br J Surg. 2005;92(1):44–9.
16. Chandler CF, Lane JS, Ferguson P, Thompson JE, Ashley SW. Prospective evaluation of early versus delayed laparoscopic cholecystectomy for treatment of acute cholecystitis. Am Surg. 2000;66(9):896–900.
17. Jarvinen HJ, Hastbacka J. Early cholecystectomy for acute cholecystitis: a prospective randomized study. Ann Surg. 1980;191(4):501–5.
18. Johansson M, Thune A, Blomqvist A, Nelvin L, Lundell L. Management of acute cholecystitis in the laparoscopic era: results of a prospective, randomized clinical trial. J Gastrointest Surg. 2003;7(5):642–5.
19. Kolla SB, Aggarwal S, Kumar A, Kumar R, Chumber S, Parshad R, et al. Early versus delayed laparoscopic cholecystectomy for acute cholecystitis: a prospective randomized trial. Surg Endosc. 2004;18(9):1323–7.
20. Lai PB, Kwong KH, Leung KL, Kwok SP, Chan AC, Chung SC, et al. Randomized trial of early versus delayed laparoscopic cholecystectomy for acute cholecystitis. Br J Surg. 1998;85(6):764–7.
21. Lo CM, Liu CL, Fan ST, Lai EC, Wong J. Prospective randomized study of early versus delayed laparoscopic cholecystectomy for acute cholecystitis. Ann Surg. 1998;227(4):461–7.
22. Norrby S, Herlin P, Holmin T, Sjodahl R, Tagesson C. Early or delayed cholecystectomy in acute cholecystitis? A clinical trial. Br J Surg. 1983;70(3):163–5.
23. Gurusamy K, Samraj K, Gluud C, Wilson E, Davidson BR. Meta-analysis of randomized controlled trials on the safety and effectiveness of early versus delayed laparoscopic cholecystectomy for acute cholecystitis. Br J Surg. 2010;97(2):141–50.
24. Gutt CN, Encke J, Koninger J, Harnoss JC, Weigand K, Kipfmuller K, et al. Acute cholecystitis: early versus delayed cholecystectomy, a multicenter randomized trial (ACDC study, NCT00447304). Ann Surg. 2013;258(3):385–93.
25. Akyurek N, Salman B, Yuksel O, Tezcaner T, Irkorucu O, Yucel C, et al. Management of acute calculous cholecystitis in high-risk patients: percutaneous cholecystotomy followed by early laparoscopic cholecystectomy. Surg Laparosc Endosc Percutan Tech. 2005;15(6):315–20.
26. Ito K, Fujita N, Noda Y, Kobayashi G, Kimura K, Sugawara T, et al. Percutaneous cholecystostomy versus gallbladder aspiration for acute cholecystitis: a prospective randomized controlled trial. AJR Am J Roentgenol. 2004;183(1):193–6.
27. Gomi H, Solomkin JS, Takada T, Strasberg SM, Pitt HA, Yoshida M, et al. TG13 antimicrobial therapy for acute cholangitis and cholecystitis. J Hepatobiliary Pancreat Sci. 2013;20(1):60–70.
28. Hauer-Jensen M, Karesen R, Nygaard K, Solheim K, Amlie EJ, Havig O, et al. Prospective randomized study of routine intraoperative cholangiography during open cholecystectomy: long-term follow-up and multivariate analysis of predictors of choledocholithiasis. Surgery. 1993;113(3):318–23.
29. Ford JA, Soop M, Du J, Loveday BP, Rodgers M. Systematic review of intraoperative cholangiography in cholecystectomy. Br J Surg. 2012;99(2):160–7.
30. Reinhold C, Taourel P, Bret PM, Cortas GA, Mehta SN, Barkun AN, et al. Choledocholithiasis: evaluation of MR cholangiography for diagnosis. Radiology. 1998;209(2):435–42.
31. Tzovaras G, Baloyiannis I, Zachari E, Symeonidis D, Zacharoulis D, Kapsoritakis A, et al. Laparoendoscopic rendezvous versus preoperative ERCP and laparoscopic cholecystectomy for the management of cholecysto-choledocholithiasis: interim analysis of a controlled randomized trial. Ann Surg. 2012;255(3):435–9.
32. Gurusamy K, Sahay SJ, Burroughs AK, Davidson BR. Systematic review and meta-analysis of intraoperative versus preoperative endoscopic sphincterotomy in patients with gallbladder and suspected common bile duct stones. Br J Surg. 2011;98(7):908–16.
33. Rogers SJ, Cello JP, Horn JK, Siperstein AE, Schecter WP, Campbell AR, et al. Prospective randomized trial of LC + LCBDE vs ERCP/S + LC for common bile duct stone disease. Arch Surg. 2010;145(1):28–33.
34. Li MK, Tang CN, Lai EC. Managing concomitant gallbladder stones and common bile duct stones in the laparoscopic era: a systematic review. Asian J Endosc Surg. 2011;4(2):53–8.
35. Barie PS, Eachempati SR. Acute acalculous cholecystitis. Gastroenterol Clin N Am. 2010;39(2):343–57. 2.
36. Cello JP. AIDS-Related biliary tract disease. Gastrointest Endosc Clin N Am. 1998;8(4):963.
37. Tseng JY, Yang MJ, Yang CC, Chao KC, Li HY. Acute cholecystitis during pregnancy: what is the best approach? Taiwan J Obstet Gynecol. 2009;48 (3):305–7.
38. Date RS, Kaushal M, Ramesh A. A review of the management of gallstone disease and its complications in pregnancy. Am J Surg. 2008;196(4):599–608.
39. Silvestri MT, Pettker CM, Brousseau EC, Dick MA, Ciarleglio MM, Erekson EA. Morbidity of appendectomy and cholecystectomy in pregnant and nonpregnant women. Obstet Gynecol. 2011;118(6):1261–70.
40. Othman MO, Stone E, Hashimi M, Parasher G. Conservative management of cholelithiasis and its complications in pregnancy is associated with recurrent symptoms and more emergency department visits. Gastrointest Endosc. 2012;76(3):564–9.
41. Kimura Y, Takada T, Strasberg SM, Pitt HA, Gouma DJ, Garden OJ, et al. TG13 current terminology, etiology, and epidemiology of acute cholangitis and cholecystitis. J Hepatobiliary Pancreat Sci. 2013;20(1):8–23.
42. Higuchi R, Takada T, Strasberg SM, Pitt HA, Gouma DJ, Garden OJ, et al. TG13 miscellaneous etiology of cholangitis and cholecystitis. J Hepatobiliary Pancreat Sci. 2013;20(1):97–105.
43. Lai EC, Mok FP, Tan ES, Lo CM, Fan ST, You KT, et al. Endoscopic biliary drainage for severe acute cholangitis. N Engl J Med. 1992;326(24):1582–6.
44. Lau WY, Chu KW, Yuen WK, Poon GP, Hwang JS, Li AK. Operative choledochoscopy in patients with acute cholangitis: a prospective, randomized study. Br J Surg. 1991;78(10):1226–9.
45. Lee DW, Chan AC, Lam YH, Ng EK, Lau JY, Law BK, et al. Biliary decompression by nasobiliary catheter or biliary stent in acute suppurative cholangitis: a prospective randomized trial. Gastrointest Endosc. 2002;56(3):361–5.
46. Miura F, Takada T, Strasberg SM, Solomkin JS, Pitt HA, Gouma DJ, et al. TG13 flowchart for the management of acute cholangitis and cholecystitis. J Hepatobiliary Pancreat Sci. 2013;20(1):47–54.
47. Schmidt CM. Introduction: SSAT/AGA/ASGE State-of-the-Art Conference: necrotizing pancreatitis: novel minimally invasive strategies. J Gastrointest Surg. 2011;15(7):1086–8.
48. Bradley 3rd EL. A clinically based classification system for acute pancreatitis. Summary of the International Symposium on Acute Pancreatitis, Atlanta, Ga, September 11 through 13, 1992. Arch Surg. 1993;128(5):586–90.
49. Kimura Y, Arata S, Takada T, Hirata K, Yoshida M, Mayumi T, et al. Gallstone-induced acute pancreatitis. J Hepatobiliary Pancreat Sci. 2010;17(1):60–9.
50. Dellinger EP, Forsmark CE, Layer P, Levy P, Maravi-Poma E, Petrov MS, et al. Determinant-based classification of acute pancreatitis severity: an international multidisciplinary consultation. Ann Surg. 2012;256(6):875–80.
51. Howard TJ, Temple MB. Prophylactic antibiotics alter the bacteriology of infected necrosis in severe acute pancreatitis. J Am Coll Surg. 2002;195 (6):759–67.
52. Bakker OJ, van Santvoort HC, van Brunschot S, Geskus RB, Besselink MG, Bollen TL, et al. Endoscopic transgastric vs surgical necrosectomy for infected necrotizing pancreatitis: a randomized trial. JAMA. 2012;307(10):1053–61.
53. Mamlouk MD, van Sonnenberg E. Interventional radiology for necrotizing pancreatitis. J Gastrointest Surg. 2011;15(7):1101–3.
54. van Santvoort HC, Besselink MG, Bakker OJ, Hofker HS, Boermeester MA, Dejong CH, et al. A step-up approach or open necrosectomy for necrotizing pancreatitis. N Engl J Med. 2010;362(16):1491–502.

55. van Santvoort HC, Bakker OJ, Bollen TL, Besselink MG, Ahmed Ali U, Schrijver AM, et al. A conservative and minimally invasive approach to necrotizing pancreatitis improves outcome. Gastroenterology. 2011;141(4):1254–63.
56. Howard TJ. As good as it gets: the study of prophylactic antibiotics in severe acute pancreatitis. Ann Surg. 2007;245(5):684–5.
57. Fernandez-del CC. Open pancreatic necrosectomy: indications in the minimally invasive era. J Gastrointest Surg. 2011;15(7):1089–91.
58. Fink D, Soares R, Matthews JB, Alverdy JC. History, goals, and technique of laparoscopic pancreatic necrosectomy. J Gastrointest Surg. 2011;15(7):1092–7.
59. Fogel EL. Endoscopic pancreatic necrosectomy. J Gastrointest Surg. 2011;15(7):1098–100.
60. Acosta JM, Katkhouda N, Debian KA, Groshen SG, Tsao-Wei DD, Berne TV. Early ductal decompression versus conservative management for gallstone pancreatitis with ampullary obstruction: a prospective randomized clinical trial. Ann Surg. 2006;243(1):33–40.
61. Petrov MS, van Santvoort HC, Besselink MG, van der Heijden GJ, van Erpecum KJ, Gooszen HG. Early endoscopic retrograde cholangiopancreatography versus conservative management in acute biliary pancreatitis without cholangitis: a meta-analysis of randomized trials. Ann Surg. 2008;247(2):250–7.
62. Petrov MS, Correia MI, Windsor JA. Nasogastric tube feeding in predicted severe acute pancreatitis. A systematic review of the literature to determine safety and tolerance. JOP. 2008;9(4):440–8.
63. Dellinger EP, Tellado JM, Soto NE, Ashley SW, Barie PS, Dugernier T, et al. Early antibiotic treatment for severe acute necrotizing pancreatitis: a randomized, double-blind, placebo-controlled study. Ann Surg. 2007;245(5):674–83.
64. Garcia-Barrasa A, Borobia FG, Pallares R, Jorba R, Poves I, Busquets J, et al. A double-blind, placebo-controlled trial of ciprofloxacin prophylaxis in patients with acute necrotizing pancreatitis. J Gastrointest Surg. 2009;13(4):768–74.
65. Isenmann R, Runzi M, Kron M, Kahl S, Kraus D, Jung N, et al. Prophylactic antibiotic treatment in patients with predicted severe acute pancreatitis: a placebo-controlled, double-blind trial. Gastroenterology. 2004;126(4):997–1004.
66. Mazaki T, Ishii Y, Takayama T. Meta-analysis of prophylactic antibiotic use in acute necrotizing pancreatitis. Br J Surg. 2006;93(6):674–84.
67. Jiang K, Huang W, Yang XN, Xia Q. Present and future of prophylactic antibiotics for severe acute pancreatitis. World J Gastroenterol. 2012;18(3):279–84.
68. Villatoro E, Mulla M, Larvin M. Antibiotic therapy for prophylaxis against infection of pancreatic necrosis in acute pancreatitis. Cochrane Database Syst Rev (Online). 2010;12(5):CD002941.
69. Al-Omran M, Albalawi ZH, Tashkandi MF, Al-Ansary LA. Enteral versus parenteral nutrition for acute pancreatitis. Cochrane Database Syst Rev. 2010;1:CD002837.
70. Fan ST, Lai EC, Mok FP, Lo CM, Zheng SS, Wong J. Early treatment of acute biliary pancreatitis by endoscopic papillotomy. N Engl J Med. 1993;328(4):228–32.
71. Folsch UR, Nitsche R, Ludtke R, Hilgers RA, Creutzfeldt W. Early ERCP and papillotomy compared with conservative treatment for acute biliary pancreatitis. The German Study Group on Acute Biliary Pancreatitis. N Engl J Med. 1997;336(4):237–42.
72. Moretti A, Papi C, Aratari A, Festa V, Tanga M, Koch M, et al. Is early endoscopic retrograde cholangiopancreatography useful in the management of acute biliary pancreatitis? A meta-analysis of randomized controlled trials. Dig Liver Dis. 2008;40(5):379–85.
73. Neoptolemos JP, Carr-Locke DL, London NJ, Bailey IA, James D, Fossard DP. Controlled trial of urgent endoscopic retrograde cholangiopancreatography and endoscopic sphincterotomy versus conservative treatment for acute pancreatitis due to gallstones. Lancet. 1988;2(8618):979–83.
74. Oria A, Cimmino D, Ocampo C, Silva W, Kohan G, Zandalazini H, et al. Early endoscopic intervention versus early conservative management in patients with acute gallstone pancreatitis and biliopancreatic obstruction: a randomized clinical trial. Ann Surg. 2007;245(1):10–7.
75. van Santvoort HC, Besselink MG, de Vries AC, Boermeester MA, Fischer K, Bollen TL, et al. Early endoscopic retrograde cholangiopancreatography in predicted severe acute biliary pancreatitis: a prospective multicenter study. Ann Surg. 2009;250(1):68–75.
76. Besselink MG, van Santvoort HC, Buskens E, Boermeester MA, van Goor H, Timmerman HM, et al. Probiotic prophylaxis in predicted severe acute pancreatitis: a randomised, double-blind, placebo-controlled trial. Lancet. 2008;371(9613):651–9.
77. Uhl W, Buchler MW, Malfertheiner P, Beger HG, Adler G, Gaus W. A randomised, double blind, multicentre trial of octreotide in moderate to severe acute pancreatitis. Gut. 1999;45(1):97–104.
78. Bauer TW, Morris JB, Lowenstein A, Wolferth C, Rosato FE, Rosato EF. The consequences of a major bile duct injury during laparoscopic cholecystectomy. J Gastrointest Surg. 1998;2(1):61–6.
79. Csendes A, Navarrete C, Burdiles P, Yarmuch J. Treatment of common bile duct injuries during laparoscopic cholecystectomy: endoscopic and surgical management. World J Surg. 2001;25(10):1346–51.
80. McPartland KJ, Pomposelli JJ. Iatrogenic biliary injuries: classification, identification, and management. Surg Clin North Am. 2008;88(6):1329–43. 6.
81. Way LW, Stewart L, Gantert W, Liu K, Lee CM, Whang K, et al. Causes and prevention of laparoscopic bile duct injuries: analysis of 252 cases from a human factors and cognitive psychology perspective. Ann Surg. 2003;237(4):460–9.
82. Waage A, Nilsson M. Iatrogenic bile duct injury: a population-based study of 152 776 cholecystectomies in the Swedish Inpatient Registry. Arch Surg. 2006;141(12):1207–13.
83. Bektas H, Schrem H, Winny M, Klempnauer J. Surgical treatment and outcome of iatrogenic bile duct lesions after cholecystectomy and the impact of different clinical classification systems. Br J Surg. 2007;94(9):1119–27.
84. Bujanda L, Calvo MM, Cabriada JL, Orive V, Capelastegui A. MRCP in the diagnosis of iatrogenic bile duct injury. NMR Biomed. 2003;16(8):475–8.
85. Ragozzino A, De Ritis R, Mosca A, Iaccarino V, Imbriaco M. Value of MR cholangiography in patients with iatrogenic bile duct injury after cholecystectomy. AJR Am J Roentgenol. 2004;183(6):1567–72.
86. Li J, Frilling A, Nadalin S, Radunz S, Treckmann J, Lang H, et al. Surgical management of segmental and sectoral bile duct injury after laparoscopic cholecystectomy: a challenging situation. J Gastrointest Surg. 2010;14(2):344–51.
87. Strasberg SM, Helton WS. An analytical review of vasculobiliary injury in laparoscopic and open cholecystectomy. HPB (Oxford). 2011;13(1):1–14.
88. Avgerinos DV, Llaguna OH, Lo AY, Voli J, Leitman IM. Management of endoscopic retrograde cholangiopancreatography: related duodenal perforations. Surg Endosc. 2009;23(4):833–8.
89. Ercan M, Bostanci EB, Dalgic T, Karaman K, Ozogul YB, Ozer I, et al. Surgical outcome of patients with perforation after endoscopic retrograde cholangiopancreatography. J Laparoendosc Adv Surg Tech A. 2012;22(4):371–7.
90. Stapfer M, Selby RR, Stain SC, Katkhouda N, Parekh D, Jabbour N, et al. Management of duodenal perforation after endoscopic retrograde cholangiopancreatography and sphincterotomy. Ann Surg. 2000;232(2):191–8.
91. Assalia A, Suissa A, Ilivitzki A, Mahajna A, Yassin K, Hashmonai M, et al. Validity of clinical criteria in the management of endoscopic retrograde cholangiopancreatography related duodenal perforations. Arch Surg. 2007;142(11):1059–64.
92. Enns R, Eloubeidi MA, Mergener K, Jowell PS, Branch MS, Pappas TM, et al. ERCP-related perforations: risk factors and management. Endoscopy. 2002;34 (4):293–8.
93. Kwon W, Jang JY, Ryu JK, Kim YT, Yoon YB, Kang MJ, et al. Proposal of an endoscopic retrograde cholangiopancreatography-related perforation management guideline based on perforation type. J Korean Surg Soc. 2012;83(4):218–26.
94. Fatima J, Baron TH, Topazian MD, Houghton SG, Iqbal CW, Ott BJ, et al. Pancreaticobiliary and duodenal perforations after periampullary endoscopic procedures: diagnosis and management. Arch Surg. 2007;142(5):448–54. discussion 54–5.
95. Wu HM, Dixon E, May GR, Sutherland FR. Management of perforation after endoscopic retrograde cholangiopancreatography (ERCP): a population-based review. HPB (Oxford). 2006;8(5):393–9.

16

Endoscopic obstruction is associated with higher risk of acute events requiring emergency operation in colorectal cancer patients

Virote Chalieopanyarwong[1], Teeranut Boonpipattanapong[1,2], Paradee Prechawittayakul[3] and Surasak Sangkhathat[1,2*]

Abstract

Introduction: Unplanned emergency operations in colorectal cancers (CRC) are generally associated with increased risk of operative complications. This study aimed to examine the association, if any, between an endoscopic finding of obstructing tumor and the subsequent need for an emergency operation, with the aim of determining if this finding could be useful in identifying CRC cases who are more likely to require an emergency operation.

Methods: The records of CRC cases operated on in our institute during the years 2002-2011 were retrospectively reviewed regarding an endoscopic obstruction (eOB), defined as a luminal obstruction of the colon or rectum severe enough to prevent the colonoscope from passing beyond the tumor. The eOBs were analyzed against outcomes in terms of need for emergency operation, surgical complications and overall survival (OS).

Results: A total of 329 CRCs which had been operated on during the study period had complete colonoscopic data. eOB was diagnosed in 209 cases (64%). Occurrence of eOB was not correlated with clinical symptoms. Colon cancer had a higher incidence of eOB (70%) than rectal cases (50%) (p-value < 0.01). eOB was significantly associated with higher tumor size and more advanced T-stage ($p < 0.01$). Twenty-two cases (7%) had required an emergency operation before their scheduled elective surgery. The cases with eOB had a significantly higher risk of requiring an emergency operation while waiting for their scheduled procedure (p-value < 0.01), and these emergency surgeries had more post-operative complications (36%) than elective procedures (13%) (p-value 0.01) and poorer OS (p-value < 0.01).

Conclusion: Regardless of the presenting symptom, luminal obstruction severe enough to prevent further passage of a colonoscope should prompt the physician to consider an urgent surgery.

Keywords: Colorectal cancers, Colonic obstruction, Surgical waiting time, Surgical outcome

Introduction

Colorectal cancer (CRC) is one of the common cancers in which surgery plays a crucial role in the definitive management. When a diagnosis of CRC is suspected, it is recommended by the UK National Health Service that the patient should be referred within 2 weeks [1] and treatment should be performed within one month of diagnosis [2]. However, due to resource constraints, this quick response is often impossible [3], resulting in 15-30% of CRC cases require emergency surgery due to development of acute symptoms while they await their surgery [4]. Identifying CRC patients who are likely to develop acute conditions in order to have the option of considering fast-track service could reduce problems associated with prolonged waits for necessary surgeries.

Unplanned operations in patients with colorectal cancer are associated with a higher incidence of operative complications and poorer surgical outcome than non-emergency procedures [4-6], and the most common condition that leads to emergency surgery in these patients is colonic obstruction [7]. CRC patients that are at risk of

* Correspondence: surasak.sa@psu.ac.th
[1]Department of Surgery, Faculty of Medicine, Prince of Songkla University, Hat Yai, Songkhla 90110, Thailand
[2]Tumor Biology Research Unit, Faculty of Medicine, Prince of Songkla University, Hat Yai, Songkhla 90110, Thailand
Full list of author information is available at the end of the article

needing emergency surgery should, therefore, be prioritized. However, the clinical presentation of CRC patients is not always correlated with the severity of obstruction, this making the scheduling of prioritized surgeries a hit-and-miss decision at best. In this study, we aimed to look for a correlation between an endoscopic finding of tumor obstruction and the risk of needing emergency surgery in CRCs.

Methods

Histologically proven colorectal adenocarcinoma patients recorded in the Cancer Registry Unit of Songklanagarind Hospital who were operated on at the institute during the period between the years 2002 and 2011 and who had a colonoscopy before their operation were included in this retrospective review. The data were retrieved from electronic medical records and reviewed regarding clinical and pathological parameters with an emphasis on the management timeline. Access and use of clinical data were approved by the Research Ethics Committee of the Faculty of Medicine, Prince of Songkla University.

Clinical management of CRC patients who were referred to our institute as an elective case usually begins with primary diagnostic confirmation by colonoscopic biopsy, followed by an appointment for an elective colectomy. Endoscopic obstruction (eOB) is diagnosed when a standard colonoscope (11.8-13.0 millimeters diameter) is unable to pass beyond the tumor. All patients were also sent for computerized tomography of their chest and abdomen as our standard pre-operative work-up while they were waiting for their surgery. During the surgical waiting period, patients who developed an emergency condition such as colonic obstruction, bleeding or tumor rupture were immediately admitted for an emergency procedure. An on-table colonic lavage technique was used in cases of left-sided colonic obstruction. Cases with an acute condition requiring immediate surgery at their initial presentation were not included in the original study. Patients who had received a prior treatment such as a colostomy from another institute or those who received neoadjuvant therapy were also excluded. In the majority of cases, laboratory tests including complete blood count, carcinoembryonic antigen and serum albumin were performed both on the first visit and on the surgical hospitalization date 4-6 weeks later. Tumor size was measured directly from the pathological specimen. Lymph node ratio (LNR) refers to the ratio between the number of positive lymph nodes and the total number of harvested nodes. A LNR cut-off of 0.35 used to determine cases with poorer prognosis in this study analysis was derived from our previous study [6]. Post-operative follow-up assessments were done through both clinical evaluation and periodic colonoscopies every 6-12 months. Adjuvant therapy was administered when indicated and the patient was physically well enough. Hospital-based follow-up data was updated until December 2012. In cases which were lost to follow-up, survival status was determined using death registry data from the regional municipal office.

Statistical analysis used Chi-squared test and logistic regression to test for any associations between eOB and the clinical parameters we were interested in. Cox's hazard analysis was used to study association between eOB and emergency surgery. Survival outcome was analyzed in terms of overall survival (OS). Log-rank test and Kaplan-Meier survival analysis were used for survival comparison. Data are presented as hazard ratios (HR) with a 95% confidence interval (95% CI), with p-values of less than 0.05 considered statistically significant.

Results

Patients data

A total of 329 consecutive cases (191 males and 138 females) who were operated on during the study period and had complete data concerning colonoscopic findings were included in the analysis. Their mean age was 62 years with 193 patients (59%) aged more than 60 years. The primary tumor was in the rectum in 94 cases (29%), the colon in 223 cases (68%) and multiple sites in 12 cases (4%). The most common presenting symptoms were abdominal pain (29%), bowel habit change (26%) and lower gastrointestinal bleeding (26%). Decreased stool frequency was the predominating symptom in 19 cases (6%). Other pathological parameters and their association with survival are presented in Table1. The average waiting time from the first hospital visit to the operation was 35 days.

Endoscopic obstruction and factors associated with this finding

On colonoscopy, the endoscope could not be passed beyond the tumor mass in 209 cases (63%). Clinical symptoms suggestive of early obstruction including decreased stool frequency or change in bowel habit were not significantly correlated with eOB (p-values 0.64 and 0.45, respectively). Although a primary tumor situated at the right colon had a significantly lower incidence of predominating obstructive symptoms (1%) than a left-sided CRC (8%) (p-value 0.02), the right-sided tumors had a higher incidence of eOB (72%) when compared to those on the left (60%, p-value 0.047). Colonic tumors had a higher incidence of eOB (70%) than rectal tumors (50%) (p value < 0.01).

Considering tumor size, CRC with eOB had a significantly larger size (5.9 cm compared with 5.2 cm, p-value < 0.01) and a higher frequency of T3-4 lesions (91% compared to 75%, p-value < 0.01). Also, eOBs were associated with lower serum albumin level (3.7 g/dl, compared to

Table 1 Selected demographic and medical parameters and their association with 5-year overall survival (OS) and modes of surgery

		Survival probability		Emergency surgery	
Parameter	No. (cases) (%)	5-year OS (%)	Log-rank p-value	(cases) (%)	p-value
All	329	64.1	-	22 (7)	-
Sex			0.5		0.73
male	191 (58)	62.4		12 (6)	
female	138 (42)	66.5		10 (7)	
Age			0.51		0.35
< 60 years	136 (41)	66.7		7 (5)	
≥ 60 years	193 (59)	62.3		15 (8)	
Co-morbidity			0.71		0.97
Absent	193 (59)	65.5		13 (7)	
Present	136 (41)	61.7		9 (7)	
Serum CEA			< 0.01		0.32
< 5 ng/ml	144 (59)	71.1		8 (6)	
≥ 5 ng/ml	102 (41)	54.8		9 (9)	
Tumor site			0.32		0.79
Rectum	94 (29)	56.8		5 (5)	
Colon	223 (68)	66.8		16 (7)	
T			0.02		0.18
T0-2	47 (14)	75.9		1 (2)	
T3-4	282 (86)	62		22 (8)	
N			< 0.01		0.34
N0	171 (53)	78.7		9 (5)	
N1-2	152 (47)	49.4		12 (8)	
M			< 0.01		0.02
M0	281 (85)	72.1		15 (5)	
M1	48 (15)	18.5		7 (15)	
Tumor differentiation			0.16		0.77
Well/Moderate	279 (92)	64.9		18 (7)	
Poor	25 (8)	58.6		2 (8)	
Lymphovascular invasion			< 0.01		0.12
Absent	276 (84)	69		16 (6)	
Present	51 (16)	35.3		6 (12)	
Lymph node ratio			< 0.01		0.53
< 0.35	273 (86)	72.7		17 (6)	
≥ 0.35	46 (14)	23.6		4 (9)	
Endoscopic obstruction			0.73		< 0.01
Absent	120 (37)	67.2		2(2)	
Present	209 (64)	62.3		20 (10)	
Mode of operation			< 0.01		-
Elective	307 (93)	66.4		-	
Emergency	22 (7)	32.3		-	

CEA carcinoembryonic antigen.

3.9 g/dl, p-value 0.04) and lower hemoglobin level (10.5 g/dl, compared to 11.2 g/dl, p-value < 0.01) (Table 2).

Significance of endoscopic obstruction on mode of operation and outcome

Twenty-two cases (7%) required an emergency operation before their scheduled elective procedure. The emergency surgery requirement was significantly higher in eOB cases (10%), compared to those without obstruction (2%). Cases with an eOB had a significantly higher chance of requiring an emergency operation at a Cox's hazard ratio of 6.9 (95% confidence interval 1.6-29.7). Among cases with eOB, the frequency of cases requiring emergency surgery was not significantly different between rectal cases (9%) and colonic cases (10%) (p-value 0.8). The median time from colonoscopy to operation in the emergency cases was 14 days. The cumulative incidences of emergency surgery in all cases at 15, 30 and 60 days of surgical waiting were 3%, 5% and 9%, respectively (Figure 1). The 60-day cumulative emergency operation rate was 14% in those with an obstructing tumor, compared to 3% in cases in which an endoscope could be passed beyond the tumor (p-value < 0.01). The reasons for the emergency surgery included complete colonic obstruction presenting as abdominal pain, vomiting and obstipation in 20 cases and 1 case each of gastrointestinal bleeding and tumor perforation. The emergency procedure was a definitive colorectal resection in all 22 cases. Patients who underwent emergency surgery had a higher incidence of distant metastasis (32% compared to 13% in elective cases, p-value 0.02).

Table 2 Association between selected clinicopathological parameters and endoscopic obstruction

Parameter	No. (cases) (%)	Endoscopic obstruction (%)	p-value
All	329	120 (37)	-
Tumor site			< 0.01
Rectum	94 (29)	47 (50)	
Colon	223 (68)	155 (70)	
Tumor side			0.047
Left colon and rectum	224 (68)	135 (60)	
Right colon	93 (28)	67 (72)	
serum CEA			0.31
< 5 ng/ml	144 (59)	87 (60)	
≥ 5 ng/ml	102 (41)	68 (67)	
Tumor size			< 0.01
< 5.5 cm	181 (57)	104 (57)	
≥ 5.5 cm	136 (43)	98 (72)	
T			< 0.01
T0-2	47 (14)	18 (38)	
T3-4	282 (86)	191 (68)	
N			0.90
N0	171 (53)	108 (63)	
N1-2	152 (47)	97 (64)	
M			0.07
M0	281 (85)	173 (61)	
M1	48 (15)	36 (75)	
Tumor differentiation			0.63
Well/Moderate	279 (92)	181 (64)	
Poor	25 (8)	15 (60)	
Lymphovascular invasion			0.18
Absent	276 (84)	179 (64)	
Present	51 (16)	28 (59)	

CEA carcinoembryonic antigen.

Operative complications occurred in 48 cases (15%). Patients who underwent an emergency operation had a higher rate of post-operative complications (36%) than those who had surgery according to their elective schedule (13%, p-value < 0.01). (Table 3) On survival analysis, although eOB was not directly associated with overall survival, requiring emergency operation had a statistically significant impact on poorer overall survival (p-value < 0.01).

Discussion

Previous studies have suggested that CRCs that present with acute symptoms and require emergency surgery have more aggressive behavior and higher tumor stages [4,8]. Consistent with those findings, our study found that CRC patients who underwent emergency surgery had a more advanced stage tumor, which may partly explain the poorer survival. In addition, unplanned emergency operations are inferior to elective surgeries in terms of inadequate control of any underlying co-morbidities. For these reasons, it could be expected that procedures done in an emergency setting post a higher risk of operative complications. Obstruction and perforation are common problems that bring CRC patients to an emergency surgery before their scheduled surgery [5,7,9]. The number of emergency surgeries in our series was relatively lower than other previous reports [4,5,7-9], which might be explained by the fact that we did not include cases who first presented with emergency conditions in our analysis.

Providing fast-track service for these higher risk CRC patients may help in reducing acute events that require emergency surgery and its related higher morbidity [10]. Our study found that clinical symptoms alone were not adequate in determining such high-risk patients, especially when the tumor was situated on the right colon. The pre-operative colonoscopy is an objective study that should be performed in all cases suspected of CRC, as in addition to a tissue biopsy for histological confirmation of malignancy, severity of luminal obstruction can be

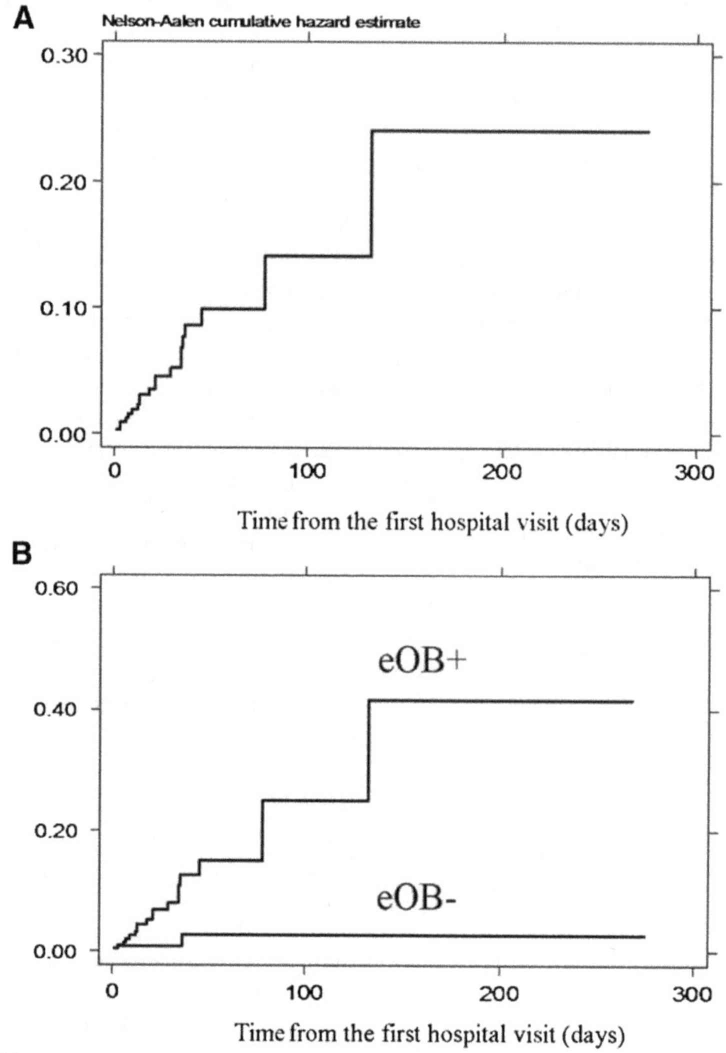

Figure 1 Probability of requiring an emergency operation A: overall B: comparing between cases with and without endoscopic obstruction.

evaluated. We also found that a luminal obstruction was associated with larger tumor size and T-stage, but not histological grade. Moreover, eOB was also correlated with poorer nutritional status in our cases, as evidenced by lower serum albumin and hemoglobin. Above all, the evidence of eOB was associated with required emergency surgery. Overall, the data from our study suggest that patients with eOB should be reevaluated carefully and considered for fast-track urgent surgery. The average surgical waiting time in the study CRC cases was 35 days. If all of our cases are considered as on the same elective list, 10% of cases with eOB and 2% of non-eOB cases required an emergency operation. However, if the patients with eOB had been scheduled for surgery within 2 weeks of their first hospital visit, the overall number of emergency surgeries would have been reduced to 5%.

Table 3 Post-operative complications according to mode of surgery (some cases had more than one complication)

	Emergency (N:22)	Elective (N:307)
Wound infection	5 (23%)	13 (4%)
Wound dehiscence/evisceration	2 (9%)	5 (2%)
Anastomotic leakage/fistula	2 (9%)	10 (3%)
Intestinal obstruction	0 (0%)	5 (2%)
Other (collection, seroma, etc.)	1 (5%)	10 (3%)

Use of a self-expandible metallic stent as a bridge-to -surgery method has been recently proposed, not only as a time-buying strategy, but also to allow for more adequate pre-operative staging and bowel preparation [11]. The stent procedure has one notable technical limitation, however, in that it can be applied only for an obstruction in the left colon and rectum. Although various retrospective case series have reported the benefits of this intervention [12-14], there are yet no good quality data to support its clinical advantage over emergency surgery.

In conclusion, our study found that a luminal obstruction detected by endoscopy was significantly associated with locally advanced tumor. This group of CRC patients had a higher risk of requiring an unplanned operation. The data suggest that this endoscopic finding should be regarded as an indication that these patients should be considered for fast-track surgical scheduling list.

Competing interests

The authors declare that they have no competing interests.

Authors' contribution

VC initiated the research project and collected all data. TB provided clinical data and reviewed the quality of data collection. PP provided community based follow-up data. SS managed the project, analyzed data and prepared the manuscript draft. All authors read and approved the final manuscript.

Acknowledgements

The authors thank the Medical Records Unit, Songklanagarind Hospital for their assistance in retrieving the archived patient records. Dave Patterson of the International Affair Unit, Faculty of Medicine, Prince of Songkla University, offered editorial suggestions for the English in the manuscript.

Author details

[1]Department of Surgery, Faculty of Medicine, Prince of Songkla University, Hat Yai, Songkhla 90110, Thailand. [2]Tumor Biology Research Unit, Faculty of Medicine, Prince of Songkla University, Hat Yai, Songkhla 90110, Thailand. [3]Cancer Registry Unit, Songklanagarind Hospital, Faculty of Medicine, Prince of Songkla University, Hat Yai, Songkhla 90110, Thailand.

References

1. Department of Health: *The NHS Cancer Plan*. London: Department of Health; 2000.
2. Duff SE, Wood C, McCredie V, Levine E, Saunders MP, O'Dwyer ST: **Waiting times for treatment of rectal cancer in North West England.** *J R Soc Med* 2004, **97**:117–118.
3. Hanna SJ, Muneer A, Khalil KH: **The 2-week wait for suspected cancer: time for a rethink?** *Int J Clin Pract* 2005, **59**:1334–1339.
4. Wong SK, Jalaludin BB, Morgan MJ, Berthelsen AS, Morgan A, Gatenby AH, Fulham SB: **Tumor pathology and long-term survival in emergency colorectal cancer.** *Dis Colon Rectum* 2008, **51**:223–230.
5. Bass G, Fleming C, Conneely J, Martin Z, Mealy K: **Emergency first presentation of colorectal cancer predicts significantly poorer outcomes: a review of 356 consecutive Irish patients.** *Dis Colon Rectum* 2009, **52**:678–684.
6. Kritsanasakul A, Boonpipattanapong T, Wanitsuwan W, Phukaoloun M, Prechawittayakul P, Sangkhathat S: **Impact of lymph node retrieval on surgical outcomes in colorectal cancers.** *J Surg Oncol* 2012, **106**:238–242.
7. Cuffy M, Abir F, Audisio RA, Longo WE: **Colorectal cancer presenting as surgical emergencies.** *Surg Oncol* 2004, **13**:149–157.
8. Ghazi S, Berg E, Lindblom A, Lindforss U, Low-Risk Colorectal Cancer Study Group: **Clinicopathological analysis of colorectal cancer: a comparison between emergency and elective surgical cases.** *World J Surg Oncol* 2013, **11**:133.
9. Chen HS, Sheen-Chen SM: **Obstruction and perforation in colorectal adenocarcinoma: an analysis of prognosis and current trends.** *Surgery* 2000, **127**:370–376.
10. Scott MA, Knight A, Brown K, Novell JR: **A single common urgent pathway for all colorectal referrals reduces time to diagnosis and treatment.** *Colorectal Dis* 2006, **8**:766–771.
11. Baik SH, Kim NK, Cho HW, Lee KY, Sohn SK, Cho CH, Kim TI, Kim WH: **Clinical outcomes of metallic stent insertion for obstructive colorectal cancer.** *Hepatogastroenterol* 2006, **53**:183–187.
12. Ng KC, Law WL, Lee YM, Choi HK, Seto CL, Ho JW: **Self-expanding metallic stent as a bridge to surgery versus emergency resection for obstructing left-sided colorectal cancer: a case-matched study.** *J Gastrointest Surg* 2006, **10**:798–803.
13. van Hooft JE, Bemelman WA, Oldenburg B, Marinelli AW, Holzik MF, Grubben MJ, Sprangers MA, Dijkgraaf MG, Fockens P, collaborative Dutch Stent-in study group: **Colonic stenting versus emergency surgery for acute left-sided malignant colonic obstruction: a multicentre randomised trial.** *Lancet Oncol* 2011, **12**:344–352.
14. Zhang Y, Shi J, Shi B, Song CY, Xie WF, Chen YX: **Self-expanding metallic stent as a bridge to surgery versus emergency surgery for obstructive colorectal cancer: a meta-analysis.** *Surg Endosc* 2012, **26**:110–119.

17

Emergency surgery due to diaphragmatic hernia

Mario Testini[1*], Antonia Girardi[1], Roberta Maria Isernia[1], Angela De Palma[2], Giovanni Catalano[1], Angela Pezzolla[3] and Angela Gurrado[1]

Abstract

Background: Congenital diaphragmatic hernia (CDH) is a congenital abnormality, rare in adults with a frequency of 0.17–6%. Diaphragmatic rupture is an infrequent consequence of trauma, occurring in about 5% of severe closed thoraco-abdominal injuries. Clinical presentation ranges from asymptomatic cases to serious respiratory or gastrointestinal symptoms. Diagnosis depends on anamnesis, clinical signs and radiological investigations.

Methods: From May 2013 to June 2016, six cases (four females, two males; mean age 58 years) of diaphragmatic hernia were admitted to our Academic Department of General Surgery with respiratory and abdominal symptoms. Chest X-ray, barium studies and CT scan were performed.

Results: Case 1 presented left diaphragmatic hernia containing transverse and descending colon. Case 2 showed left CDH which allowed passage of stomach, spleen and colon. Case 3 and 6 showed stomach in left hemithorax. Case 4 presented left diaphragmatic hernia which allowed passage of the spleen, left lobe of liver and transverse colon. Case 5 had stomach and spleen herniated into the chest. Emergency surgery was always performed. The hernia contents were reduced and defect was closed with primary repair or mesh. In all cases, post-operative courses were uneventful.

Conclusion: Overlapping abdominal and respiratory symptoms lead to diagnosis of diaphragmatic hernia, in patients with or without an history of trauma. Chest X-ray, CT scan and barium studies should be done to evaluate diaphragmatic defect, size, location and contents. Emergency surgical approach is mandatory reducing morbidity and mortality.

Keyword: Congenital diaphragmatic hernia, Diaphragmatic rupture, Mesh, Emergency surgery, Laparotomy, Thoracotomy

Background

Congenital diaphragmatic hernia (CDH) is an abnormality found in 1/2500 newborns, with a survival rate of 67% [1]. A primary characterization of CDH is that the diaphragm fails to form properly during embryogenesis. This incomplete formation of the diaphragm allows abdominal contents to herniate into the chest creating a mass-like effect that impedes lung development. Clinical presentation ranges from asymptomatic cases to serious respiratory or gastrointestinal symptoms, and sometimes haemodynamic instability. The broad spectrum of severity in patients with CDH is dependent on the degree of pulmonary hypoplasia and pulmonary hypertension. Posterolateral hernias (*Bochdalek* hernias) are the most common hernia type (>80%) with the majority occurring on the left side (85%), less frequently on the right side (13%) or bilateral (2%) [2].

Diaphragmatic rupture (DR) is an infrequent complication of trauma that occurs during 5% of trauma, including vehicle accidents [3–5]. Diagnosis is usually delayed; patients may be asymptomatic for years after trauma, until complications occur. Traumatic rupture of the diaphragm is considered an indication for surgical repair, especially in symptomatic patients [6].

However, there is no consensus on the absolute indications to surgery and about the timing. The onset of complications carries highest mortality and morbidity rates; therefore, it makes emergency surgery mandatory. During the past decades, primary suture repair or covering the defect with a synthetic mesh has been the

* Correspondence: mario.testini@uniba.it
[1]Unit of Endocrine, Digestive, and Emergency Surgery, Department of Biomedical Sciences and Human Oncology, University Medical School "Aldo Moro" of Bari, Bari, Italy
Full list of author information is available at the end of the article

standard procedures. More recently, biologic meshes have been thought to be effective in closing the diaphragmatic defect, inducing limited inflammatory response and minimizing adhesion formation [7]. Laparotomy or thoracotomy are the traditional treatments for patients with DR. Moreover, laparoscopic approaches for repair of hernias have recently gained in popularity [8]. Robotic approach is not yet described as effective approach in emergency, and it is reported in literature in only one case [9] in elective surgery.

This paper includes the surgical experience of congenital or traumatic diaphragmatic hernia of a surgical unit in emergency setting and reports the literature.

Methods

Six cases of diaphragmatic hernia were observed in emergency at our Academic Department, with respiratory and abdominal symptoms. No breath sounds were detected in the left chest area, but bowel sounds were audible. Emergency surgery was performed in all cases. The hernia contents were reduced, and the defect was closed with primary repair or mesh.

Case 1: A 63-year-old woman was admitted with complaints of bowel obstruction and dyspnoea. Anamnesis revealed chronic abdominal pain, mental retardation and strabismus. In the physical examination, no breath sounds were detected in the left chest area; however, bowel sounds were audible. Chest X-ray and barium enema showed the transverse colon displaced into the left hemithorax above the splenic flexure. Computed tomography suggested collapse of the lung and the mediastinal shift towards the right. The left diaphragmatic hernia contained the transverse and descending colon (Fig. 1a). Emergency laparotomy was performed, and a left diaphragm agenesis, mega colon (diameter 10 cm) and left liver agenesis were found. An intra-operative bronchoscopy revealed hypoplasia of the left lung (Fig. 1b). A subtotal colectomy with ileo-rectal anastomosis was performed, and primary repair of diaphragm was done. The post-operative course was uneventful, and the patient was discharged on the 15th post-operative day. The research of abnormalities of the karyotype, phenotype and genetic pattern was negative for all the known congenital syndromes.

Case 2: A 50-year-old woman was admitted with complaints of dyspnoea, chest and abdominal pain. No breath sounds were detected in the left chest area. There was no history of trauma. Chest X-ray revealed mediastinal shift towards the right and bowel gas in the left chest. CT scan showed large annular diaphragmatic defect which allowed passage of the stomach, spleen and colon (Fig. 2). An emergency combined chest-abdominal approach was performed, and contents were reduced repairing the defect with *Mersilene* mesh®. Thoracotomy approach was used to release the thoracic dense adhesion between the chest and the abdominal contents. Before placing the mesh, the anaesthesiologist increased the tidal volume to expand the collapsed left lower lobe of the lung and a chest drain was placed in the left pleural space. Immediate post-operative chest X-ray showed expansion of the left lung with minimal pleural effusion. Post-operative course was uneventful, and post-operative stay was 13 days.

Case 3: A 73-year-old woman arrived with complaint of breathlessness and dysphagia. No history of trauma was evident in anamnesis. Her current medical history included hypertension and hypothyroidism. Chest X-ray and barium studies demonstrated the presence of stomach in left hemithorax. CT scan revealed the presence of large diaphragmatic hernia which allowed the stomach

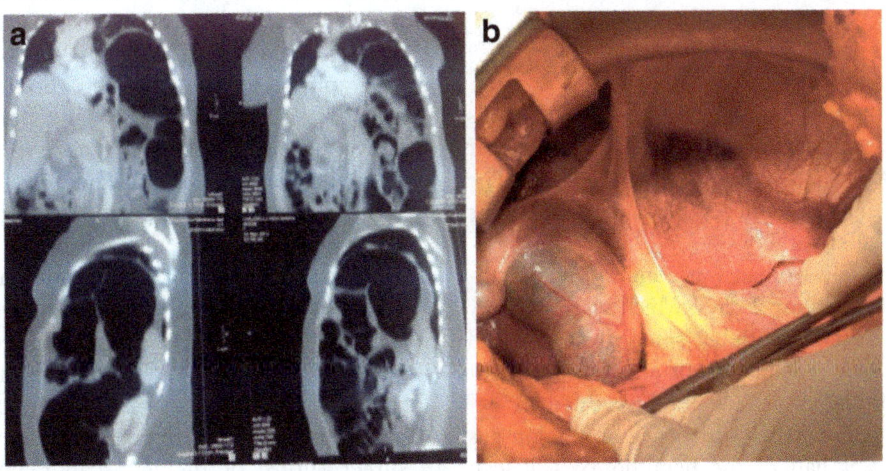

Fig. 1 **a** CT scan shows collapse of the lung and the mediastinal shift towards to the *right side*. The *left* diaphragmatic hernia contained the transverse and descending colon. **b** Intraoperative evidence: diaphragmatic defect allows migration of viscera

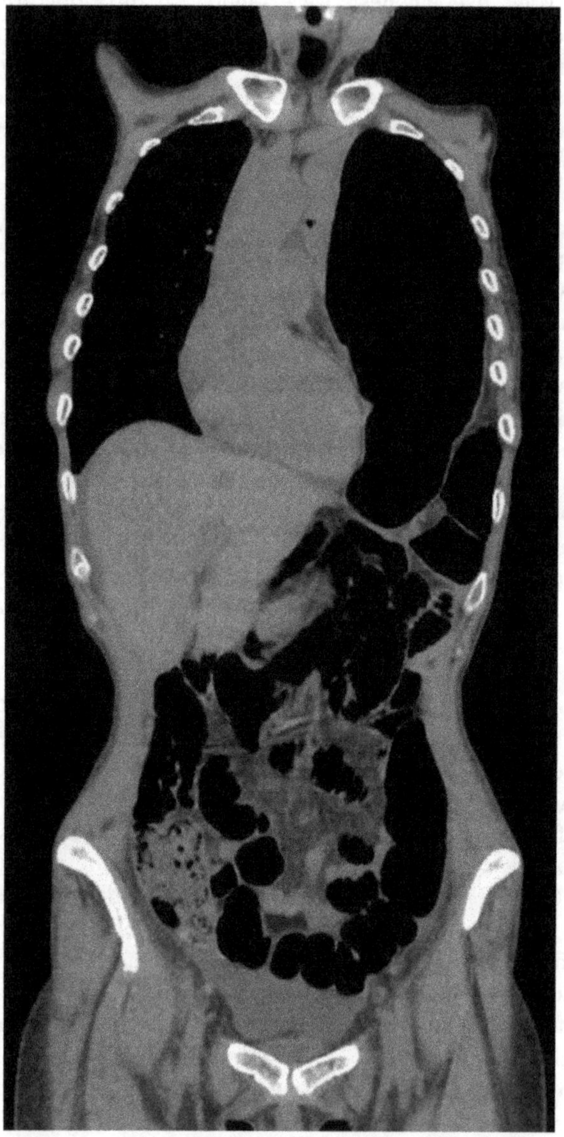

Fig. 2 CT scan shows in *left side*, large diaphragmatic defect which allows passage of the stomach, spleen and colon (referred to as *Bochdalek* hernias) and complete collapse of left lung

to herniate into the chest. Emergency laparoscopy was performed; hernia contents were reduced; and a repair of the defect with *Proceed* mesh® was done (Fig. 3). The post-operative course was uneventful, and patient was discharged 7 days after surgery.

Case 4: A 63-year-old woman was admitted with complaints of breathlessness for 2 days, which was gradually progressive and associated with left-sided chest pain and a dry cough. There was a history of a vehicle accident 6 years ago. The initial chest radiograph revealed an elevated left hemi diaphragm with presence of a colon gas shadow in the lower half of the hemithorax. CT scan suggested left diaphragmatic hernia which allowed passage of the spleen, left lobe of liver and transverse colon (Fig. 4a). Surgery was performed in emergency, reducing contents and repairing the defect with biological mesh (Fig. 4b; *Tutomesh, bovine pericardium mesh*®). The patient was discharged on the 10th post-operative day, without complications.

Case 5: A 50-year-old man was involved in a work accident. He was managed in accordance with *Advanced Trauma Life Support* protocol. He arrived in the emergency room with decreased breath sounds on the left side, dyspnoea, fever, left hypochondrium hematoma, subcutaneous emphysema, and chest and abdominal pain. His current medical history included obesity and treated hypertension. Initial chest radiography and barium studies demonstrated stomach in the left hemithorax. CT scan revealed stomach and spleen in left hemithorax, consistent with a traumatic diaphragmatic rupture with complete disruption of all muscular layers, collar sign and multiple rib fractures, fractured left humerus and scapula (Fig. 5a, b). At exploratory laparotomy, traumatic defect in the left diaphragm was found, with stomach and spleen in the left thorax (Fig. 5c). The hernia contents were reduced and the defect was closed with biologic mesh *(Tutomesh bovine pericardium mesh*®). Post-operatively, the patient was placed in an intensive care unit. He was transferred from the ICU on the 8th post-operative day and discharged on the 20th day.

Case 6 [10]: A 51-year-old man, referred to a history of 5 months of dyspnea, abdominal pain, nausea and vomiting. These symptoms had increased in severity during the previous 2 weeks. Anamnesis revealed left splenopancreatectomy 4 years earlier for non-*Hodgkin's* lymphoma. The physical examination revealed a moderate peritoneal effusion without a peritoneal reaction. The introduction of a nasogastric tube remarkably improved symptoms. The chest X-ray showed a large fluid level beneath an apparently raised left hemi diaphragm (Fig. 6a) hypothesizing a left hemi diaphragmatic rupture with gastric herniation; diagnosis was confirmed by barium studies and a thoracic-abdominal computed tomography. An emergency left thoracotomy was performed, revealing a volvulus of the stomach, with some intestinal loops. Part of the transverse colon was incarcerated herniating through the torn diaphragm. The hernia was localized into the posterior side of the left hemi diaphragm with a diameter of 12 cm. During surgery, dense adhesions between the herniated organs and the left pleura-lung, as well as a marked reduction in left lung volume and an inflammatory mass in the greater omentum adherent to the diaphragm, were found. Thus, a reduction of the volvulus, an adhesiolysis and a resection of the mass were performed. Finally, a direct suture of the left diaphragmatic defect was employed (Fig. 6b, c). The patient had an uneventful recovery and histology showed Hodgki's lymphoma.

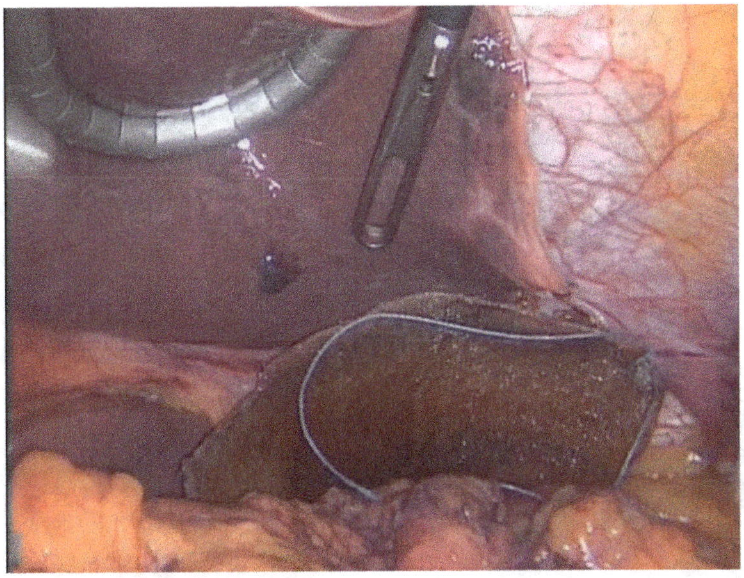

Fig. 3 Laparoscopic image during correction of defect with synthetic mesh

Review of the literature

A systematic review was performed by consulting PubMed/MEDLINE from 1983 to 2017 using the terms "emergency surgery", associated with "traumatic diaphragmatic rupture", and "congenital diaphragmatic hernia". The search returned 555 papers (Fig. 7). Three hundred twenty-three publications were excluded because these articles were not written in English ($N = 87$), presented cases in childhood (<19 years old; $N = 178$) or were not interesting human species ($N = 58$); 32 papers were excluded because regarded hiatal hernia, 40 paraesophageal hernia and 59 elective setting. Consequently, the full texts of 101 articles were assessed for eligibility: the ethiopathogenesis was traumatic in 697 patients and congenital in 38 (Table 1).

Pathogenetic mechanism

Diaphragmatic rupture with abdominal organ herniation was first described in 1541 by *Sennertus* [11]. Congenital diaphragmatic hernias are prenatally or during the neonatal period diagnosed. On the contrary, CDH in adulthood are exceedingly rare and can occur through an anterior parasternal *Morgagni* foramen or through a posterolateral, mainly left-sided, named as Bochdalek hernia, firstly described in 1848 [12]. The aetiology is still under study, but the disease is due to the failure of closure of the canal between the *septum transversum* and the oesophagus during the 8th week of gestation. Morgagni hernia is a rare disease caused by the defective development of the sternal attachments to the diaphragm. Traumatic diaphragmatic hernias are thought to be produced by a sudden increase in the pleuroperitoneal pressure gradient occurring at areas of potential weakness along embryological points of fusion [13].

DR usually result from blunt or penetrating injuries or iatrogenic causes and result in entry of an abdominal hollow viscus or the omentum into the pleural cavity, which may lead to incarceration and even strangulation with a fatal outcome. Traumatic diaphragmatic hernias are frequently caused by a penetrating injury (10–19%), sometimes by blunt thoracic-abdominal trauma (5%) [14, 15]. Moreover, some authors described rare and particularly cases of DR after surgery or pregnancy; that is Sano A. et al. reported a case of a pregnant woman in the 28th week of pregnancy, who was underwent to emergency caesarean section and repair of the diaphragm [16]; Moussa G. et al., described a right DR in a patient with previous history of window fenestration and sarcoidosis [17]; Nakamura T. et al., reported a case of right DR in patient with a history of hepatic carcinoma treated with radiofrequency ablation [18]. Furthermore, there was an association between Marfan's syndrome and CDH as *Barakat* et al. reported [19].

Site of rupture

CDH formation is found 80% on the left side [20]. Also, 88–95% of diaphragmatic ruptures occurred on the left side [21], especially, blunt trauma causes large diaphragmatic defects, commonly involving (>80%) the left posterolateral diaphragm [22]. The right haemidiaphragm is stronger than the left one because of the size of the liver which has a protective effect. For this reason, the side ruptures are very rare and associated with high mortality and morbidity rate [23].

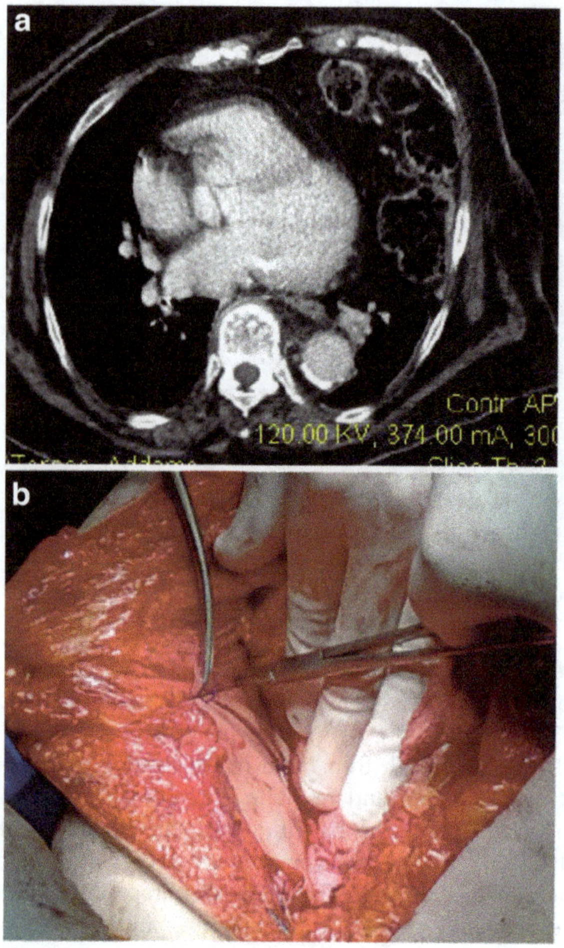

Fig. 4 **a** CT scan suggests *left* diaphragmatic hernia which allowed migration of colon in *left* chest. **b** Intraoperatively, biological mesh repairing defect

The review of literature reported in this study confirmed the high frequency of left defect 80%, and only two cases of bilateral DR were reported.

Presenting symptom and investigations

Nayak et al. described severe symptoms, in 46% of CDH cases with 32% of mortality due to visceral strangulation [24]. Moreover, the literature analysis shows a variable rate of delayed symptoms (5–45.5%) [25, 26]. Late-presenting CDH of left sided typically produces acute, obstructive, gastrointestinal symptoms, chronic dyspnea, chest pain, recurrent abdominal pain, postprandial fullness and vomiting, evolving to cardiorespiratory failure [27]. Indeed, right-sided CDH is usually associated with only respiratory issues because partial liver displacement may block the further herniation of hollow viscera [1]. Although the presence of bowel sounds within the chest and the absence of breath sounds are typical findings associated with a CDH, a misdiagnosis rate of 38% has

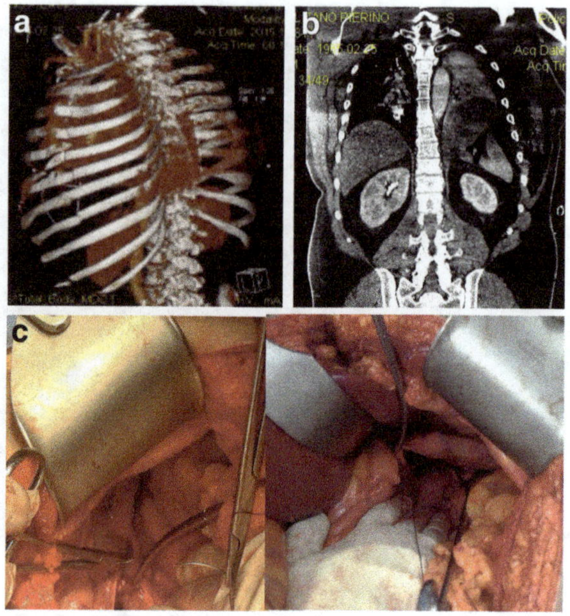

Fig. 5 **a** 3D-CT scan shows rib fractures. **b** CT scan shows stomach and spleen in the *left* hemi-thorax, complete disruption of all muscular layers. **c** Intraoperatively, repair of traumatic defect in the *left* diaphragm

been reported [28]. Obviously, in totally asymptomatic cases, diagnosis is very hard. On the contrary, when acute presentations occur because of the increasing of abdominal pressure and consequent rapid visceral displacement into the chest or due to rapid distension of previously herniated viscera, diagnosis is clear [29, 30].

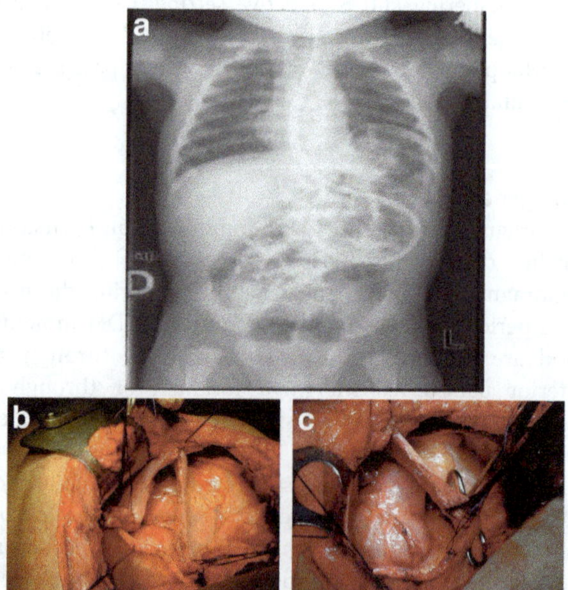

Fig. 6 **a** X-ray shows herniated stomach into the chest. **b** Thoracotomy shows large diaphragmatic defect. **c** Repair of defect

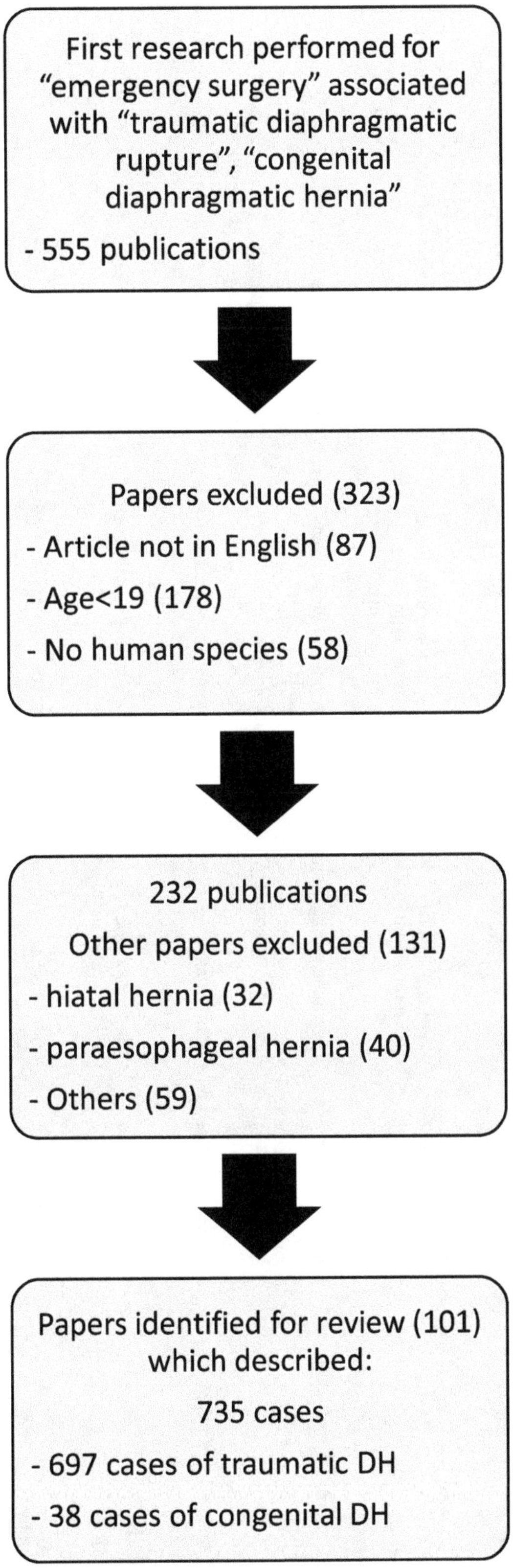

Fig. 7 Flow chart of the literature selection process

Chest X-ray and barium studies are useful for determining which viscera have herniated into the thorax. The most common reported radiological finding of CDH is the opaqueness of the hemithorax usually associated with mediastinal shift to the contralateral side. Moreover, the position of the nasogastric tube in the chest cavity will provide an important indicator and prompt correct diagnosis. Computed tomography can be considered the *gold standard* technique for diagnosis, offering the unique opportunity to evaluate the presence, size and location of a diaphragmatic defect, as well as the contents of various types of diaphragmatic hernias [31] and showing sensitivity and specificity of 14–82% and 87%, respectively [32]. MRI is also useful, but usually it is not performable in emergency. However, it is usually employed in stable patients or where the CT scan is equivocal [33]. According with literature, in this reported experience, a definitive diagnosis was made with CT scan and barium studies.

Late-presenting CDH is considered as a benign condition but it can rapidly becomes a life-threatening disease [1, 27, 28, 31, 33]; consequently, an immediate surgical treatment is mandatory. Associated anomalies in late-presenting CDH patients, such as congenital heart disease, *Fryns* syndrome and trisomy 18, have been reported in 8.6–80% of cases [1, 2, 27, 28], significantly increasing the mortality rate. At this proposal, in case 1, even if there was a high suspicion of congenital syndrome, surprisingly it was not confirmed by genetic studies.

Surgical treatment

Surgical repair typically involves primary or patch closure of the diaphragm through an open abdominal approach. When the diagnosis is delayed, due to suspicions of adhesions between viscera and chest, thoracotomy or combined thoracic-abdominal approach is preferred, as in the reported case 2. Some authors have reported success with thoracoscopic approach but vitiated by an increased incidence of hernia recurrence [34–36]. Furthermore, during thoracoscopy, an intraoperative pulmonary hypertension with subsequent hemodynamic instability could develop; moreover, the placement and management of a patch results in substantially longer operating times. For these reasons, thoracoscopic repair of CDH is preferred in the presence of small diaphragmatic defects and/or mild pulmonary hypertension [37]. Nowadays, the laparoscopic approach is safe and feasible for CDH and it could be an excellent option [37], as in case 3.

However, emergency surgery is the treatment of choice for diaphragmatic rupture. In delayed cases, thoracic approach is recommended to reduce viscera-pleural adhesions and to avoid intra-thoracic visceral perforation

Table 1 Review of literature showing demographics data, diagnosis and treatment

Authors, references	Number of patient, sex, age (years)	Aetiology	Diagnosis	Treatment	Type of hernia	Herniated organs
Lu J et al. Medicine 2016 [41]	1, M, 51	Traffic accident	Barium enema CT scan	Splenectomy	Left hemi diaphragm	Splenic flexure of the colon
	1, M, 45	Traffic accident	Chest X-ray, gastrografin contrast	Splenectomy	Left hemi diaphragm	Stomach and small bowel
	1, M, 47	Traffic accident	Chest X-ray, gastrografin contrast	Splenectomy	Left hemi diaphragm	Stomach and omentum
	1, M, 30	Traffic accident	Chest X-ray, Gastrografin contrast	Nonoperative treatment	Left hemi diaphragm	Stomach and omentum
	1, M, 33	Traffic accident	Chest X-ray, gastrografin contrast	Nonoperative treatment	Left hemi diaphragm	Stomach and omentum
	1, M, 29	Penetrating injury	Chest X-ray, gastrografin contrast	Nonoperative treatment	Left hemi diaphragm	Stomach and omentum
Manabu Harada, Int J Surg Case Rep. 2016 [42]	1, M, 78	Bochdalek hernia	Chest radiography and computed tomography	Laparoscopic Primary closure	Left hemi diaphragm	Omentum, transverse colon, and small intestine
De la Cour CD; Ugeskr Laeger. 2016 [43]	1, F, 27	Partum	Chest radiography and computed tomography	Primary closure	Left hemi diaphragm	
Razi K; J Surg Case Rep. 2016 [44]	1, F, 83	Morgagni hernia	Chest radiography and computed tomography	Mesh closure	Left hemi diaphragm	Transverse colon, greater curvature of the stomach and a partial gastric volvulus
Manson HJ Ann R Coll Surg Engl. 2016 [45]	1, F, 30	Bochdalek hernia	Chest radiography and computed tomography	Total gastrectomy with primary Roux-en-Y reconstruction, splenectomy and insertion of a feeding jejunostomy	Left hemi diaphragm	Gangrenous stomach and spleen, cardiac arrest
Massloom HS; N Am J Med Sci. 2016. [46]	1, M, 50	Bochdalek hernia	Computed tomography	Laparotomy and thoracotomy for repairing of defect	Left hemi diaphragm	Bowel
Kumar, J Surg Case Rep. 2016 [47]	1, M, 80	Morgagni hernia	Computed tomography	Laparotomy primary suture	Left hemi diaphragm	Gastric outlet obstruction
Manipadam JMJ Clin Diagn Res. 2016 [48]	1, M, 23	Bochdalek hernia	Chest X-ray	Laparotomy, sleeve resection of the gangrenous portion of the stomach	Left hemi diaphragm	Organoaxial volvulus of the stomach
Harada M, Int J Surg Case Rep. 2016 [49]	1, M, 78	Bochdalek hernia	Chest radiography and computed tomography	laparoscopic repair with primary closure	Left hemi diaphragm	Omentum, transverse colon, and small intestine
Siow SL; J Med Case Rep. 2016 [50]	1, M, 32	Traffic accident	Computed tomographic scan	Laparoscopic surgery with synthetic mesh repair	Left hemi diaphragm	

Table 1 Review of literature showing demographics data, diagnosis and treatment *(Continued)*

A.L. Andreev JSLS 2010 [51]	1, M, 40	Traffic accident 12 years earlier	CT scan	Laparoscopic primary suture	Left hemi diaphragm	Large intestine and greater omentum and acute colon obstruction
	1, M, 46	Surgery for a stab wound to the chest with injury to the heart 5 months before	Chest X-ray	Laparoscopic primary suture	Left hemi diaphragm	Transverse colonic segment
Bhatt NR, Trauma Mon. 2016 [52]	1, M, 23	Multitrauma 2 y before	Chest X-ray and CT scan	Laparotomy, adhesiolisis and primary repair	Left hemi diaphragm	Small bowel, omentum and large bowel obstruction
Abdullah M, Stonelake P BMJ case rep 2016 [53]	1, F 65	Trauma	Chest X-ray, CT scan	Emergency operation, laparotomy	Left hemi diaphragm	Perforated colon
Razi K; Journal of Surgical Case Reports, 2016 [54]	1, F, 83	Diaphragmatic Morgagni Hernia	Chest X-ray and CT scan	Laparoscopic repair with a composite mesh with an absorbable tic fixation on the diaphragm	Left hemi diaphragm	Transverse colon, the greater curvature of the stomach with a partial gastric volvulus
A Wigley J Ann R Coll Surg Engl 2014 [55]	1, F, 72	Traffic accident				
Atef Mejri Medicine 2015 [56]	1, M, 56	Bochdalek hernia	Chest X-ray, barium studies and CT scan	Primary repair Laparoscopy was converted laparotomy	Left hemi diaphragm	Gastric volvulus
Mahmut Tokur Ulus Travma Acil Cerrahi Derg, July 2015 [57]	1, F, 27	Congenital DH	Chest X-ray, CT scan	Thoracotomy, primary repair	Left hemi diaphragm	Gastro thorax
Topuz Mustafa Ulus Travma Acil Cerrahi Derg. 2014 [58]	1, F, 55	Traffic accident	Chest X-ray, CT scan	Laparotomy primary repair	Right hemi diaphragm	Liver causing mechanic compression on ventricle
Moussa G Ann R Coll Surg Engl. 2014 [17]	1, F, 65	Previous history of pericardial window fenestration and sarcoidosis	Chest X-ray, CT scan	Laparoscopy, mesh repair	Right hemi diaphragm	Left lobe of liver, stomach and colon
Nakamura T, Ulus Travma Acil Cerrahi Derg. 2014 [18]	1, M, 81	History of HCC treated with Radiofrequency ablation	Chest US, CT scan	Laparotomy, primary hernia repair, small bowel resection	Right hemi diaphragm	Liver, incarcerated small bowel
Haratake Naoki Surgery today 2015 [59]	1, F, 50		CT scan	Laparotomy, primary hernia repair	Right hemi diaphragm	Heterotopic endometriosis in a patient with Chilaiditi syndrome
Gali BM, Niger J Med. 2014 [60]	1, M, 28	Penetrating injury years before	CT scan	Laparotomy, primary repair	Left hemi diaphragm	Bowel

Table 1 Review of literature showing demographics data, diagnosis and treatment *(Continued)*

Michael Joseph Newman, BMJ Case Rep 2014 [61]	1, M, 25	Bochdalek hernia	Chest X-ray, CT scan	Laparotomy, primary repair, gastric resection	Left hemi diaphragm	Stomach and bowel
Tyagi Sam, Ann Thorac Surg. 2014 [62]	1, M, 36	Morgagni hernia	Chest X-ray, CT scan	Laparoscopy Gore-Tex fixed with a spiral tacker	Left hemi diaphragm	Omentum and transverse colon
Kurniawan N, Acta Chir Belg. 2013 [32]	1, M, 17	Bochdalek hernia	Chest X-ray, CT scan	Laparoscopy primary sutture	Left hemidiaphragm	Stomach, spleen colon
Ota H Ann Thorac Cardiovasc Surg. 2014 [63]	1, M, 62	Fall accident	ECO FAST, Chest X-ray, CT scan	Video assisted mini thoracotomy Primary suture	Right hemi diaphragm	Hemothorax
G, et al. BMJ Case Rep 2013 [64]	1, M, 60	Fall	Chest X-ray, CT scan	Laparoscopy and laparotomy	Left diaphragm	Stomach, bowel and spleen
Sonthalia N, J Emerg Med. 2013 [65]	1, F, 78	Morgagni hernia	Chest X-ray, CT scan, barium studies	Thoracotomy	Left diaphragm	Gastric volvulus
Nayak HK BMJ Case Rep. 2012 [66]	1, M, 50	Blunt trauma	EGDS, barium studies, CT SCAN	Laparoscopic repair	Left hemi diaphragm	Gastric volvulus and duodenum
Vernadakis S, Transplant Proc. 2012 [67]	1, F, 46	Liver donor	Chest X-ray, CT scan, barium studies	Laparotomy	Right diaphragm	Bowel
Ngai I, BMJ Case Rep. 2012 [68]	1, F, 31	Pregnancy	MRI	Nasogastric tube	Left hemi diaphragm	Spleen, bowel, stomach and pancreas
Elangovan A J Emerg Med. 2013 [69]	1, M, 30	Accident	Chest X-ray and CT scan	Laparoscopy	Left hemi diaphragm	Stomach
Kuppusamy A, Ulus Trauma Acil Cherrai Derg 2012 [70]	1, M, 28	Trauma	CT scan	Thoracotomy	Right hemi diaphragm	Liver
Ismail Okan, Ulus Travma Acil Cerrahi Derg. 2011 [71]	10 cases, 44,3 y	Trauma	CT scan	7 laparotomy 1 thoracic-abdominal approach 2 thoracic	9 left side	
Ioannis Baloyiannis General Thoracic and Cardiovascular Surgery 2011 [72]	1, M, 56	Trauma		Laparotomy		

Table 1 Review of literature showing demographics data, diagnosis and treatment *(Continued)*

Vassileva CM Ann Thorac Cardiovasc Surg. 2012 [73]	1, F, 25	Morgagni hernia	Chest X-ray, CT scan	Laparoscopic repair	Right hemi diaphragm	Omentum
Agrafiotis AC Acta Chir Belg. 2011 [74]	1, F, 52	Bochdalek hernia	Chest X-ray, CT scan	Laparoscopic approach, and mini laparotomy prosthetic polypropylene mesh	Left hemi diaphragm	Small bowel loops and the right colon
Tan K K, Singapore Med J 2009 [75]	14, median age 38 y	Trauma	Chest X Ray, CT Scan, RMN	Laparotomy, thoracotomy or VATS Primary repair (85.7%) patients or patch repair	five (35.7%) right-sided and nine (64.3%) left-sided diaphragmatic ruptures	
Akhtar K, Br J Hosp Med (Lond). 2009 [76]	1, M, 27	Bochdalek hernia	Chest X Ray, Upper gastrointestinal endoscopy, CT scan	Laparoscopy Goretex dual mesh	Left hemi diaphragm	Small bowel, ascending and transverse colon, and spleen
Ozpolat B, Ulus Travma Acil Cerrahi Derg. Nov; 2009 [77]	1, M, 52	Tube thoracostomy at the seventh left intercostal	Chest X-ray, MRI	Left standard thoracotomy, primary suture	Left hemi diaphragm	Omentum
Altinkaya N Hernia. 2010 [78]	12 patients mean age of 60 years, ten were female.	Morgagni hernia	CT scan	Six patients had surgery. 1 emergency surgery for hernia, 2 laparoscopic hernia repair, 3 trans-abdominal repair and 1 transthoracic repair	Right hemi diaphragm	Omentum and colon
Syed Murfad Peer, Int J Surg. 2009 [79]	2496 patients 25 (86%) males 4 (14%) females mean age 33.6 y	Trauma	Chest X-ray diagnostic in 20 (69%) patients CT scan in 4 (14%) patients. Intra-operative diagnosis of rupture diaphragm was made in 5 (17%) patients.	29 (1.1%) underwent to surgery 20 thoracotomy (69%) 8 laparotomy (27.5%) 1 Thoracoabdominal approach (3.5%)	Right defect: 6 left defect:23	
Sung HY J Korean Med Sci. 2009 [80]	1, F, 49	Congenital hernia	Chest radiography	Thoracotomy	Left hemi diaphragm	Stomach, spleen, splenic flexure of the colon bowel loops
Ouazzani A Acta Chir Belg. 2009 [81]	1, M, 24	Trauma	Chest X-ray computed tomography	Laparoscopically, with mesh	Left diaphragm	Stomach
Kavanagh D Acta Chir Belg. 2008 [82]	1, M, 76	Bochdalek hernia	Chest radiograph and computed tomogram	Laparotomy, primary repair	Right diaphragm	Strangulation of a portion of transverse colon
Yeh-Huang Hung; J Chin Med Assoc. 2008 [83]	1, M, 74 1, F, 75	Bochdalek hernia Bochdalek hernias	Chest X-ray CT scan MRI	Laparotomy Transthoracic repair	Left diaphragm Right diaphragm	Intestinal obstruction Small and large bowels
Sano A Surg Today. 2008 [16]	1, F, 25	Diaphragm hernia during pregnancy	Chest radiograph and computed tomography	Emergency caesarean section sutures and a Gore-Tex sheet	Left diaphragm	Bowel loop

Table 1 Review of literature showing demographics data, diagnosis and treatment *(Continued)*

Gourgiotis S, Turkish Journal of Trauma & Emergency Surgery 2008 [84]	1, M, 25	Trauma	Chest X-ray CT scan	Laparoscopic primary repair	Left diaphragm	
Walchalk LR, J Emerg Med. 2010 [85]	1, F, 57	Trauma				
Mohammadhosseini B, J Coll Physicians Surg Pak. 2008 [86]	1, M	Bochdalek hernia				
Boyce S, Obes Surg. 2008 [87]		Diaphragmatic hernia post surgery	CT of the chest and abdomen	Laparotomy an repair of hernia	Left diaphragmatic hernia	Ischemic small bowel
Tsuboi K, Surg Today. 2008 [88]	1, M, 50	16 months after surgery	Computed tomography of the chest	Laparotomy	Left diaphragmatic hernia	Stomach had herniated into the thoracic cavity
Vogelaar Obes Surg. 2008 [89]	1, F, 37	Six months after gastric banding	Chest X-ray computed tomography scan	Laparotomy	Left diaphragm	Intra thoracic stomach distended, rotated, and perforated at the orifice of the hernia
Young-Shun Wu; Am J Emerg Med. 2008 [90]		History of left-sided upper abdominal blunt injury 2 months before	CT scan	Thoracotomy and primary repair	Left traumatic diaphragm rupture	
Igai H, Y Gen Thorac Cardiovasc Surg. 2007 [91]	1, M, 48	Trauma	Chest X-ray, CT scan		Right diaphragm rupture	Hepatothorax
Rifki Jai S Arch Gynecol Obstet. 2007 [92]	1, F, 27	32-week gestation no history of trauma	Chest X-ray CT scan	Emergency laparotomy	Left hemi diaphragm.	Stomach, transverse colon and greater omentum herniated in the left hemithorax
Rout S Hernia. 2007 [93]	1, F, 35	Bochdalek hernias	Chest X-ray CT scan	Emergency laparotomy defect was repaired using non-absorbable sutures	Right-sided Bochdalek hernia	Colon
Campbell AS Hernia. 2007 [94]	1, M, 85		Chest X-ray CT scan	Emergency laparotomy identified a massive diaphragmatic defect which was not amenable to primary closure. A colopexy procedure was performed	Left hemi diaphragm.	Diaphragmatic herniation of bowel
Testini M Surg Today. 2006 [10]	1, M, 51	Left splenopancreatectomy 4 years earlier	Chest X-ray, CT scan, MRI	Left thoracotomy	Left hemi diaphragm	Stomach
Luu TD, Ann Thorac Surg 2006 [95]	1, F, 34	33 weeks' gestation	Chest roentgenogram, CT scan, barium study Esophagoscopy	the patient went into preterm labour and had a spontaneous vaginal delivery of a healthy new-born at 34 weeks' gestation. left thoracotomy	Left hemi diaphragm	Necrotic stomach

Table 1 Review of literature showing demographics data, diagnosis and treatment *(Continued)*

Iso Y., Hernia 2006 [96]	1, F, 81	Morgagni's hernia	Chest X-ray	The diaphragm defect was sutured first, and partial resection of the transverse colon	Right thorax	transverse colon
Eglinton T, ANZ J Surg. 2006 Jul [97]	3 cases	During third trimester of pregnancy	Chest X-ray	Laparotomy and thoracotomy in one case. Delivery was by Caesarean section at the time of emergency surgery		
Barbetakis N, World J Gastroenter ol. 2006 Apr 21 [98]	1, F, 31	Bochdalek hernias during pregnancy (23-week gestation)	Chest X-ray, chest ultrasound	Left thoraco- abdominal incision, segmental resection of the involved portion of large bowel. The diaphragmatic defect was repaired with interrupted sutures	Left hemi thorax	Strangulated Right and transverse colon, necrotic the greater omentum and stomach
Barret J, J Emerg Med. 2006 [99]	1,M, 50	Trauma	Electrocardiogram and CT scan		Left hemi thorax and pericardium	
Abboud B, J Med Liban. 2004 [100]	1 M	Trauma	Chest X-ray, exploratory laparotomy	Laparotomy, colectomy resection of ileum with anastomosis	left hemi thorax	Transverse colon and a proximal small bowel
Hsu YP, Hepatogastroenterology. 2005 [101]	78 patients	Trauma	Chest roentgenogram	Only 20% of elderly patients were operated on within 24 h of trauma, 87% of young patients		
P Ransom Emerg Med J 2005 [102]	1, M, 21	Trauma	Chest radiograph, ultrasound, oesophago-gastro-duodenoscopy	Thoracotomy	Left diaphragm	Stomach and a loop of colon had herniated through a 6 cm defect
Tiberio GA Acta Chir Belg. 2005 Feb [103]	33 p	Blunt (22 patients) or penetrating injury	Chest X-ray, CT scan	Laparotomy		
Barakat MJ, BMC Surg. 2005 [19]	1, F, 43	CDH in Marfan's syndrome	Chest X-ray, CT scan	Laparoscopy	Right hemi diaphragm	Perforated gangrenous appendix
Gupta V Eur J Emerg Med. 2005 [104]	1, M, 43	Spontaneous rupture	CT scan		Left hemi diaphragm	
Kara E Ann Acad Med Singapore 2004 [105]	1, M, 28	Trauma	Chest X-ray, CT scan	Left thoracotomy	Left hemi diaphragm	Gastric fundus
Sirbu H Hernia. 2005 [106]	1, M, 67	Trauma	CT scan	Laparotomy and right thoracotomy	Delayed bilateral diaphragmatic ruptures	
Dalton AM Emerg Med J. 2004 [107]	1, M, 43	Bochdalek hernia	Chest radiograph	Thoracotomy	Left hemi thorax	Stomach, transverse colon, and spleen in to the chest.
Niwa T Respiration. 2003 [108]	1, F, 53	Bochdalek hernia	Chest X-ray	Thoracotomy	Left hemithorax	Stomach and greater omentum
Genc MR, Obstet Ginecol 2003 [109]	1, M, 29	Bochdalek hernia during pregnancy	Chest X-ray, CT scan	Antepartum repair	Left hemithorax	Bowel obruction

Table 1 Review of literature showing demographics data, diagnosis and treatment *(Continued)*

Sato M, Jpn J Thorac Cardiovasc Surg. 2002 [110]	1, M, 57	Traffic accident	Chest X-ray, CT scan, MRI	Toracoscopy	Right hemidiaphragm	Liver
Guven H, Acta CHir Belg 2002 [111]	2 cases	Morgagni hernia				Bowel perforation Upper gastrointestinal bleeding
Kanazawa A, Surg Today 2002 [112]	1 F 63 y	Bochdalek hernia	Chest X-ray, CT scan,	Thoraco-Laparotomy Primary suture	Right hemidiaphragm	Colon and right kidney
Fisichella PM, Ann Ital CHIR 2001 [113]	1 F 55 y	Bochdalek hernia	Computed tomography	Thoracotomy and laparotomy	Right hemidiaphragm	Liver intestinal maloration
Bergeron E, J Trauma 2002 [15]	160 cases	Trauma				
Carreno G, Surg Endosc 2001 [114]	1, M, 52	Bochdalek hernia	CT scan	Laparoscopic approach	Left hemi thorax	Colon and volvulated stomach
Prieto Nieto I, Acta chir Belg 2001 [115]	1, M, 36	8 months after trauma	CT scan	Laparotomy, repair of defect, gastric perforation were closed	Left hemi diaphragm	Gastric incarceration and perforation
Nursal TZ, Hernia 2001 [116]	26 cases	Trauma	Chest X-ray, CT scan,	92% Primary repair	92% left hemi diaphragm	31.8% stomach 27,2 colon
Bujanda L, J Clin Gastroenterol 2001 [117]	1	Bochdalek hernia			Left hemi diaphragm	Gastric volvulus
Pross M, J Laparoendosc Adv Surg Tech A 2000 [118]	1, M, 20	Trauma	Diagnostic laparoscopy	Laparoscopy primary repair	Left hemi diaphragm	Stomach
Saito Y, Surg Today 2000 [119]	1, M, 51	3 years after pleuropneumectomy for mesotelioma		Laparotomy	Left hemi thorax	Ulcer of stomach, which was displaced into the thorax, had perforated aorta
De Waele JJ, J Accid Emerg Med 1999 [120]	1, M, 45	Trauma	Chest X-ray, Chest tube; ultrasound,	Laparotomy, resection of spleen	Left hemi thorax	Spleen completely disrupted
Colliver C, J Trauma 1997 [121]	1, M, 80	Trauma	Echocardiograph, ultrasonography		Left hemi diaphragm	Stomach Intrapericardial hernia
Zantut LF, Rev Paul Med 1993 [122]	1, M, 33	Trauma	Chest X-Ray, liver scintigraphy, CT scan, MRI, diagnostic laparoscopy	Laparoscopy	Bilateral diaphragmatic rupture	
Allen MS, J Thorac Cardiovasc Surg 1993 [123]	147 cases 5 emergency setting		Chest X-ray CT scan		Left hemi diaphragm	Stomach
Girzadas DV Jr Ann Emerg Med. 1991 [124]	1, F, 71	Trauma	Chest radiograph		Pericardial sac	Omentum and transverse colon

Table 1 Review of literature showing demographics data, diagnosis and treatment *(Continued)*

Thomas S Jpn J Surg. 1991 [125]	2 cases	Bochdalek hernia	X-ray of the chest and contrast studies of the gastrointestinal tract	Laparotomy	Left hemi diaphragm	Intestinal obstruction
Bush CA, South Med J 1990 [126]	2 cases	Trauma	Chest X-ray, barium studies of the gastrointestinal tract, CT scans, ultrasonography, laparoscopy, and radionuclide scanning	Laparoscopy	Left hemi diaphragm	Intestinal obstruction
Feliciano DV, J Trauma 1988 [127]	16 cases	Penetrating trauma	Chest X-ray	Laparotomy		
Chidamdaram M Thorac Cardiovasc Surg. 1988 [128]	1, M, 32	Trauma	Chest X-ray	Thoracotomy	Left hemi diaphragm	Stomach
Symbas PN, Ann Thorac Surg 1986 [129]	194 cases	Trauma	Chest X-ray, barium studies exploratory laparotomy	Laparotomy Primary repair In a case Prolene mesh		
Saber WL, J Emerg Med 1986 [130]	111 cases 8 emergency surgery	Trauma	Chest X-ray		7 left 1 right hemi diaphragm	
Gardezi SA, J Pak Med Assoc 1986 [131]	2 cases 1, M, 43	Bochdalek hernia	Chest X-ray	Laparotomy	Left hemi diaphragm	Transverse colon and splenic flexure
	1 M 26 y	CDH	Chest X-ray	Laparotomy	Left hemi diaphragm	Greater curvature of stomach, a small part of jejunum, left part of transverse colon and greater omentum
Brown GL, Ann Thorac Surg 1985 [132]	41 cases	Trauma	Chest X-ray	23 laparotomy, 13 thoracotomy, 5 combined	29 Left, 14 Right-sided, hemi diaphragm.	
Clark DE, Surgery 1983 [133]	10 cases median age 40	Trauma	Chest X-ray		Left hemi diaphragm	

***M* male, *F* female *Y* years**

with catastrophic complications [38]. When the suspicion of intestinal obstruction is evident, an abdominal approach may also be required to control organs. Although the type of closure used for diaphragmatic hernias is still a matter of debate, it is generally accepted that most defects can be primarily closed with a non-absorbable suture [39]. Mesh repair usually is used when the defect is too large to be primarily closed and the use of tension free mesh is vital to the success of the procedures. Recently, biologic mesh has been introduced to replace the synthetic one because of its lower rate of hernia recurrence, higher resistance to infections and lower risk of displacement [7, 40]; however, limited evidence in literature yet exists about their superiority. Indeed, in our previous experience, biologic meshes have also been used in contaminated surgical fields with favourable results [40]. However, because of the rarity of this condition, clinicians should be encouraged to publish their experience with biologic meshes in diaphragmatic hernia repair [7].

Conclusions

When a diaphragmatic hernia is diagnosed, surgery is the treatment of choice, above all in emergency setting. A multidisciplinary approach in dedicated centres is advisable.

Abbreviations

CDH: Congenital diaphragmatic hernia; CT: Computed tomography; DR: Diaphragmatic rupture; MRI: Magnetic resonance imaging

Acknowledgements

The authors would like to thank Dr Channielle Mascarenhas and Dr Luke Palma for the English language revision.

Funding

This study did not receive funding.

Authors' contributions

Authors contributed to this study as follows: MT contributed to the conception and design. AG contributed to the writing acquisition of the data. RMI contributed to writing. GC and AD contributed to the critical revision. AP contributed to the review of literature. AG contributed to the conception and design and critical revision. All authors read and approved the final manuscript.

Competing interests

The authors declare that they have no competing interests.

Author details

[1]Unit of Endocrine, Digestive, and Emergency Surgery, Department of Biomedical Sciences and Human Oncology, University Medical School "Aldo Moro" of Bari, Bari, Italy. [2]Department of Thoracic Surgery, University of Bari, Bari, Italy. [3]Unit of Laparoscopic Surgery, Department of Emergency and Organ Transplantation, University Medical School "A. Moro" of Bari, Bari, Italy.

References

1. Baerg J, Kanthimathinathan V, Gollin G. Late-presenting congenital diaphragmatic hernia: diagnostic pitfalls and outcome. Hernia. 2012;16:461–6.
2. Torfs CP, Curry CJ, Bateson TF, Honoré LH. A population-based study of congenital diaphragmatic hernia. Teratology. 1992;46:555–65.
3. Pancholi CK, Hombalkar NN, Dalvi SB, Gurav PDY. Left sided hydro-pneumothorax in a operated case of left diaphragmatic hernia repair: a diagnostic dilemma. J Clin Diagn Res. 2015;9:PD03-4.
4. Meyers BF, McCabe CJ. Traumatic diaphragmatic hernia. Occult marker ofserious injury. Ann Surg. 1993;218:783–90.
5. Kozak O, et al. Late presentation of blunt right diaphragmatic rupture (hepatic hernia). Am J Emerg Med. 2008;26(5):638. e3-5.
6. DeAlwis K, Mitsunaga EM. Sudden death due to nontraumatic diaphragmatic hernia in an adult. Am J Forensic Med Pathol. 2009;30:366–8.
7. Antoniou SA, Rudolph P. The use of biological meshes in diaphragmatic defects an evidence-based review of the literature. In: Frontiers in surgery October 2015. 2015.
8. Izzo BG, Maffettone V, et al. Laparoscopic treatment of Bochdalek hernia without the use of a mesh. Surg Endosc. 2003;17:1497–8.
9. Chen B, Finnerty BM, Schamberg NJ, Watkins AC, DelPizzo J, Zarnegar R. Transabdominal robotic repair of a congenital right diaphragmatic hernia containing an intrathoracic kidney: a case report. J Robot Surg. 2015;9(4): 357–60.
10. Testini M, Vacca A, Lissidini G, Di Venere B, Gurrado A, Loizzi M. Acute intrathoracic gastric volvulus from a diaphragmatic hernia after left splenopancreatectomy: report of a case. Surg Today. 2006;36(11):981–4.
11. Farhan Rashid, Mallicka M Chakrabart, Rajeev Singh and Syed Y Iftikhar. A review on delayed presentation of diaphragmatic rupture. World J Emerg Surg 2009, 4:32 doi:10.1186/1749-7922-4-32
12. Yeh-Huang H, Yu-Hon C, Sheng-Lei Y, Ming-Feng C. Adult Bochdalek hernia with bowel incarceration. J Chin Med Assoc. 2008;71:10.
13. Jing Lu, MDa, Bo Wang, MDb, Xiangming Che, MD, PhDa, Xuqi Li, MDa, Guanglin Qiu, MDa, Shicai He, MDa, Lin Fan, MDa. Delayed traumatic diaphragmatic hernia: a case-series report and literature review. Medicine 2016
14. Mariadason JG, Parsa MH, Ayuyao A, Freeman HP. Management of stab wounds to the thoracoabdominal region. A clinical approach. Ann Surg. 1988;207:335–40.
15. Bergeron E, Clas D, Ratte S, Beauchamp G, Denis R, Evans D, et al. Impact of deferred treatment of blunt diaphragmatic rupture: a 15-year experience in six trauma centers in Quebec. J Trauma. 2002;52(4):633–40.
16. Sano A, Kato H, Hamatani H, Sakai M, Tanaka N, Inose T, Kimura H, Kuwano H. Diaphragmatic hernia with ischemic bowel obstruction in pregnancy: report of a case. Surg Today. 2008;38(9):836–40.
17. Moussa G, Thomson PM. Bohra A Volvulus of the liver with intrathoracic herniation. Ann R Coll Surg Engl. 2014;96(7):e27–29.
18. Nakamura T, Masuda K, Thethi RS, Sako H, Yoh T, Nakao T, Yoshimura N. Successful surgical rescue of delayed onset diaphragmatic hernia following radiofrequency ablation for hepatocellular carcinoma. Ulus Travma Acil Cerrahi Derg. 2014;20(4):295–9. doi:10.5505/tjtes.2014.03295.
19. Barakat MJ, Vickers JH. Necrotic gangrenous intrathoracic appendix in a marfanoid adult patient: a case report. BMC Surg. 2005;5:4.
20. Brown SR, Horton JD, Trivette E, et al. Bochdalek hernia in the adult: demographics, presentation, and surgical management. Hernia. 2011;15: 23–30.
21. Goh BK, Wong AS, Tay KH, Hoe MN. Delayed presentation of a patient with a ruptured diaphragm complicated by gastric incarceration and perforation after apparently minor blunttrauma. Canad J Emerg Med. 2004;6(4):277–80.
22. Ravinder Kaur, Anuj Prabhakar1, Suman Kochhar1, Usha Dalal2 Blunt traumatic diaphragmatic hernia: pictorial review of CT signs. Indian J Rad Imaging / August 2015 / Vol 25 / Issue 3
23. Kelly J, Condon E, Kirwan W, Redmond H. Post-traumatic tension faecopneumothorax in a young male: case report. World J Emerg Surg. 2008;3:20.
24. Nayak HK, Maurya G, Kapoor N, Kar P. Delayed presentation of congenital diaphragmatic hernia presenting with intrathoracic gastric volvulus: a case report and review. BMJ Case Rep. 2012 Nov 28;2012. pii: bcr2012007332.
25. Kitano Y, Lally KP, Lally PA. Congenital diaphragmatic hernia study group: late presenting congenital diaphragmatic hernia. J Pediatr Surg. 2005;40: 1839–43.
26. Baglaj M. Late-presenting congenital diaphragmatic hernia in children: a clinical spectrum. Pediatr Surg Int. 2004;20:658–69.

27. Hosgor M, Karaca I, Karkiner A, Ucan B, Temir G, Erdag G, et al. Associated malformations in delayed presentation of congenital diaphragmatic hernia. J Pediatr Surg. 2004;39:1073–6.
28. Elhalaby EA, Abo Sikeena MH. Delayed presentation of congenital diaphragmatic hernia. Pediatr Surg Int. 2002;18:480–5.
29. Lawrence B, David S, Sigmund H, Barry S. The late-presenting pediatric bochdalek hernia: a 20-year review. J Ped Surg. 1988;23:735–39.
30. Joel AF, John L, Samuel E, James F, Louis MB. Diaphragmatic hernia masquerading as pneumothorax in two toddlers case report. Ann Emerg Med. 1993;22:1221–4.
31. Chao PH, Chuang JH, Lee SY, Huang HC. Acta Paediatr. 2011;100:425–8.
32. Kurniawan N, Verheyen L, Ceulemans. Acute chest pain while exercising: a case report of Bochdalek hernia in an adolescent. J Acta Chir Belg. 2013; 113(4):290–2.
33. Ravinder Kaur, Anuj Prabhakar1, Suman Kochhar1, Usha Dalal2. Blunt traumatic diaphragmatic hernia: pictorial review of CT signs Indian Journal of Radiology and Imaging / August 2015 / Vol 25 / Issue 3
34. Gander JW, Fisher JC, Gross ER, et al. Early recurrence of congenital diaphragmatic hernia is higher after thoracoscopic than open repair: a single institutional study. J Pediatr Surg. 2011;46(7):1303–8.
35. Lansdale N, Alam S, Losty PD, Jesudason EC. Neonatal endosurgical congenital diaphragmatic hernia repair: a systematic review and meta-analysis. Ann Surg. 2010;252(1):20–6.
36. Tsao K, Lally PA, Lally KP. Minimally invasive repair of congenital diaphragmatic hernia. J Pediatr Surg. 2011;46(6):1158–64.
37. Badillo A, Gingalewski C. Congenital diaphragmatic hernia: treatment and outcomes. Semin Perinatol. 2014;3(8):92–6.
38. Mansour KA. Trauma to the diaphragm. Chest Surg Clin N Am. 1997;7(2): 373–83.
39. Soper NJ, Teitelbaum EN. Laparoscopic paraesophageal hernia repair: current controversies. Surg Laparosc Endosc Percutan Tech. 2013;23(5):442–5.
40. Coccolini F, Agresta F, Bassi A, Catena F, Crovella F, Ferrara R, Gossetti F, Marchi D, Munegato G, Negro P, Piccoli M, Melotti G, Sartelli M, Schianodi Visconte M, Testini M, Bertoli P, Capponi MG, Lotti M, Manfredi R, Pisano M, Poiasina E, Poletti E, Ansaloni L. Italian Biological Prosthesis Work-Group (IBPWG): proposal for a decisional model in using biological prosthesis. World J Emerg Surg. 2012;7:34.
41. Lu J, Wang B, Che X, Li X, Qiu G, He S, Fan L. Delayed traumatic diaphragmatic hernia: a case-series report and literature review. Medicine (Baltimore). 2016;95(32):e4362.
42. Manabu H, Harada M, Tsujimoto H, Nagata K, Ito N, Yamazaki K, Kanematsu K, Horiguchi H, Kajiwara Y, Hiraki S, Aosasa S, Yamamoto J, Hase K. Successful laparoscopic repair of an incarcerated Bochdalek hernia associated with increased intra-abdominal pressure during use of blow gun: A case report. Int J Surg Case Rep. 2016;23:131–3.
43. De la Cour CD, Teklay B. Acute post-partum presentation of Bochdalek hernia in a grown-up woman Ugeskr Laeger. 2016 Oct 31;178(44).
44. Razi K1, Light D2, Horgan L. Emergency repair of Morgagni hernia with partial gastric volvulus: our approach. J Surg Case Rep. 2016 Aug 31;2016(8).
45. Manson HJ, Goh YM, Goldsmith P, Scott P, Turner P. Congenital diaphragmatic hernia causing cardiac arrest in a 30-year-old woman. Ann R Coll Surg Engl. 2017;99(2):e75–7.
46. Massloom HS. Acute bowel obstruction in a giant recurrent right Bochdalek's hernia: a report of complication on both sides of the diaphragm. N Am J Med Sci. 2016;8(6):252–5.
47. Kumar, J. Morgagni hernia presenting as gastric outlet obstruction in an elderly male. Surg Case Rep. 2016 2016 Jul 18;2016(7).
48. Manipadam JM, Sebastian GM, Ambady V, Hariharan R. Perforated gastric gangrene without pneumothorax in an adult Bochdalek hernia due to volvulus. J Clin Diagn Res. 2016;10(4):D09–10.
49. Harada M, Tsujimoto H, Nagata K, Ito N, Yamazaki K, Kanematsu K, Horiguchi H, Kajiwara Y, Hiraki S, Aosasa S, Yamamoto J, Hase K. Successful laparoscopic repair of an incarcerated Bochdalek hernia associated with increased intra-abdominal pressure during use of blow gun: a case report. Int J Surg Case Rep. 2016;23:131–3.
50. Siow SL1,2, Wong CM3,4, Hardin M5, Sohail M6. Successful laparoscopic management of combined traumatic diaphragmatic rupture and abdominal wall hernia: a case report. J Med Case Rep. 2016 Jan 18;10:11. doi: 10.1186/ s13256-015-0780-8.
51. Andreev AL, Protsenko AV, Globin AV. Laparoscopic repair of a posttraumatic left-sided diaphragmatic hernia complicated by strangulation and colon obstruction. JSLS. 2010;14:410-3.
52. Bhatt NR, McMonagle M. Recurrence in a laparoscopically repaired traumatic diaphragmatic hernia: case report and literature review. Trauma Mon. 2016; 21:e20421.
53. Abdullah M1, Stonelake P2. Tension pneumothorax due to perforated colon. BMJ Case Rep. 2016 May 31;2016.
54. Razi K, Light D2, Horgan L2. Emergency repair of Morgagni hernia with partial gastric volvulus: our approach. Journal of Surgical Case Reports, 2016 J Surg Case Rep. 2016 Aug 31;2016(8).
55. Wigley J, Noble F, King A. Thoracoabdominal herniation—but not as you know it. Ann R Coll Surg Engl. 2014;96:e1–2.
56. Atef M, Emna T. Bochdalek Hernia with gastric volvulus in an adult: common symptoms for an original diagnosis. Medicine (Baltimore). 2015;94:e2197.
57. Tokur M, Demiröz ŞM, Sayan M. Non-traumatic tension gastrothorax in a young lady. Ulus Travma Acil Cerrahi Derg. 2015;21(4):306–8.
58. Topuz M, Ozek MC. Right ventricle collapse secondary to hepatothorax caused by diaphragm rupture due to blunt trauma. Ulus Travma Acil Cerrahi Derg. 2014;20:463–5.
59. Haratake N, Yamazaki K, Shikada Y. Diaphragmatic hernia caused by heterotopic endometriosis in Chilaiditi syndrome: report of a case. Surg Today. 2015;45(9):1194–6.
60. Gali BM, Bakari AA, Wadinga DW, Nganjiwa US. Missed diagnosis of a delayed diaphragmatic hernia as intestinal obstruction: a case report. Niger J Med. 2014;23(1):83–5.
61. Newman MJ1. A mistaken case of tension pneumothorax. BMJ Case Rep. 2014 May 16;2014. pii: bcr2013203435.
62. Tyagi S, Steele J, Patton B, Fukuhara S, Cooperman A, Wayne M. Laparoscopic repair of an intrapericardial diaphragmatic hernia. Ann Thorac Surg. 2014;97(1):332–3.
63. Ota H, Kawai H, Matsuo T. Video-assisted minithoracotomy for blunt diaphragmatic rupture presenting as a delayed hemothorax. Ann Thorac Cardiovasc Surg. 2014;20(Suppl):911–4. doi:10.5761/atcs.cr.13-00201. Epub 2013 Nov 8.
64. Safdar G, Slater R, Garner JP. Laparoscopically assisted repair of an acute traumatic diaphragmatic hernia. BMJ Case Rep. 2013 Jun 24;2013.
65. Sonthalia N, Ray S, Khanra D, Saha A,Maitra S, Talukdar A; Gastric volvulus through morgagni hernia: an easily overlooked emergency. J Emerg Med. 2013
66. Nayak HK, Maurya G, Kapoor N, Kar P. Delayed presentation of congenital diaphragmatic hernia presenting with intrathoracic gastric volvulus: a case report and review. BMJ Case Rep. 2012;28:2012.
67. Vernadakis S, Paul A, Kykalos S, Fouzas I, Kaiser GM, Sotiropoulos GC. Incarcerated diaphragmatic hernia after right hepatectomy for living donor liver transplantation: case report of an extremely rare late donor complication. Transplant Proc. 2012;44(9):2770–2.
68. Ngai I, Sheen JJ, Govindappagari S, Garry DJ. Bochdalek hernia in pregnancy. BMJ Case Rep. 2012;11:2012.
69. Elangovan A, Chacko J, Gadiyaram S, Moorthy R. Ra traumatic tension gastrothorax and pneumothorax. J Emerg Med. 2013;44(2):e279–80.
70. Kuppusamy A, Ramanathan G, Gurusamy J, Ramamoorthy B, Parasakthi K. Delayed diagnosis of traumatic diaphragmatic rupture with herniation of the liver: a case report. Ulus Travma Acil Cerrahi Derg. 2012;18(2):175–7.
71. Okan I, Baş G, Ziyade S, Alimoğlu O, Eryılmaz R, Güzey D, Zilan A. Delayed presentation of posttraumatic diaphragmatic hernia. Ulus Travma Acil Cerrahi Derg. 2011;17(5):435–9.
72. Baloyiannis I, Kouritas VK, Karagiannis K, Spyridakis M, Efthimiou M. Isolated right diaphragmatic rupture following blunt trauma. Gen Thorac Cardiovasc Surg. 2011;59(11):760–2. doi:10.1007/s11748-010-0759-8. Epub 2011 Nov 15.
73. Vassileva CM, Shabosky J, Boley T, Hazelrigg S. Morgagni hernia presenting as a rigright middle lobe compression. Ann Thorac Cardiovasc Surg. 2012; 18(1):79–81. Epub 2011 Sep 29.
74. Agrafiotis AC, Kotzampassakis N, Boudaka W. Complicated right-sided Bochdalek hernia in an adult. Acta Chir Belg. 2011;111(3):171–3.
75. Tan KK, Yan ZY, Vijayan A, Chiu MT. Management of diaphragmatic rupture from blunt trauma. Singap Med J. 2009;50(12):1150–3.
76. Akhtar K, Qurashi K, Rizvi A, Isla R. Emergency laparoscopic repair of an obstructed Bochdalek hernia in an adult. Br J Hosp Med (Lond). 2009;70(12):718–9.
77. Ozpolat B, Doğan OV, Yücel E. Delayed diaphragmatic hernia: an unusual complication of tube thoracostomy. Ulus Travma Acil Cerrahi Derg. 2009; 15(6):617–8.

78. Altinkaya N, Parlakgümüş A, Koc Z, Ulusan S. Morgagni hernia: diagnosis with multidetector computed tomography and treatment. Hernia. 2010;14(3):277–81.
79. Peer SM, Devaraddeppa PM, Buggi S. Traumatic diaphragmatic hernia—our experience. Int J Surg. 2009;7(6):547–9.
80. Sung HY, Cho SH, Sim SB, Kim JI, Cheung DY, Park SH, Han JY, Lee SM, Noh CH, Park YB, Jung SE, Lee SH, Choi KY. Congenital hemidiaphragmatic agenesis presenting as reversible mesenteroaxial gastric volvulus and diaphragmatic hernia: a case report. J Korean Med Sci. 2009;24(3):517–9.
81. Ouazzani A, Guerin E, Capelluto E, Landolfo G, Roman A, Bruyns J, Cadiere GB. A laparoscopic approach to left diaphragmatic rupture after blunt trauma. Acta Chir Belg. 2009;109(2):228–31.
82. Kavanagh DO, Ryan RS, Waldron R. Acta Chir Belg. Acute dyspnoea due to an incarcerated right-sided Bochdalek's hernia. 2008 Sep-Oct;108(5):604–6.
83. Hung YH, Chien YH, Yan SL, Chen MF. Adult Bochdalek hernia with bowel incarceration. J Chin Med Assoc. 2008;71(10):528–31.
84. Gourgiotis S, Rothkegel S, Germanos S. Combined diaphragmatic and urinary bladder rupture after minor motorcycle accident (report of a case and literature review). Ulus Travma Acil Cerrahi Derg. 2008;14(2):163–6.
85. Walchalk LR, Stanfield SC. Delayed presentation of traumatic diaphragmatic rupture. J Emerg Med. 2010;39(1):21–4.
86. Mohammadhosseini B, Shirani S. Incarcerated Bochdalek hernia in an adult. J Coll Physicians Surg Pak. 2008;18(4):239–41.
87. Boyce S, Burgul R, Pepin F, Shearer C. Late presentation of a diaphragmatic hernia following laparoscopic gastric banding. Obes Surg. 2008;18(11):1502–4.
88. Tsuboi K, Omura N, Kashiwagi H, Kawasaki N, Suzuki Y, Yanaga K. Delayed traumatic diaphragmatic hernia after open splenectomy: report of a case. Surg Today. 2008;38(4):352–4.
89. Vogelaar FJ, Adhin SK, Schuttevaer HM. Delayed intrathoracic gastric perforation after obesity surgery: a severe complication. Obes Surg. 2008;18(6):745–6.
90. Wu YS, Lin YY, Hsu CW, Chu SJ, Tsai SH. Massive ipsilateral pleural effusion caused by transdiaphragmatic intercostal hernia. Am J Emerg Med. 2008; 26(2):252. doi:10.1016/j.ajem.2007.04.018. e3-4.
91. Igai H, Yokomise H, Kumagai K, Yamashita S, Kawakita K, Kuroda Y. Delayed hepatothorax due to right-sided traumatic diaphragmatic rupture. Gen Thorac Cardiovasc Surg. 2007;55(10):434–6.
92. Rifki Jai S, Bensardi F, Hizaz A, Chehab F, Khaiz D, Bouzidi A. A late post-traumatic diaphragmatic hernia revealed during pregnancy by post-partum respiratory distress. Arch Gynecol Obstet. 2007;276(3):295–8. Epub 2007 Apr 4.
93. Rout S, Foo FJ, Hayden JD, Guthrie A, Smith AM. Right-sided Bochdalek hernia obstructing in an adult: case report and review of the literature. Hernia. 2007;11(4):359–62. Epub 2007 Mar 7.
94. Campbell AS, O'Donnell ME, Lee J. Mediastinal shift secondary to a diaphragmatic hernia: a life-threatening combination. Hernia. 2007;11(4): 377–9. Epub 2007 Feb 13.
95. Luu TD, Reddy VS, Miller DL, Force SD. Gastric rupture associated with diaphragmatic hernia during pregnancy. Ann Thorac Surg. 2006;82(5):1908–10.
96. Iso Y, Sawada T, Rokkaku K, Furihata T, Shimoda M, Kita J, Kubota K. A case of symptomatic Morgagni's hernia and a review of Morgagni's hernia in Japan (263 reported cases). Hernia. 2006;10(6):521–4. Epub 2006 Aug 16.
97. Eglinton T, Coulter GN, Bagshaw P, Cross L. Diaphragmatic hernias complicating pregnancy. ANZ J Surg. 2006;76(7):553–7.
98. Barbetakis N, Efstathiou A, Vassiliadis M, Xenikakis T, Fessatidis. Bochdaleck's hernia complicating pregnancy: case report. World J Gastroenterol. 2006; 12(15):2469–71.
99. Barrett J, Satz W. Traumatic, pericardio-diaphragmatic rupture: an extremely rare cause of pericarditis. J Emerg Med. 2006;30(2):141–5.
100. Abboud B, Jaoude JB, Riachi M, Sleilaty G, Tabet G. Intrathoracic transverse colon and small bowel infarction in a patient with traumatic diaphragmatic hernia. Case report and review of the literature. J Med Liban. 2004;52(3): 168–70. Review.
101. Hsu YP, Chen RJ, Fang JF, Lin BC. Blunt diaphragmatic rupture in elderly patients. Hepatogastroenterology. 2005;52(66):1752–8.
102. Ransom P, Cornelius P. Stabbing chest pain: a case of intermittent diaphragmatic herniation. Emerg Med J. 2005;22(6):460–1.
103. Tiberio GA, Portolani N, Coniglio A, Baiocchi GL, Vettoretto N, Giulini SM. Traumatic lesions of the diaphragm. Our experience in 33 cases and review of the literature. Acta Chir Belg. 2005;105(1):82–8.
104. Gupta V, Singhal R, Ansari MZ. Spontaneous rupture of the diaphragm. Eur J Emerg Med. 2005;12(1):43–4.
105. Kara E, Kaya Y, Zeybek R, Coskun T, Yavuz C. A case of a diaphragmatic rupture complicated with lacerations of stomach and spleen caused by a violent cough presenting with mediastinal shift. Ann Acad Med Singapore. 2004;33(5):649–50.
106. Sirbu H, Busch T, Spillner J, Schachtrupp A, Autschbach R. Late bilateral diaphragmatic rupture: challenging diagnostic and surgical repair. Hernia. 2005;9(1):90–2. Epub 2004 Sep 3.
107. Dalton AM, Hodgson RS, Crossley C. Bochdalek hernia masquerading as a tension pneumothorax. Emerg Med J. 2004;21(3):393–4.
108. Niwa T, Nakamura A, Kato T, Kutsuna T, Tonegawa K, Kawai A, Itoh M. An adult case of Bochdalek hernia complicated with hemothorax. Respiration. 2003;70(6):644–6.
109. Genc MR, Clancy TE, Ferzoco SJ, Norwitz E. Maternal congenital diaphragmatic hernia complicating pregnancy. Obstet Gynecol. 2003;102(5 Pt 2):1194–6.
110. Sato M, Minimally invasive diagnosis and treatment of traumatic rupture of the right hemidiaphragm with liver herniation. Jpn J Thorac Cardiovasc Surg. 2002
111. Guven H, Malazgirt Z, Dervisoglu A, Danaci M, Ozkan K. Morgagni hernia: rare presentations in elderly patients. Acta Chir Belg. 2002;102(4):266–9.
112. Kanazawa A, Yoshioka Y, Inoi O, Murase J, Kinoshita H. Acute respiratory failure caused by an incarcerated right-sided adult bochdalek hernia: report of a case. Surg Today. 2002;32(9):812–5. Review.
113. Fisichella PM, Perretta S, Di Stefano A, Di Carlo I, La Greca G, Russello D, Latteri F. Chronic liver herniation through a right Bochdalek hernia with acute onset in adulthood. Ann Ital Chir. 2001;72(6):703–5.
114. Carreño G, Sánchez R, Alonso RA, Galarraga MA, Moriyón C, Magarzo A, Bouzón F, Makdissi Z, Obregón RA. Laparoscopic repair of Bochdalek's hernia with gastric volvulus. Surg Endosc. 2001;15(11):1359. Epub 2001 Aug 16.
115. Prieto Nieto I, Pérez Robledo JP, Rosales Trelles V, De Miguel IR, Fernández Prieto A, Calvo Celada A. Gastric incarceration and perforation following posttraumatic diaphragmatic hernia. Acta Chir Belg. 2001;101(2):81–3.
116. Nursal TZ, Ugurlu M, Kologlu M, Hamaloglu E. Traumatic diaphragmatic hernias: a report of 26 cases. Hernia. 2001;5(1):25–9.
117. Bujanda L, Larrucea I, Ramos F, Muñoz C, Sánchez A, Fernández I. Bochdalek's hernia in adults. J Clin Gastroenterol. 2001;32(2):155–7.
118. Pross M, Manger T, Mirow L, Wolff S, Lippert H. Laparoscopic management of a late-diagnosed major diaphragmatic rupture. J Laparoendosc Adv Surg Tech A. 2000;10(2):111–4.
119. Saito Y, Yamakawa Y, Niwa H, Kiriyama M, Fukai I, Kondo S, Fujii Y. Left diaphragmatic hernia complicated by perforation of an intrathoracic gastric ulcer into the aorta: report of a case. Surg Today. 2000;30(1):63–5.
120. De Waele JJ, Vermassen FE. Splenic herniation causing massive haemothorax after blunt trauma. J Accid Emerg Med. 1999;16(5):383–4.
121. Colliver C, Oller DW, Rose G, Brewer D, 1. Traumatic intrapericardial diaphragmatic hernia diagnosed by echocardiography. J Trauma. 1997;42(1):115–7.
122. Zantut LF, Machado MA, Volpe P, Poggetti RS, Birolini D. Bilateral diaphragmatic injury diagnosed by laparoscopy. Rev Paul Med. 1993;111(3):430–2.
123. Allen MS, Trastek VF, Deschamps C, Pairolero PC. Intrathoracic stomach. Presentation and results of operation. J Thorac Cardiovasc Surg. 1993;105(2): 253–8. discussion 258–9.
124. Girzadas Jr1 DV, Fligner DJ. Delayed traumatic intrapericardial diaphragmatic hernia associated with cardiac tamponade. Ann Emerg Med. 1991;20(11):1246–7.
125. Thomas S, Kapur B. Adult Bochdalek hernia—clinical features, management and results of treatment. Jpn J Surg. 1991;21(1):114–9.
126. Bush CA, Margulies R. Traumatic diaphragmatic hernia and intestinal obstruction due to penetrating trunk wounds. South Med J. 1990;83(11):1347–50. Review.
127. Feliciano DV, Cruse PA, Mattox KL, Bitondo CG, Burch JM, Noon GP, Beall Jr AC. Delayed diagnosis of injuries to the diaphragm after penetrating wounds. J Trauma. 1988;28(8):1135–44.
128. Chidamdaram M, Eyres KS, Szabolcs Z, Ionescu MI. Management problems of coincident traumatic diaphragmatic hernia and myocardial infarction. Thorac Cardiovasc Surg. 1988;36(3):167–9.
129. Symbas PN, Vlasis SE, Hatcher Jr C. Blunt and penetrating diaphragmatic injuries with or without herniation of organs into the chest. Ann Thorac Surg. 1986;42(2):158–62.
130. Saber WL, Moore EE, Hopeman AR, Aragon WE. Delayed presentation of traumatic diaphragmatic hernia. J Emerg Med. 1986;4(1):1–7.
131. Gardezi SA, Chaudhry AM, Sial GA, Ahmad I, Rashid M, Yusuf A, Siddique S, Gardezi JR, Shafique T. Congenital diaphragmatic hernia in the adult. J Pak Med Assoc. 1986;36(1):16–20.
132. Brown GL, Richardson JD. Traumatic diaphragmatic hernia: a continuing challenge. Ann Thorac Surg. 1985;39(2):170–3.

18

Acute care and emergency general surgery in patients with chronic liver disease: how can we optimize perioperative care?

Michael S. Bleszynski[1], Alexsander K. Bressan[2], Emilie Joos[1], S. Morad Hameed[1] and Chad G. Ball[2*]

Abstract

The increasing prevalence of advanced cirrhosis among operative candidates poses a major challenge for the acute care surgeon. The severity of hepatic dysfunction, degree of portal hypertension, emergency of surgery, and severity of patients' comorbidities constitute predictors of postoperative mortality. Comprehensive history taking, physical examination, and thorough review of laboratory and imaging examinations typically elucidate clinical evidence of hepatic dysfunction, portal hypertension, and/or their complications. Utilization of specific scoring systems (Child-Pugh and MELD) adds objectivity to stratifying the severity of hepatic dysfunction. Hypovolemia and coagulopathy often represent major preoperative concerns. Resuscitation mandates judicious use of intravenous fluids and blood products. As a general rule, the most expeditious and least invasive operative procedure should be planned. Laparoscopic approaches, advanced energy devices, mechanical staplers, and topical hemostatics should be considered whenever applicable to improve safety. Precise operative technique must acknowledge common distortions in hepatic anatomy, as well as the risk of massive hemorrhage from porto-systemic collaterals. Preventive measures, as well as both clinical and laboratory vigilance, for postoperative hepatic and renal decompensation are essential.

Keywords: Chronic liver disease, Cirrhosis, Acute care surgery, General surgery, Portal hypertension

Background

Approximately one in every ten patients with chronic liver disease requires surgery in the final 2 years of life [1]. This commonly quoted estimation was originally reported over four decades ago, and it does not account for the expanding surgical eligibility of cirrhotic patients due to advances in both perioperative care and operative techniques for non-hepatic and hepatic operations (i.e., resection of hepatocellular carcinoma and liver transplantation). In the greater context, non-hepatic surgery is far more common and typically presents within the everyday scope of acute care surgery.

Chronic liver disease, however, imposes a significantly increased risk of postoperative morbi-mortality, largely due to sepsis and hepatic failure. In a systematic review conducted by de Goede et al., the overall risk of perioperative morbidity and mortality were 30.1 and 11.6% respectively and the coexistence of portal hypertension was found to be associated with a twofold increase in mortality [2]. In another study identifying 772 cirrhotic patients, the severity of hepatic dysfunction and emergency surgery were both major risk factors for postoperative mortality [3]. An analysis of Nationwide Inpatient Sample data describing over 22,000 patients with cirrhosis also showed an increase in adjusted mortality rates in a stepwise manner with the severity of hepatic dysfunction [4]. This was observed even for elective procedures and in the absence of portal hypertension.

Assessment and management of chronic liver disease in operative patients thus represent a relevant topic for general surgeons. More specifically, understanding the pathophysiology and clinical aspects of hepatic dysfunction and portal hypertension has a direct impact in the perioperative care of this patient population. The goal of

* Correspondence: ball.chad@gmail.com
[2]Department of Surgery, University of Calgary, Foothills Medical Centre, 1403 - 29 Street NW, Calgary, Alberta, Canada
Full list of author information is available at the end of the article

this study is therefore to provide an updated review of relevant aspects of cirrhosis for the acute care surgeon.

A brief description of pertinent pathophysiology provides the basis of this review upon which surgical topics are expanded to include state-of-the art evidence, where available. The literature search was limited to English publications from two databases (EMBASE and PubMed) and manual search of additional references. A narrative format was utilized to better accommodate a broad comprehensive coverage of major topics of interest for the general surgeon. Our literature search was not limited to a specific question or strategy.

Pathophysiology

Chronic hepatocyte injury is characterized by inflammation, fibrosis, and ultimately cirrhosis. Cirrhosis thus results from distortion of hepatic architecture and increased resistance to portal venous flow secondary to progressive fibrotic replacement of hepatocytes. Portal hypertension and loss of metabolic functions are the main factors that determine the clinical manifestations of cirrhosis.

The most important clinical manifestations of portal hypertension are varices and ascites. An increased pressure gradient from the post-hepatic venous system opens collateral portosystemic shunts in the esophagogastric and anorectal regions, umbilical vein, and retroperitoneum. As this process advances, visceral congestion increases, ascites accumulates, varices enlarge, and portal venous flow decelerates, or even reverses. Diminished delivery of hepatotrophic factors further impairs hepatic function via ongoing hepatocyte loss.

In surgical patient, hepatic dysfunction translates into an increased risk of infection, hemorrhage, thrombosis, and a prolonged half-life of numerous drugs (e.g., opioids and benzodiazepines). The associated imbalance of neuroendocrine mediators (e.g., vasopressin, renin-angiotensin-aldosterone system, and nitric oxide) also potentiates sodium and fluid retention, resulting in a background hyperdynamic circulation with splanchnic venous congestion and systemic vasodilation [5].

In emergency surgery, stress response to the underlying condition, anesthesia, and surgical trauma increase the risk of hepatic decompensation and associated multi-system failure. Changes in hepatic perfusion with shock and fluid shifts further compromise hepatocellular synthetic and excretory functions. In addition, endotoxemia from gram-negative sepsis potentiates platelet aggregation and creates a state of low-grade disseminated intravascular coagulation [6].

Renal system

Activation of the renin-angiotensin-aldosterone system with hypersecretion of vasopressin acts as compensatory mechanisms to preserve arterial pressure and replenish effective circulating volume when blood is pooled in the splanchnic territory. With the progression of cirrhosis, avidity for water and sodium increases, and dilutional hyponatremia results from water retention. In advanced cases, exacerbation of these abnormalities leads to hepatorenal syndrome (HRS). HRS is characterized by rapid decline in renal function with low urinary excretion of sodium due to severe renal vasoconstriction and diminished or absent cortical perfusion. This syndrome is potentially reversible, but carries an extremely poor prognosis [7].

Cardiovascular system

The bypass of bacterial endotoxins from the splanchnic to the systemic circulation and an increased production of nitric oxide cause peripheral vasodilation and increased cardiac output in cirrhotic patients. Along with this vasodilator-mediated hyperdynamic circulatory state, decreased myocardial contractility, accentuated in cases of chronic alcohol use, has been described. These events compromise mean arterial pressure and also impair the cardiac adaptive response to resuscitative intravenous fluid expansion.

Respiratory system

Patients are at increased risk of hypoxia secondary to restrictive lung disease (due to ascites and pleural effusions), diffusion abnormalities due to pulmonary arterial and venous vasodilation and shunting, and pulmonary hypertension. Patients with large-volume ascites are also predisposed to bronchopulmonary aspiration.

Central nervous system

Hepatic encephalopathy is a reversible neurological condition associated with hepatic failure and portal hypertension that may present with varying degrees of cognitive impairment, ranging from minimal changes to deep coma. This pathophysiology is driven by cerebral edema and an increased passage of ammonia through the blood-brain barrier [8]. Ammonia is produced via glutamine metabolism by enterocytes, and urea breakdown by gut flora. With impaired hepatocellular function and portosystemic shunting, ammonia is less likely to be converted to urea and therefore accumulates within the bloodstream. It eventually crosses the blood-brain barrier where it contributes to cerebral edema and other pathological processes [9].

Coagulation

Primary hemostasis is impaired in advanced cirrhosis due to thrombocytopenia and platelet dysfunction, but it is associated with a compensatory increase in von Willebrand factor levels. Platelet abnormalities result from splenic sequestration, bone marrow suppression (secondary to alcohol, folic acid deficiency, or viral hepatitis C), decreased hepatic production of thrombopoietin, infection, and renal failure.

When activated, platelets trigger secondary hemostasis, generating thrombin to convert fibrinogen to fibrin. With the exception of von Willebrand factor, all plasma clotting factors, anticoagulants, and fibrinolytic proteins are synthesized by the liver and susceptible to advancing hepatic disease. Deficient excretion of bile salts impairs absorption of liposoluble vitamins and the synthesis of vitamin K-dependent clotting factors (factors II, VII, IX, and X). The liver also clears activated clotting factors, anticoagulants, and fibrinolytic proteins. Such widespread effects on coagulation and anticoagulation translate into an unpredictably increased risk of both bleeding and thrombosis.

Preoperative assessment and management

Hypovolemia, coagulopathy, and thrombocytopenia are the major concerns during preoperative assessment and resuscitation. Goal-directed fluid administration and use of blood products (Table 1) should be guided, where possible, by hemodynamic monitoring [10]. Low urine output should be interpreted with caution. Oliguria from hormonal and inflammatory changes associated with cirrhosis and the underlying emergency might mislead the clinician to volume overload the patient. Excessive crystalloid and blood product infusion, in turn, can precipitate respiratory failure and variceal hemorrhage.

Conventional coagulation tests, which commonly focus on measuring defects in specific hemostatic pathways, often do not provide an accurate picture of the overall clotting ability within cirrhosis. Furthermore, these tests are poor predictors of the risk of hemorrhage versus thrombosis [11]. Given that thromboelastography evaluates the viscoelastic properties of blood and therefore provides a comprehensive evaluation of the clotting process, its use has been recommended in the global assessment of clot formation, strength, and dissolution. In a prospective study, thromboelastography differentiated cirrhotic patients from healthy volunteers (AUC = 0.921, $p < 0.001$), while conventional coagulation tests did not [12]. A growing body of literature supports the use of thromboelastography in liver transplantation [13, 14], but more studies are still necessary for many other diagnostic tests [15]. Other coagulation studies such as sonorheometry, international normalized ratio calibrated for cirrhosis, and coagulation-like thrombin generation time have also been recommended, but still lack definitive prospective validation for cirrhotic patients [11].

Electrolyte imbalances (hypokalemia, hypocalcemia, hypomagnesemia, and dilutional hyponatremia) should be monitored and corrected. A high index of suspicion for malnutrition and micronutrient deficiencies (folate, vitamins A, D, E, K, and complex B) needs to be maintained. Early supplementation of these nutrients is also recommended, particularly in alcoholic liver disease. Hypoglycemia, from impaired gluconeogenesis, should also be expected and promptly corrected. Blood lactate level, a specific marker of tissue ischemia, can be significantly elevated in the context of chronic liver disease

Table 1 Management of perioperative coagulopathy in chronic liver disease

Treatment	Comment	Dosing principles
Vitamin K	IV vitamin K can be given for patients who are severely malnourished or have malabsorption, secondary to biliary obstruction, bile salt deficiency, or use of broad spectrum antibiotics.	The recommended dose in 10 mg IV daily for 3 days prior to surgery.
Fresh frozen plasma (FFP)	The correction of INR with FFP has not been shown to decrease the risk of bleeding in cirrhotics. It is not recommended to empirically transfuse FFP for elevated INR or prothrombin time. Excessive use of FFP can lead to significant complications such as volume expansion, infection, and transfusion-associated lung injury (TRALI).	If the patient is clinically bleeding, it is recommended to transfuse FFP, at a dose of 10–15 ml/kg.
Platelets	Platelet transfusion should be considered in active bleeding if platelet levels are below 50,000.	The recommended dose is 1 unit per 10 kg body weight.
Cryoprecipitate	Hypofibrinogenemia (≤ 100 mg/dl) should be corrected with cryoprecipitate.	The recommended dose is one bag (10 units) per 10 kg of body weight.
Tranexemic acid	Tranexemic acid, an anti-fibrinolytic agent, should be used in patients with hyperfibrinolysis diagnosed by thromboelastography or patients with intractable bleeding.	A loading dose of 10 mg/kg is given, repeated three times for 2–8 days.
DDAVP	DDAVP is an analogue of vasopressin. It releases vWF and factor VIII. Despite the high levels of vWF in cirrhosis, DDAVP has been shown to decrease bleeding time in those patients.	The recommended dose is 300 µg IV.
rfVIIa	rfVIIa has a high cost, transient effect, and thrombotic complications. It has been shown to reduce bleeding in the placement of intracranial pressure monitoring devices but not in any other surgical procedure. Its clinical indications are limited.	If used, the dose is 40 µg/kg.

due to impaired hepatic clearance. Nevertheless, the trend in serial measurements in serum lactate in response to resuscitation may be a useful adjunct in hemodynamic assessment. Mild increases in aminotransferases (AST and ALT) are commonly noted in chronic liver disease, reflecting active hepatic injury. Marked elevation (greater than 1000 IU/l), however, suggests acute viral, alcoholic, or ischemic hepatitis. In asymptomatic patients with three or more fold increases in ALT/AST levels or any elevation in bilirubin, the incidence of undiagnosed cirrhosis ranges from 6 to 34%.

The precise etiology of the underlying hepatic disease mandates specific treatment measures. Thiamine replacement with glucose infusion is indicated to prevent progression of Wernicke encephalopathy. The risk of symptoms from alcohol withdrawal also mandates supportive measures, as well as multivitamins. Patients on chronic steroids for autoimmune hepatitis should receive a stress-dose adjustment in the perioperative period. Finally, delays in restarting anti-viral therapy for hepatitis should be avoided.

Scoring systems for cirrhosis: Child and MELD systems

The Child-Turcotte classification system was initially proposed in 1964 to predict mortality after portosystemic shunt surgery [16]. It was then modified in 1972 by Pugh et al., when the nutritional status criterion was replaced by prothrombin time (or INR) [17]. The Child-Pugh classification relies on three objective laboratory (albumin level, bilirubin level, and prothrombin time) and two subjective clinical (severity of ascites and encephalopathy) criteria to stratify patients into three classes (A, B, or C; with C representing the most advanced cases). It is currently utilized in a variety of surgical and medical scenarios. Predicted mortality varies from 10% for Child-Pugh A, 30% for Child-Pugh B, and up to 80% for Child-Pugh C [18, 19]. Its discriminatory ability, however, is extremely compromised by inter-observer variability of the subjective criteria, and the stratification of a wide range of laboratory values into only three risk groups.

The sentinel publication of the Model of End-Stage Liver Disease (MELD) in 2000 introduced a more accurate scoring system to predict mortality after insertion of transjugular intra-hepatic portosystemic shunts (TIPS), based on bilirubin, creatinine, and international normalized ratio (INR) values [20]. In the original publication, a MELD score < 8 was predictive of good post-TIPS survival, whereas a MELD score > 18 translated into significantly greater mortality. Since then, a number of series have validated the MELD system for different operations, with slightly variable reported cutoff values for poor outcomes. In a review of the literature, Hanje and colleagues concluded that elective abdominal surgery could be recommended for MELD scores < 10, but should be strongly discouraged for a MELD scores > 15 [21]. The current major utility of the MELD system, however, has been demonstrated in prioritizing patients on liver transplantation waiting lists [22]. Recently, the superiority of a revised MELD system incorporating sodium levels has been suggested [23], but is awaiting further validation [24].

In non-transplant patients, MELD risk stratification is also often preferred to Child-Pugh scoring due to its more objective and detailed risk stratification with a continuum of possible scores. Unfortunately, and similar to the limitations associated with the Child-Pugh score, the MELD is not specific to patients with surgical emergencies.

Imaging exams

Morphologic findings of early cirrhosis include hepatomegaly, as well as widening of the *porta hepatis*, umbilical fissure, and pericholecystic space. As cirrhosis advances, hepatomegaly evolves into the typical nodular shrunken liver with atrophy of segment 4 and the right lobe, as well as hypertrophy of segments 2 and 3 and the caudate lobe. Bright and coarse nodular texture with surface nodularity (most commonly noticed on the undersurface of the liver) can be demonstrated on bedside ultrasonography [25]. Dysplastic and regenerative nodules are difficult to appreciate on CT due to their small size and isointensity. However, the identification of nodules, particularly if they are hyper-enhancing, on the arterial phase, should raise suspicion for an incidental hepatocellular carcinoma [26].

Vascular manifestations of cirrhosis include signs of hepatic perfusion abnormalities and portal hypertension. Progressive hepatic fibrosis increases resistance to both arterial and venous inflow. While the portal venous system may decompress through portosystemic collaterals, there is no equivalent alternative for hepatic arterial inflow. Intra-hepatic vascular communications thus develop in the hepatic sinusoids, *vasa vasorum* of portal vein, and peribiliary capillaries to shunt arterial blood into the portal venous system [27]. These changes present on cross-sectional imaging as heterogeneous delayed enhancement of hepatic parenchyma, sometimes mixed with geographic areas of arterialization. Evidence of overt portal hypertension can also be found on imaging (esophageal, gastric, and umbilical varices, prominent left gastric vein and tributaries, splenomegaly, and ascites).

Intraoperative considerations

Surgical access (open or laparoscopic) and placement of retractors should be planned to avoid engorged abdominal wall veins and to optimize surgical exposure in anticipation to the most critical operative steps. Despite the lack of definitive evidence [28], the authors believe that bipolar and ultrasonic energy devices, mechanical vascular staplers, and topical hemostatics are useful adjuncts in attempting to decrease both operating time and blood loss. This seems particularly true for the surgeon coming through the abdominal wall with associated dilated veins. Use of a concurrent ligating and cutting energy instrument in a careful and cautious manner can help prevent undue blood loss. Postoperative coagulopathy can easily facilitate bleeding from initially minor sources, so extra attention to hemostasis is required.

Utilization of intra-abdominal drains to help control postoperative ascites and prevent surgical wound complications is a controversial topic. While a more restrict policy for placement of surgical abdominal drains has gained growing support in the literature [29], its safety in the context of cirrhosis yet remains poorly explored. Better control of postoperative ascites and potential associated surgical wound complications presents a compelling rationale for prophylactic drainage, but the risk of contamination of ascites and increased postoperative fluid shifts should be taken into account. In fact, increased morbidity due to wound complications was demonstrated in cirrhotic patients randomized to prophylactic drainage after liver resection in a small clinical trial conducted in the early 2000s [30]. It is the opinion of the authors of this review that routine use of surgical drains should be avoided in cirrhotic patients, and if indicated, early removal should be aggressively pursued.

As a general rule, the most expeditious and least invasive operation should be utilized, including a laparoscopic approach where feasible and safe. The safety of laparoscopy in cirrhotic patients has been historically challenged due to the theoretical risks of hemorrhage from abdominal wall varices during port placement, detrimental effects of pneumoperitoneum on hepatic perfusion, and technical limitations to approaching intraoperative hemorrhage. These concerns, however, have been vastly mitigated over the years, with multiple reports now attesting to the safety of laparoscopy, as well as suggesting some useful technical tips (Table 2).

The superiority of laparoscopic over open cholecystectomy in cirrhotic patients has been demonstrated in terms of operative blood loss, surgical time, postoperative pain, morbidity, and hospital length of stay [31, 32]. Technical difficulties must be expected in retracting the liver and identifying anatomic landmarks due to hepatic distortion.

In cirrhotic patients, an increased risk of intraoperative hemorrhage should be expected. In laparoscopic surgery, utilization of additional ports and meticulous operative technique assist in preventing iatrogenic injuries. Venous hemorrhage can be temporized by brief increases in pneumoperitoneum pressure and compression with sponges. If application of electrocautery is contemplated for gallbladder bed bleeding, a high setting (100 units on spray) and precise contact to the site of bleeding is recommended. In cases where this technique does not arrest ongoing bleeding, placement of a clip immediately beside the site of hemorrhage (i.e., into the liver in a perpendicular manner) can be helpful as an ignition tool for cauterization.

Laparoscopy has also been recommended for cirrhotic patients with appendicitis. Tsugawa and colleagues compared open (25 patients) to laparoscopic appendectomy (15 patients) in a retrospective series. Laparoscopy compared favorably with open surgery with respect to blood loss, ascites formation, wound complications, hospital length of stay, postoperative pain, and liver function [33].

Ascites predisposes patients with chronic liver disease to ventral hernias. Up to 20% of all patients with cirrhotic ascites develop umbilical hernias [34]. Surgical indications are debatable in non-complicated cases due to the high risk of postoperative morbidity and recurrence (60%) in patients with persistent ascites [35]. Conservative management, however, imposes a risk of hernia strangulation and rupture of overlying skin, with even

Table 2 Laparoscopic strategies in advanced liver disease

Port placement	As a general rule, an open Hasson technique is recommended for entry into the peritoneal cavity [31]. To avoid abdominal wall varices from the umbilical vein and falciform ligament, several authors have recommended port placement to the right of the midline, especially the subxiphoid port in laparoscopic cholecystectomy [32, 33].
Pneumoperitoneum	Blunting of the hepatic arterial buffer response is a theoretical risk. There is no report in the literature of liver failure related to pneumoperitoneum in a cirrhotic patient [34, 35]. Some authors reduce their intra-abdominal pressure in cirrhotic patients [36].
Bleeding risk	There are few reports of bleeding during laparoscopic procedures in cirrhotic patients. Cobb et al. describes an 8% transfusion rate, with only one patient requiring transfusion for bleeding [37]. In a retrospective study of 68 patients undergoing laparoscopic cholecystectomy, only one patient received a blood transfusion [35]. Laparoscopic hemostatic devices such as ultrasound knife, ligasure, and harmonic scalpel can significantly improve hemostasis and are recommended by many authors [32, 36].
Conversion	The published conversion rate for laparoscopic cholecystectomy is between 4 and 6%, which is similar to the non-cirrhotic patient population [32, 35–37].
Immune function	Li et al. report a reduced risk of bacterial seeding with laparoscopy, with subsequent decreased risk in spontaneous bacterial peritonitis [36].

poorer surgical outcomes. Once an emergency occurs, prompt surgical treatment and clinical management of ascites are mandatory. Concerns about the increased risk of surgical site infection, ascites leakage, and mesh displacement mandate judicious planning of the repair technique by the acute care surgeon. To minimize the risk of these complications, when a repair with mesh is indicated, pre-peritoneal placement has been favored over an onlay technique. A laparoscopic approach has also been proven safe in multiple surgical series [35–37].

Postoperative issues

Much of the resuscitative and therapeutic effort initiated preoperatively, including volume resuscitation, correction of electrolyte abnormalities, and coagulopathy, must be continued in the postoperative period. The surgical team should also maintain a high degree of vigilance for evidence of hepatic decompensation. Hepatic failure might simply result from the inflammatory response to surgery and underlying emergency condition, but the possibility of precipitating factors (e.g., constipation, fluid and electrolyte abnormalities, gastrointestinal hemorrhage, and spontaneous bacterial peritonitis) should always be considered.

Ascites

Large-volume ascites after abdominal surgery increases the risk of abdominal wall dehiscence and herniation. It also predisposes the patient to atelectasis, aspiration, and pneumonia. Associated fluid shifts might precipitate electrolyte imbalances, hypovolemia, and acute kidney injury. Management is based on sodium restriction and judicious use of diuretics, with close monitoring of electrolytes and renal function. Therapeutic paracentesis should be reserved for refractory cases and limited to symptomatic relief. A high index of suspicion for spontaneous bacterial peritonitis is also required.

Hepatic encephalopathy

Other possible etiologies of global neurologic decline should be investigated (e.g., hypoxia, hypercapnia, hypoglycemia, uremia, medications, *delirium tremens*, hypoactive delirium, seizures, intracranial hemorrhage). Elevated blood ammonia level (found in over 90% of cases) corroborates the clinical diagnosis, but correlation with the actual disease severity is poor. It should also be noted that monitoring blood ammonia levels is inferior to clinical assessment, and it is not recommended in asymptomatic patients [37]. Benzodiazepines should be avoided and replaced with haloperidol when chemical restraint is indicated.

The classic protein-restricted diet does not find support in the current literature [38] because most patients do not tolerate high-food/calorie intake. Furthermore, malnutrition is a much more significant concern. Despite ongoing debate, branched amino acid supplementation may also be beneficial [39]. Other adjuncts, such as cathartics and oral antibiotics, are recommended in an attempt to decrease the intestinal production of ammonia due to bacterial overgrowth.

Lactulose, a non-absorbable sugar that causes osmotic diarrhea, has been traditionally used to treat hepatic encephalopathy. It acidifies the colon and promotes the conversion of ammonia to ammonium, which is not reabsorbed [40]. Lactulose dosing should be titrated to two to three bowel movements per day. Known side effects of this therapy include electrolyte imbalances, nausea, and bloating.

Rifaximin, a semisynthetic drug derivative of rifampin, was originally employed as a second-line treatment for hepatic encephalopathy. In 2012, a meta-analysis of 12 randomized controlled trials stated that rifaximin had similar effectiveness compared to lactulose, with fewer side effects [41]. A more recent, larger meta-analysis has also further supported its use [42], although the dominant limitation remains its high cost when compared to lactulose.

Hepatorenal syndrome

Euvolemia and electrolyte homeostasis should be maintained under strict clinical and laboratory monitoring. Acute kidney injury in the absence of hemodynamic instability, use of nephrotoxic drugs, or parenchymal renal disease suggests the diagnosis of hepatorenal syndrome. Additional diagnostic criteria include no improvement in renal function after volume expansion with albumin and diuretic withdrawal. Treatment of hepatorenal syndrome requires the use of splanchnic vasoconstrictors (terlipressin, noradrenalin, or midodrine) and albumin infusion. Improved renal function has been demonstrated with medical treatment [10], but a mortality benefit is only ultimately achieved with liver transplantation. TIPS placement and renal and hepatic replacement therapies can be indicated as bridging strategies.

Variceal hemorrhage

Perioperative volume overload can increase portal pressure and precipitate bleeding from esophageal varices. Other possible contributing factors include postoperative hepatic dysfunction and portal venous thrombosis. Variceal hemorrhage represents a medical emergency to be managed in the intensive care unit [43].

Resuscitative measures to preserve the respiratory and circulatory systems should be promptly initiated. A restrictive transfusion strategy aiming at hemoglobin levels of 7–9 g/dl has been associated with decreased re-bleeding and mortality rates [44]. Antibiotic prophylaxis with ceftriaxone for up to 7 days is indicated to address the increased risk of bacterial infections and also to decrease the risk of re-bleeding and mortality [45]. Infusion of vasoactive agents (somatostatin, terlipressin, and octreotide) for 2 to 5 days has been associated with lower mortality and transfusion requirements [46].

An urgent endoscopy should be completed no longer than 12 h from presentation [43]. Elastic band ligation represents the first-line endoscopic intervention for esophageal varices, but sclerotherapy is an excellent alternative for difficult cases [47]. Elastic band ligation has proven more effective than sclerotherapy in terms of the number of required sessions, as well as re-bleeding and mortality rates [48, 49]. A non-specific beta-blocker (propranolol or nadolol) is indicated after the vasoactive infusion is discontinued.

Balloon tamponade is reserved for temporary control of ongoing variceal bleeding while definitive therapy is being arranged. TIPS should be considered pre-emptively in high-risk patients, or in refractory or recurrent hemorrhage, as improved mortality rates have been observed [50].

Table 3 summarizes current recommendations for the management of hemorrhage from esophageal varices.

Venous thromboembolism prophylaxis

Coagulation disorders of cirrhosis confer an increased risk of both venous thromboembolism and hemorrhage. As previously indicated, conventional coagulation tests do not reflect these risks, and an increased INR is not necessarily protective for thromboembolic events. Although detailed guidelines remain unavailable, thromboprophylaxis is recommended in most patients, and certainly in high-risk situations.

Conclusions

Chronic liver disease in the surgical patient directly affects perioperative care. In acute care surgery, cirrhosis and the postoperative inflammatory response confound the boundaries between low effective circulating volume with renal failure and anasarca with respiratory failure. Perioperative care should contemplate specific topics such as (1) severity stratification for hepatic dysfunction, (2) imaging findings of portal hypertension, (3) management of coagulation disorders, and (4) vigilance for postoperative hepatic failure (e.g., ascites, jaundice, hepatic encephalopathy, hepatorenal syndrome, and variceal hemorrhage) and possible precipitating factors.

Table 3 Management of variceal hemorrhage

Blood product transfusion: aim at hemoglobin levels between 7 and 9 g/dl.
Antibiotic prophylaxis: ceftriaxone 1 g/dl, no longer than 7 days.
Vasoactive agents (octreotide, terlipressin, somatostatin): bolus followed by infusion for 2 to 5 days.
Endoscopy: no longer than 12 h from presentation.
Start non-specific beta-blocker (propranolol, nadolol): once vasoactive agent is discontinued.
Consider TIPS: high-risk patients, refractory or recurrent hemorrhage.

Abbreviations

ALT: Alanine aminotransferase; AST: Aspartate aminotransferase; CT: Computed tomography; HRS: Hepatorenal syndrome; INR: International normalized ratio; MELD: Model of End-Stage Liver Disease; TIPS: Transjugular intra-hepatic portosystemic Shunt

Authors' contributions

CGB, SMH, and EJ designed this study. MSB and AKB drafted the manuscript. All authors (MSB, AKB, EJ, SMH, and CGB) critically revised and approved the final version to be submitted.

Competing interests

The authors declare that they have no competing interests.

Author details

[1]Department of Surgery, University of British Columbia, Vancouver, Canada. [2]Department of Surgery, University of Calgary, Foothills Medical Centre, 1403 - 29 Street NW, Calgary, Alberta, Canada.

References

1. Jackson FC, Christophersen EB, Peternel WW, Kirimli B. Preoperative management of patients with liver disease. Surg Clin North Am. 1968;48(4): 907–30.
2. de Goede MSc B, MD PJK, Professor JFLM, Professor HJMM, Professor GKM. Morbidity and mortality related to non-hepatic surgery in patients with liver cirrhosis: a systematic review. Best Pract Res Clin Gastroenterol. 2012;26(1):47–59.
3. Teh SH, Nagorney DM, Stevens SR, Offord KP, Therneau TM, Plevak DJ, Talwalkar JA, Kim WR, Kamath PS. Risk factors for mortality after surgery in patients with cirrhosis. Gastroenterology. 2007;132(4):1261–9.
4. Csikesz NG, Nguyen LN, Tseng JF, Shah SA. Nationwide volume and mortality after elective surgery in cirrhotic patients. J Am Coll Surg. 2009; 208(1):96–103.
5. Moore CM. Cirrhotic ascites review: pathophysiology, diagnosis and management. World J Health. 2013;5(5):251–13.
6. Blasi A. Coagulopathy in liver disease: lack of an assessment tool. World J Gastroenterol. 2015;21(35):10062–71.
7. Arroyo V, Terra C, Gines P. Advances in the pathogenesis and treatment of type-1 and type-2 hepatorenal syndrome. J Hepatol. 2007;46(5):935–46.
8. Patidar KR, Bajaj JS. Covert and overt hepatic encephalopathy: diagnosis and management. Clin Gastroenterol Hepatol. 2015;13(12):2048–61.
9. Dhiman RK. Gut microbiota and hepatic encephalopathy. Metab Brain Dis. 2013;28(2):321–6.
10. Davenport A, Ahmad J, Al-Khafaji A, Kellum JA, Genyk YS, Nadim MK. Medical management of hepatorenal syndrome. Nephrol Dial Transplant. 2012;27(1):34–41.
11. Amarapurkar PD, Amarapurkar DN. Management of coagulopathy in patients with decompensated liver cirrhosis. Int J Hepatol. 2011;2011: 695470.
12. Branco BC, Inaba K, Ives C, Okoye O, Shulman I, David JS, Schöchl H, Rhee P, Demetriades D. Thromboelastogram evaluation of the impact of hypercoagulability in trauma patients. Shock. 2014;41(3):200–7.
13. Coakley M, Reddy K, Mackie I, Mallett S. Transfusion triggers in orthotopic liver transplantation: a comparison of the thromboelastometry analyzer, the thromboelastogram, and conventional coagulation tests. J Cardiothorac Vasc Anesth. 2006;20(4):548–53.
14. Feltracco P, Barbieri S, Cillo U, Zanus G, Senzolo M, Ori C. Perioperative thrombotic complications in liver transplantation. World J Gastroenterol. 2015;21(26):8004–13.
15. De Pietri L, Bianchini M, Montalti R, De Maria N, Di Maira T, Begliomini B, Gerunda GE, di Benedetto F, Garcia-Tsao G, Villa E. Thrombelastography-guided blood product use before invasive procedures in cirrhosis with severe coagulopathy: A randomized, controlled trial. Hepatology. 2016;63(2): 566–73.

16. Child CG, Turcotte JG. Surgery and portal hypertension. In: Child CG, editor. The liver and portal hypertension. Philadelphia: Saunders; 1964. p. 50–64.
17. Pugh RN, Murray-Lyon IM, Dawson JL, Pietroni MC, Williams R. Transection of the oesophagus for bleeding oesophageal varices. Br J Surg. 1973;60(8): 646–9.
18. Garrison RN, Cryer HM, Howard DA, Polk HC Jr. Clarification of risk factors for abdominal operations in patients with hepatic cirrhosis. Ann Surg. 1984; 199(6):648–55.
19. Mansour A, Watson W, Shayani V, Pickleman J. Abdominal operations in patients with cirrhosis: still a major surgical challenge. Surgery. 1997;122(4): 730–5. discussion 5-6
20. Malinchoc M, Kamath PS, Gordon FD, Peine CJ, Rank J, ter Borg PC. A model to predict poor survival in patients undergoing transjugular intrahepatic portosystemic shunts. Hepatology. 2000;31(4):864–71.
21. Hanje AJ, Patel T. Preoperative evaluation of patients with liver disease. Nat Clin Pract Gastroenterol Hepatol. 2007;4(5):266–76.
22. Wiesner RH, McDiarmid SV, Kamath PS, Edwards EB, Malinchoc M, Kremers WK, Krom RA, Kim WR. MELD and PELD: application of survival models to liver allocation. Liver Transpl. 2001;7(7):567–80.
23. Biggins SW, Kim WR, Terrault NA, Saab S, Balan V, Schiano T, Benson J, Therneau T, Kremers W, Wiesner R, et al. Evidence-based incorporation of serum sodium concentration into MELD. Gastroenterology. 2006;130(6): 1652–60.
24. Causey MW, Steele SR, Farris Z, Lyle DS, Beitler AL. An assessment of different scoring systems in cirrhotic patients undergoing nontransplant surgery. Am J Surg. 2012;203(5):589–93.
25. Yeom SK, Lee CH, Cha SH, Park CM. Prediction of liver cirrhosis, using diagnostic imaging tools. World J Hepatol. 2015;7(17):2069–79.
26. Sangster GP, Previgliano CH, Nader M, Chwoschtschinsky E, Heldmann MG. MDCT imaging findings of liver cirrhosis: spectrum of hepatic and extrahepatic abdominal complications. HPB Surg. 2013;2013:129396.
27. Wachsberg RH, Bahramipour P, Sofocleous CT, Barone A. Hepatofugal flow in the portal venous system: pathophysiology, imaging findings, and diagnostic pitfalls. Radiographics. 2002;22(1):123–40.
28. Moggia E, Rouse B, Simillis C, Li T, Vaughan J, Davidson BR, et al. Methods to decrease blood loss during liver resection: a network meta-analysis. Cochrane Database Syst Rev. 2016;10:Cd010683.
29. Wong-Lun-Hing EM, van Woerden V, Lodewick TM, Bemelmans MHA, Olde Damink SWM, Dejong CHC, et al. Abandoning prophylactic abdominal drainage after hepatic surgery: 10 years of no-drain policy in an enhanced recovery after surgery environment. Dig Surg. 2017;34(5):411–20.
30. Liu CL, Fan ST, Lo CM, Wong Y, Ng IO, Lam CM, et al. Abdominal drainage after hepatic resection is contraindicated in patients with chronic liver diseases. Ann Surg. 2004;239(2):194–201.
31. El-Awadi S, El-Nakeeb A, Youssef T, Fikry A, El-Hamed TMA, Ghazy H, Foda E, Farid M. Laparoscopic versus open cholecystectomy in cirrhotic patients: a prospective randomized study. Int J Surg. 2009;7(1):66–9.
32. Puggioni A, Wong LL. A metaanalysis of laparoscopic cholecystectomy in patients with cirrhosis. J Am Coll Surg. 2003;197(6):921–6.
33. Tsugawa K, Koyanagi N, Hashizume M, Tomikawa M, Ayukawa K, Akahoshi K, Sugimachi K. A comparison of an open and laparoscopic appendectomy for patients with liver cirrhosis. Surg Laparosc Endosc Percutan Tech. 2001;11(3): 189–94.
34. Belghiti J, Durand F. Abdominal wall hernias in the setting of cirrhosis. Semin Liver Dis. 1997;17(3):219–26.
35. Belli G, D'Agostino A, Fantini C, Cioffi L, Belli A, Russolillo N, Langella S. Laparoscopic incisional and umbilical hernia repair in cirrhotic patients. Surg Laparosc Endosc Percutan Tech. 2006;16(5):330–3.
36. Yu BC, Chung M, Lee G. The repair of umbilical hernia in cirrhotic patients: 18 consecutive case series in a single institute. Ann Surg Treat Res. 2015; 89(2):87–5.
37. James J, Liou IW. Comprehensive care of patients with chronic liver disease. Med Clin North Am. 2015;99(5):913–33.
38. Cabral CM, Burns DL. Low-protein diets for hepatic encephalopathy debunked: let them eat steak. Nutr Clin Pract. 2011;26(2):155–9.
39. Gluud LL, Dam G, Les I, Cordoba J, Marchesini G, Borre M, Aagaard NK, Vilstrup H. Branched-chain amino acids for people with hepatic encephalopathy. Cochrane Database Syst Rev. 2015;9:Cd001939.
40. Patil DH, Westaby D, Mahida YR, Palmer KR, Rees R, Clark ML, Dawson AM, Silk DB. Comparative modes of action of lactitol and lactulose in the treatment of hepatic encephalopathy. Gut. 1987;28(3):255–9.
41. Eltawil KM. Rifaximin vs conventional oral therapy for hepatic encephalopathy: a meta-analysis. World J Gastroenterol. 2012;18(8):767–11.
42. Kimer N, Krag A, Møller S, Bendtsen F, Gluud LL. Systematic review with meta-analysis: the effects of rifaximin in hepatic encephalopathy. Aliment Pharmacol Ther. 2014;40(2):123–32.
43. Garcia-Tsao G, Abraldes JG, Berzigotti A, Bosch J. Portal hypertensive bleeding in cirrhosis: risk stratification, diagnosis, and management: 2016 practice guidance by the American Association for the study of liver diseases. Hepatology. 2017;65(1):310–35.
44. Villanueva C, Colomo A, Bosch A, Concepcion M, Hernandez-Gea V, Aracil C, et al. Transfusion strategies for acute upper gastrointestinal bleeding. N Engl J Med. 2013;368(1):11–21.
45. Chavez-Tapia NC, Barrientos-Gutierrez T, Tellez-Avila F, Soares-Weiser K, Mendez-Sanchez N, Gluud C, et al. Meta-analysis: antibiotic prophylaxis for cirrhotic patients with upper gastrointestinal bleeding—an updated Cochrane review. Aliment Pharmacol Ther. 2011;34(5):509–18.
46. Wells M, Chande N, Adams P, Beaton M, Levstik M, Boyce E, et al. Meta-analysis: vasoactive medications for the management of acute variceal bleeds. Aliment Pharmacol Ther. 2012;35(11):1267–78.
47. Bari K, Garcia-Tsao G. Treatment of portal hypertension. World J Gastroenterol. 2012;18(11):1166–75.
48. Avgerinos A, Armonis A, Stefanidis G, Mathou N, Vlachogiannakos J, Kougioumtzian A, Triantos C, Papaxoinis C, Manolakopoulos S, Panani A, et al. Sustained rise of portal pressure after sclerotherapy, but not band ligation, in acute variceal bleeding in cirrhosis. Hepatology. 2004;39(6):1623–30.
49. Villanueva C, Piqueras M, Aracil C, Gomez C, Lopez-Balaguer JM, Gonzalez B, Ballego A, Torras X, Soriano G, Sáinz S, et al. A randomized controlled trial comparing ligation and sclerotherapy as emergency endoscopic treatment added to somatostatin in acute variceal bleeding. J Hepatol. 2006;45(4):560–7.
50. Garcia-Pagan JC, Di Pascoli M, Caca K, Laleman W, Bureau C, Appenrodt B, Luca A, Zipprich A, Abraldes JG, Nevens F, et al. Use of early-TIPS for high-risk variceal bleeding: results of a post-RCT surveillance study. J Hepatol. 2013;58(1):45–50.

19

Proceedings of resources for optimal care of acute care and emergency surgery consensus summit Donegal Ireland

M. Sugrue[1*], R. Maier[2,3], E. E. Moore[4], M. Boermeester[5], F. Catena[6], F. Coccolini[7], A. Leppaniemi[8], A. Peitzman[9], G. Velmahos[10], L. Ansaloni[11], F. Abu-Zidan[12], P. Balfe[13], C. Bendinelli[14], W. Biffl[15], M. Bowyer[16], M. DeMoya[17], J. De Waele[18], S. Di Saverio[19], A. Drake[20], G. P. Fraga[21], A. Hallal[22], C. Henry[23], T. Hodgetts[24], L. Hsee[25], S. Huddart[26], A. W. Kirkpatrick[27], Y. Kluger[28], L. Lawler[29], M. A. Malangoni[30], M. Malbrain[31], P. MacMahon[32], K. Mealy[33], M. O'Kane[34], P. Loughlin[35], M. Paduraru[36], L. Pearce[37], B. M. Pereira[38], A. Priyantha[39], M. Sartelli[40], K. Soreide[41,46], C. Steele[42], S. Thomas[43], J. L. Vincent[44] and L. Woods[45]

Abstract

Background: Opportunities to improve emergency surgery outcomes exist through guided better practice and reduced variability. Few attempts have been made to define optimal care in emergency surgery, and few clinically derived key performance indicators (KPIs) have been published. A summit was therefore convened to look at resources for optimal care of emergency surgery. The aim of the Donegal Summit was to set a platform in place to develop guidelines and KPIs in emergency surgery.

Methods: The project had multidisciplinary global involvement in producing consensus statements regarding emergency surgery care in key areas, and to assess feasibility of producing KPIs that could be used to monitor process and outcome of care in the future.

Results: Forty-four key opinion leaders in emergency surgery, across 7 disciplines from 17 countries, composed evidence-based position papers on 14 key areas of emergency surgery and 112 KPIs in 20 acute conditions or emergency systems.

Conclusions: The summit was successful in achieving position papers and KPIs in emergency surgery. While position papers were limited by non-graded evidence and non-validated KPIs, the process set a foundation for the future advancement of emergency surgery.

Keywords: Emergency surgery, Optimal care, Performance indicators, Surgical outcomes

Background

Optimal consistent emergency surgery care presents a major health challenge worldwide [1–3]. Patients requiring urgent surgical care are often critically ill with significant pre-existing comorbidities [4]. While there is a wide spectrum of potential presenting surgical conditions, there is a predictable pattern because the top seven emergency surgery conditions account for nearly 80% of presentations [5]. Modern surgical care requires a multi-disciplinary approach and streamlined acute pathways are critical to ensure optimal outcomes [6].

Historically, it is not uncommon to manage emergency surgical patients interspersed with daily elective activities within a given hospital system [7]. The lack of timely appropriate access to emergency surgical care is often multi-factorial and may include shortage of emergency surgeons, inadequate access to the operating room, lack of a dedicated team, and a paucity of clinical pathways [8].

Over the past decade, the importance of a comprehensive system in managing emergency surgical care has become evident, resulting in training bodies and health

* Correspondence: michaelesugrue@gmail.com
[1]Department of Surgery, Letterkenny University Hospital and Donegal Clinical Research Academy, Donegal, Ireland
Full list of author information is available at the end of the article

ministries publishing multiple consensus papers and statements on this topic [6, 9–13].

Monitoring emergency surgery performance and outcomes is essential and clinicians themselves need to be involved in determining key performance indicators (KPIs). KPIs in emergency surgery have not been widely developed. For this reason, under the leadership of the World Society of Emergency Surgery, with support from the Abdominal Compartment Society and Donegal Clinical Research Academy key opinion leaders in the field of emergency surgery care across many disciplines were invited to contribute to a Performance Summit in Donegal in 2016.

The Emergency Surgery Performance Summit aimed to develop key performance indicators in clinical and systems delivery that would lay the foundation for future optimal surgery development.

Methods

Common aspects of emergency surgery were identified into 14 categories (Table 1), 44 key opinion leaders were invited to participate and co-author individual chapters. There were 14 position papers and 20 topics for KPI development (Table 2). A review of published articles and consensus statements relating to the establishment and design of emergency, acute care surgery, and emergency general services was performed. Emergency surgery position statements from the surgical colleges, surgical institutions and key government organisations were assessed. The key performance indicators were proposed according to a standardised pro forma (Table 3). Each KPI had to be easily measured and reproducible. Due to the extent and complexity of topics and number of authors, the original intent to grade level was not uniform and thus reporting was confined to consensus opinion.

Table 1 Key position topics for summit

Resources and designation of emergency surgery
Acute care unit structure
Reception and triage
Data systems, registry and evaluation
Rural emergency care and transfer
Paediatric emergency care
Geriatric emergency care
Interaction and laboratory, radiology, ICU gastroenterology
Quality assurance and performance improvement
Sepsis control in emergency room
Research in acute care surgery
Education in emergency surgery
Accreditation review and consultative program
Patient related outcomes measures

Table 2 Key performance indicators topics

Appendicitis
Cholecystitis
Pancreatitis
Perforated ulcer
Gastrointestinal bleeding
Bowel obstruction
Diverticulitis
Mesenteric ischaemia
Abdominal vascular emergencies
Coagulation
Complex pneumothorax and empyema
Septic shock in emergency; ICU
Fluid resuscitation in septic shock
Abdominal compartment syndrome
Geriatric care
Triage; ICU admission
Laboratory
Wound care
Emergency theatre
Health care systems

Results

The summit was held in Lough Eske Castle Donegal Ireland on 25 July 2016, attended by 80 people of which 44 contributed to writing the Proceeding's chapters, and associated KPIs. The key opinion leaders were from seven disciplines, predominantly surgery, but also including critical care, internal medicine, emergency medicine, radiology and nursing. There were 119 KPIs

Table 3 Example of KPI of 1 of the 112 KPI generated

Title	Negative appendectomy rate
Description	Percentage of negative appendectomies performed
Rationale	It is an indicator of diagnostic efficiency. In order to avoid unnecessary surgery and decrease costs and complications.
Target	< 10% appendixes removed are normal
KPI collection frequency	Annually
KPI reporting frequency	Annually
KPI calculation	Numerator divided by denominator expressed as a percentage Numerator: number of patients underwent appendectomy with negative appendectomy Denominator: number of all patients underwent appendectomy
Reporting aggregation	Hospital, hospital group
Data source(s)	OR registry, medical records, patients chart, hospital discharge data, emergency surgery database

described for the 20 conditions, a sample is shown in Table 3. The entire proceedings for the summit are available on line [14]. The summit provided a platform for discussion and agreed consensus on the key position topics. Future resources for advancing systems, clinical care, research and reporting were debated and supported. Consensus was reached that the KPIs for use in emergency surgery care needed to be simple, with a small number for each major condition.

Discussion

Globally, there is increasing interest in improving emergency surgery outcomes by health providers, learned societies, colleges and health departments [15–17]. Over a decade ago, it was estimated that more than 230 million surgical procedures were performed and within that workload, emergency general surgery accounts for a significant part [18]. In addition, emergency surgery has one of the greatest overall associated mortalities of any medical discipline [19]. It is estimated that 890,000 patients die during their emergency surgical care annually [20]. Patients undergoing laparotomy have variable mortality depending on their diagnosis, treatment and location of service provision [1, 2, 4, 21]. The American College of Surgeons National Surgical Quality Improvement Program database identified that emergency surgery patients have significantly more postoperative complications (23 vs 14%; $P < .0001$) as well as greater mortality rates (6 vs 1%; $P < .0001$) compared with non-emergency general surgery patients [22]. Ingraham recently reported that an expert panel ranked quality indicators in certain emergency surgery conditions [23]. They reviewed historic compliance with select quality indicators for four procedures (cholecystectomy, appendectomy, colectomy, small bowel resection) at four academic centres and concluded that potential adherence to quality indicators may improve the quality of emergency general surgery care provided for which current outcomes are potentially modifiable [23]. The summit reported KPIs in a much larger group, incorporating 20 conditions and sectors of health care provision.

To improve outcomes, we must not just develop quality benchmarks and standards but also understand prevalence and significance of complications [24, 25]. While there are limitations to many new systems being developed [26, 27]. It is only through engagement with all the disciplines involved in emergency surgery that care will evolve and improve. The Donegal Summit on resources for optimal care included not just surgeons, but also emergency physicians, anaesthetists, critical care, internal medicine, gastroenterology, radiology and nursing. While the summit developed and reported potential key performance indicators and outlines of basic resources required for functioning part of emergency surgery systems, it had limitations. There was inadequate patient forum representation. The process was consensus-based and did not use a formal statistical or Delphi approach for the development of KPIs. The KPIs would in time need to be validated.

The summit and this proceedings paper have however set a process in place to facilitate concepts and benchmarks in resourcing emergency surgery. It has mirrored that international desire to improve outcomes [24].

Over the last decade there has been increasing development of Acute Care Surgical Units. Some of these have developed and reported limited KPIs [7]. Trauma care has been to the forefront of KPI development in acute care. In other areas of surgery, KPIs are widely reported. This summit was unique in having many key opinion leaders in attendance and discussing the process.

Conclusion

In conclusion, the Summit on Resources for Optimal Care of Acute Care and Emergency Surgery Consensus Summit successfully identified key aspects of emergency surgery that need to be tackled to outline optimal strategy of care and definitive KPIs. Future work needs to expand on the work achieved here and in other forums, to define optimum care and robust, meaningful measurement tools of process and outcome. The WSES will lead the process in standardised KPI development. The summit acknowledged superb efforts to enhance emergency surgery care by others but felt an international collaboration and commitment was needed to implement and monitor these systems as soon as possible.

Acknowledgements
World Society of Emergency Surgery. World Society of Abdominal Compartment. Donegal Clinical Research Academy. A project supported by the EU's INERREGVA Programme managed by the Special EU Programmes Body (SEUPB).

Funding
Donegal Clinical Research Academy. It donated 10,000 euros to help run the meeting and had no influence on outcomes.

Authors' contributions
Each author contributed to writing a chapter on either position statement or key performance indicators. All authors read and approved the final manuscript.

Competing interests
Michael Sugrue Consultant Smith and Nephew. Jan J. De Waele—consultancy for Cubist, AtoxBio, Pfizer, Smith & Nephew, KCI, Bayer Healthcare and MSD.

Author details
[1]Department of Surgery, Letterkenny University Hospital and Donegal Clinical Research Academy, Donegal, Ireland. [2]Department of Surgery, University of Washington, Seattle, USA. [3]Harborview Medical Center, Seattle, USA. [4]University of Colorado, Denver, USA. [5]Department of Surgery, Academic Medical Center, Amsterdam, Netherlands. [6]Department of Emergency Surgery, Maggiore Hospital, Parma, Italy. [7]Department of Emergency, General and Transplant Surgery, Papa Giovanni XXIII Hospital, Bergamo, Italy. [8]Abdominal Center, University Hospital Meilahti, Helsinki, Finland.

[9]Department of Surgery, University of Pittsburgh School of Medicine, Pittsburgh, PA, USA. [10]Department of Trauma, Emergency Surgery and Surgical Critical Care, Massachusetts General Hospital, Boston, MA, USA. [11]General Surgery Department, Papa Giovanni XXIII Hospital, Bergamo, Italy. [12]Department of Surgery, College of Medicine and Health Sciences, UAE University, Al-Ain, United Arab Emirates. [13]Department of Surgery, St. Luke's Hospital, Kilkenny, Ireland. [14]Department of Surgery, John Hunter Hospital, Newcastle, NSW, Australia. [15]Acute Care Surgery, The Queens Medical Center, Honolulu, HI, USA. [16]Department of Surgery, Uniformed Services University and Walter Reed National Military Medical Center, Bethesda, MD, USA. [17]Department of Trauma/Critical Care, Massachusetts General Hospital, Boston, MA, USA. [18]Department of Critical Care Medicine, Ghent University Hospital, Ghent, Belgium. [19]Maggiore Hospital of Bologna, AUSL, Bologna, Italy. [20]Letterkenny University Hospital and Donegal Clinical Research Academy, Donegal, Ireland. [21]Division of Trauma Surgery, Department of Surgery, School of Medical Sciences, University of Campinas, Campinas, Brazil. [22]Department of Surgery, American University of Beirut Medical Center, Beirut, Lebanon. [23]National Clinical Advisor for the Acute Hospitals Division, Health Service Executive, Dublin, Ireland. [24]Trauma Governance, UK Defence Medical Services, Lichfield, UK. [25]Department of Trauma and Acute Care Surgery, Auckland City Hospital, Auckland, New Zealand. [26]Department of Anaesthesiology, Royal Surrey County Hospital, Guildford, UK. [27]Department of Surgery, Critical Care Medicine and Regional Trauma Service, Foothills Medical Centre, Calgary, AB, Canada. [28]Department of General Surgery, Division of Surgery, Rambam Health Care Campus, Haifa, Israel. [29]Department of Radiology, Mater Misericordiae University Hospital, Dublin, Ireland. [30]American Board of Surgery, Philadelphia, PA, USA. [31]Intensive Care Unit and High Burn Unit, ZNA "Ziekenhuis Netwerk Antwerpen" Stuivenberg and ZNA St-Erasmus hospitals, Antwerp, Belgium. [32]Department of Radiology, Mater Misericordiae University Hospital, Dublin, Ireland. [33]Department of Surgery, Wexford University Hospital, Wexford, Ireland. [34]Department of Pathology, Altnagelvin Hospital, Londonderry, UK. [35]Department of Surgery, Altnagelvin Hospital, Londonderry, UK. [36]Milton Keynes University Hospital NHS Foundation Trust, Milton Keynes, UK. [37]Northwest Research Collaborative, Manchester, UK. [38]Division of Trauma Surgery, Department of Surgery, School of Medical Sciences, University of Campinas, Campinas, Brazil. [39]Department of Gastroenterology, Teaching Hospital, South, Colombo, Sri Lanka. [40]Department of Surgery, Macerata Hospital, Macerata, Italy. [41]Department of Clinical Medicine, University of Bergen, Bergen, Norway. [42]Department of Gastroenterology, Letterkenny University Hospital and Donegal Clinical Research Academy, Donegal, Ireland. [43]Department of Trauma Services, Memorial Hospital of South Bend, Indiana, USA. [44]Department of Intensive Care, Erasme Hospital, Université libre de bruxelles, Brussels, Belgium. [45]Department of Acute Hospitals, Health Services Executive, Dublin, Ireland. [46]Department of Gastrointestinal Surgery, Stavanger University Hospital, Stavanger, Norway.

References

1. Tan BH, Mytton J, Al-Khyatt W, Aquina CT, Evison F, Fleming FJ, Griffiths E, Vohra RS. A comparison of mortality following emergency laparotomy between populations from New York state and England. Annals Surgery. 2017;266(2):280–6.
2. The Second Patient Report of the National Emergency Laparotomy Audit (NELA) December 2014 to November 2015 July 2016 http://www.nela.org.uk/reports accessed 23 Feb 2017.
3. Santry HP, Madore JC, Collins CE, Ayturk MD, Velmahos GC, Britt LD, et al. Variations in implementation of acute care surgery: results from a national survey of university-affiliated hospitals. J Trauma Acute Care Surg. 2015; 78(1):60–7.
4. Tolstrup MB, Watt SK, Gögenur I. Morbidity and mortality rates after emergency abdominal surgery: an analysis of 4346 patients scheduled for emergency laparotomy or laparoscopy. Langenbeck's Arch Surgery. 2016;9:1–9.
5. Scott JW, Olufajo OA, Brat GA, Rose JA, Zogg CK, Haider AH, SalimA HJM. Use of national burden to defineoperative emergency general surgery. JAMA Surg. 2016;151(6):e160480.
6. Royal College of Surgeons in Ireland. Model of care for acute surgery: National Clinical Programme in Surgery [Internet]. RCSI; 2013. Available at http://www.rcsi.ie/files/surgery/20131216021838_Model%20of%20Care%20for%20Acute%20Surger.pdf. Accessed 12 Apr 2017.
7. Hsee L, Devaud M, Middleberg L, Jones W, Civil I. Acute surgical unit at Auckland City Hospital: a descriptive analysis. ANZ J Surg. 2012;82(9): 588–91.
8. Association of Surgeons of Great Britain and Ireland. Emergency general surgery: the future a consensus statement [Internet]. ASGBI. Available at http://www.asgbi.org.uk/consensus-statements/ accessed 12 Apr 2017.
9. Sorelli PG, El-Masry NS, Dawson PM, Theodorou NA. The dedicated emergency surgeon: towards consultant-based acute surgical admissions. Ann R Coll Surg Engl. 2008;90:104–8.
10. Hameed SM, Brenneman FD, Ball CG, Pagliarello J, Razek T, Parry N, et al. General surgery 2.0: the emergence of acute care surgery in Canada. Can J Surg. 2010;53(2):79–83.
11. Royal Australasian College of Surgeons. The case for the separation of elective and emergency surgery [Internet]. RACS; 2011. Available at http://www.surgeons.org/media/college-advocacy/submission-to-the-council-of-australian-government's-expert-panel-on-the-case-for-the-separation-of-elective-and-emergency-surgery/ accessed 12 Apr 2017.
12. The Royal College of Surgeons of England. Separating emergency and elective surgical care: recommendations for practice [Internet]. RCSENG Professional Standards and Regulation; 2007. Available https://www.rcseng.ac.uk/library-and-publications/college-publications/year/ accessed 12 Apr 2017.
13. Professional Standards and Regulation Directorate: Royal College of Surgeons of England. Standards for Unscheduled Surgical Care: Guidance for providers, commissioners and service planners [Internet]. Publications Department, The Royal College of Surgeons of England; 2011. Available at: https://www.rcseng.ac.uk/library-and-publications/college-publications/year/ accessed 12 Apr 2017.
14. Resources for optimal care of emergency surgery Letterkenny 2016 978–0–09926109 9-9 Available http://dcra.ie/images/Resources_2016_Emergency_Surgery.pdf accessed 12 Apr 2017.
15. Royal Australasian College of Surgeon (2015) Position paper of emergency surgery. Available at: https://www.surgeons.org/media/311630/2015-05-20_pos_fes-pst-050_emergency_surgery.pdf accessed 5 Oct 2017.
16. General Surgeon Association of Australia (2010) 12-Point plan on emergency surgery. Available at: https://www.generalsurgeons.com.au/media/files/Publications/PLN%202010-09-19%20GSA%2012%20Point%20Plan.pdf. Accessed 5 Oct 2017.
17. Ministry of Health New Zealand (2011) Targeting emergencies: shorter stays in emergency departments. Available at: https://www.health.govt.nz/search/results/Targeting%20emergencies%3A%20shorter%20stays%20in%20emergency%20department. Accessed 5 Oct 2017.
18. Stewart B, Khanduri P, McCord C, Ohene-Yeboah M, Uranues S, Vega Rivera F, Mock C. Global disease burden of conditions requiring emergency surgery. BJS. 2014;101:e9–e22.
19. Tolstrup MB, Watt SK, Gögenur I. Morbidity and mortality rates after emergency abdominal surgery: an analysis of 4346 patients scheduled for emergency laparotomy or laparoscopy. Langenbeck's Arch Surg. 2017;402(4):615–23.
20. Scott JW, Olufajo OA, Brat GA, Rose JA, Zogg CK, Haider AH, Salim A, Havens JM. Use of national burden to define operative emergency general surgery. JAMA surgery. 2016;151(6):e160480.
21. Ogola GO, Haider A, Shafi S. Hospitals with higher volumes of emergency general surgery patients achieve lower mortality rates: a case for establishing designated centers for emergency general surgery. J Trauma Acute Care Surg. 2017;82(3):497–504.
22. Becher RD, Hoth JJ, Miller PR, Mowery NT, Chang MC, Meredith JW. A critical assessment of outcomes in emergency versus nonemergency general surgery using the American College of Surgeons National Surgical Quality Improvement Program database. Am Surg. 2011;77:951–9.
23. Ingraham A, Nathens A, Peitzman A, Bode A, Dorlac G, Dorlac W, Miller P, Sadeghi M, Wasserman DD, Bilimoria K. Assessment of emergency general surgery care based on formally developed quality indicators. Surgery. 2017;162:397–407.
24. Clavien PA, Puhan MA. Measuring and achieving the best possible outcomes in surgery. Br J Surg. 2017;104:1121–2.
25. Scarborough JE, Schumacher J, Pappas TN, McCoy CC, Englum BR, Agarwal SK, Greenberg CC. Which complications matter most? Prioritizing quality improvement in emergency general surgery. J Am Coll Surg. 2016;222(4):515–24.
26. Nathan H, Dimick JB. Quality accounting: understanding the impact of multiple surgical complications. Ann Surgery. 2017;265(6):1051–2.
27. Quiney N, Aggarwal G, Scott M, Dickinson M. Survival after emergency general surgery: what can we learn from enhanced recovery programmes? World J Surg. 2016;40(6):1283–7.

20

Establishing position papers by the WSES

Miklosh Bala[1*], Jeffry Kashuk[2], Ernest E. Moore[3], Fausto Catena[4], Ari Leppaniemi[5], Luca Ansaloni[6], Walter Biffl[7], Federico Coccolini[6], Andrew Peitzman[8], Massimo Sartelli[9], Michael Sugrue[10], Gustavo P. Fraga[11], Salomone Di Saverio[12] and Yoram Kluger[13]

Abstract

A position paper (PP) should establish a unified voice in areas where controversy occurs based upon multiple practices and/or therapeutic choices. Typically, a position paper should elucidate the knowledge gap, followed by an evidence-based review of options, leading to an "endorsed position." A position paper should represent more than the opinion or consensus of the authors but should present current opinions and practices supported by the World Society of Emergency Surgery (WSES). Accordingly, position papers should require the approval of an expert group of WSES and in parallel be presented at an annual meeting prior to submission for publication.

It is important that a unified approach for drafting of position papers be established and endorsed by WSES in order to establish credibility and prevent misunderstandings during a smooth transition to publication.

The purpose of this article is to suggest a uniform process for the development of WSES guidelines.

Keywords: Position paper, Emergency surgery, Working group, Medical consensus

Background

By definition, a position paper (PP) is a written statement from an organization that discusses a contemporary clinical problem and suggests an established and agreed upon approach to this problem by the organization. The other term is a "medical consensus." According to the Council of Europe, "medical consensus" is a statement on a particular aspect of medical knowledge that generally is evidence-based, state-of-the-art knowledge by a representative group of experts in that area [1]. Its main objective is to recommend to colleagues the best possible and acceptable way to address an issue, and includes diagnosis, management, and operative treatment. PP fuses new information, largely from recent or ongoing research that may have implications for re-evaluation of routine medical practices.

The primary difference between a PP and a clinical practice guideline is that PP synthesizes newly available information and reinforces best medical practices but does not give detailed algorithms or guidelines for practice. Additionally, it is much easier to respond to patient needs with a PP compared with clinical practice guidelines [2]. Thus, consensus statements should provide generalized and not specific algorithms, i.e., PP statements should be independent from regional expertise, technology, and local practice.

Recently, several of the co-authors carried a PP concept from inception, development, presentation at the annual World Society of Emergency Surgery (WSES) meeting, and ultimately publication [3]. Based upon comments received on this process, the current article was formulated in order to serve as an example of how to generate a PP from the WSES.

The aim of this overview is to develop common practical steps in planning, preparing, and publishing a PP endorsed by the WSES.

Format for position papers

Title

The title should include key information to attract the reader's interest with a brief quote or detail. It should be connected to the WSES and express the ownership and endorsement of the society.

* Correspondence: rbalam@hadassah.org.il
[1]Trauma and Acute Care Surgery Unit, General Surgery Department, Hadassah Hebrew University Medical Center, Kiriat Hadassah, POB 12000, 91120 Jerusalem, Israel
Full list of author information is available at the end of the article

Authorship

Ethical guidelines for authorship have been published elsewhere [4, 5] and are included in the "information for authors" section in all peer review journals. Of note, authors should have conscientiously contributed to the formation and construct of the manuscript. The current recommendations of the WSES journal state very clearly: "We recommend adhering to the guidelines for authorship that are applicable in your research field or to the International Committee of Medical Journal Editors (ICMJE) guidelines." [6] Given the depth and breadth of a PP, there will generally be several authors working together to formulate the plans for proceeding on the process leading to publication. It is critically important that the assignment of author responsibilities be delineated clearly early in the project. Since a PP will generally involve extensive collaboration of many contributors, the best way to ensure delineation of responsibility is to divide topics into various sections, with establishment of a section author who will ultimately be responsible for writing the particular section where their work has focused. These authors will generally be responsible for presentations at the annual meeting relating to their particular section of the PP. The first three authors are responsible for collating all of the section information, presentation comments, and section manuscripts, and organizing the material in a cogent manner for drafting the initial manuscript. The order of priority of the first three authors should be determined ahead, but the first two authors are usually most intimately involved in the initial idea for the manuscript and the third author can serve as an additional advisor during the drafting process. In the example presented [2], the first three authors served in this role and, in addition, served as moderators as well as presenters during the session at the annual meeting when the topic was presented. Other authors who contribute directly to the drafting of the manuscript should be included as co-authors, and the senior author position may be reserved for a senior member who serves as a reviewer and advisor to all co-authors. This plan, as outlined, serves to ethically include all individuals who actively participate in the work; however, it should be emphasized that others who have little to no input should not be included.

Abstract

The abstract contains a synopsis of the key elements of the paper. The knowledge gap should be defined. The intent is to convey to the reader why the presentation is significant. The abstract should be written in the future tense, as the reader has not yet read the paper. Hence, it is suggesting what the reader may learn as opposed to what he may already know.

Introduction

The introduction should clearly define the topic and indicate the existing knowledge gaps. The verbiage should indicate both the specific nature of the topics well as the approach intended with the expressed purpose of generating the reader's interest.

Position statements

A position statement should be drafted based upon input from all contributing co-authors, following a comprehensive literature review and summary of current scientific evidence. A clear statement in point-form of the specific topic should be made, which cover the most important aspects of the topics with a focus on practical management.

Following the position statements, recommendations should be formulated based upon a grading system [7]. Every recommendation should be reviewed, and assigned a score based upon all co-authors and input from the WSES editorial board.

Conclusion

The conclusion should be a brief summary of the paper and the position of WSES. If applicable, particularly important recommendations may be re-stated.

Contributors listed in acknowledgments

All contributors who do not meet the criteria for authorship may be listed in an acknowledgments section at the conclusion of the manuscript.

Development of PP

The idea for a PP may be initiated by any member of WSES and should be submitted to the Board of Directors, who can provide guidance, feedback, and potential collaborations which may benefit the process. The concept generally arises from major areas of practice or examines clinical issues where there is controversy or where there are multiple practices or therapeutic options.

There are different ways of producing PP. Either the WSES board or individual members with specific interest may lead to the appointment of the lead author and panel of experts/working group (WG). The WG may be defined as WSES members having expertise in specific areas related to the topic.

The WG then reviews and synthesizes the evidence, leading to well-designed power point presentations before all attendees at an annual WSES meeting. The presentations correspond to a critical aspect of the evolution of the manuscript, it provides an opportunity for the WG to meet, collaborate, and organize their ideas, as well as a chance for the WSES membership at large to provide valuable input and feedback to the group who are formulating the PP. The presentation should include background information, relevant abbreviated literature review which should assess the quality of the scientific evidence, and an evidence-to-recommendation table with specific and clear proposed practical recommendations. Based upon this session, the WSES leadership may accept or modify the proposed recommendations, or suggest potential improvements.

Following the presentation, discussion sessions should be moderated by one or more of the proposed co-authors, where various opinions and comments should be recorded for later reference. At the conclusion of the session, one of the proposed co-authors should conclude the session with a response to all raised comments.

Based upon the presentation at the WSES meeting and collaborated material feedback received, the WG can feel confident moving forward with drafting of the initial manuscript for publication. Of note, all co-authors should have access to the power point presentations as a guide to writing their respective sessions.

The lead author, with the Board's approval, and selected experts (co-authors) generally prepare the first draft of the paper (Fig. 1). Once agreed upon by the first two or three authors, this draft may be shared via e-mail to all co-authors as well as the WSES board members for review and comment. The WG should only consider comments from respondents, who provide name, affiliation, and email.

The final draft is forwarded to all co-authors for an additional 2 weeks of review and final comments prior to submission to World Journal of Emergency Surgery (WJES).

Table 1 represents a flow diagram showing the complete process from inception to publication as described.

Conclusion

A suggested algorithm for development of a position paper for WSES is presented, with the aim of creating a uniform process which will be user friendly for the membership in an effort to streamline the process. Furthermore, by adhering to such a process, we hope to create a valuable template for use in preparation for various information sessions at the WSES yearly meeting.

The appropriate and ethical production of position papers published by WSES will benefit the society and surgical community in general with the hopes of inspiring practice improvement and up to date clinical care.

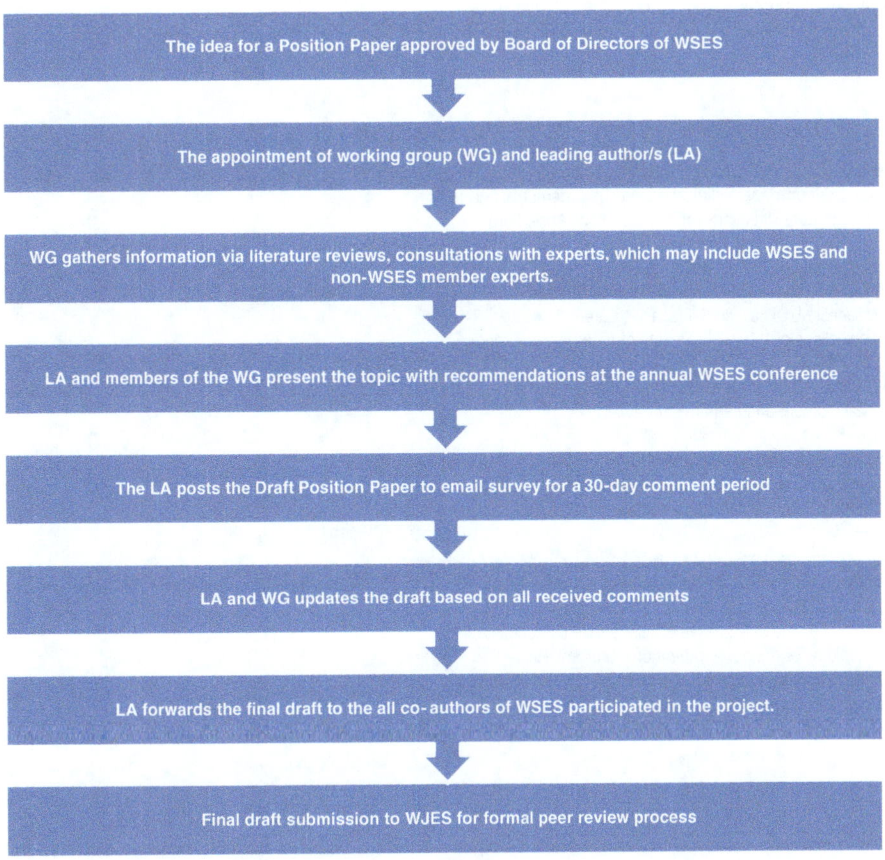

Fig. 1 Steps for the development and approval of position papers on clinical practice by WSES

Abbreviations
PP: Position paper; WG: Working group; WJES: World Journal of Emergency Surgery; WSES: World Society of Emergency Surgery

Acknowledgements
Not applicable

Funding
Not applicable

Authors' contributions
MB, JK, EM, and YK are responsible for the manuscript conception and draft; FC, AL, LA, WB, FC, AP, MS, MS, GPF, and SDS critically revised the manuscript. All authors gave the final approval.

Competing interests
The authors declare that they have no competing interests.

Author details
[1]Trauma and Acute Care Surgery Unit, General Surgery Department, Hadassah Hebrew University Medical Center, Kiriat Hadassah, POB 12000, 91120 Jerusalem, Israel. [2]Tel Aviv University Sackler School of Medicine, Assia Medical Group, Tel Aviv, Israel. [3]Department of Surgery, University of Colorado, Denver Health Medical Center, Denver, USA. [4]Emergency Department, Maggiore University Hospital, Parma, Italy. [5]Abdominal Center, University Hospital Meilahti, Helsinki, Finland. [6]General Surgery I, Papa Giovanni XXIII Hospital, Bergamo, Italy. [7]Scripps Memorial Hospital La Jolla, La Jolla, USA. [8]Department of Surgery, UPMC, University of Pittsburgh School of Medicine, Pittsburgh, PA, USA. [9]Macerata Hospital, Ancona University, Macerata Area, Italy. [10]Letterkenny University Hospital and Donegal Clinical Research Academy, Letterkenny, Ireland. [11]Division of Trauma Surgery, Hospital de Clinica, School of Medical Sciences, University of Campinas, Campinas, Brazil. [12]Department of Surgery, Maggiore Hospital, Bologna, Italy. [13]Department of General Surgery, Rambam Health Care Campus, Haifa, Israel.

References

1. Council of Europe. Developing a methodology for drawing up guidelines on best medical practice. Recommendation Rec (2001) and explanatory memorandum. Strasbourg: Council of Europe Publishing; 2002.
2. Roukis TS. White papers, position papers, clinical consensus statements, and clinical practice guidelines: future directions for ACFAS. J Foot Ankle Surg. 2015;54:151–2.
3. Bala M, Kashuk J, Moore EE, Kluger Y, Biffl W, Gomes CA, Ben-Ishay O, Rubinstein C, Balogh ZJ, Civil I, Coccolini F, Leppaniemi A, Peitzman A, Ansaloni L, Sugrue M, Sartelli M, Di Saverio S, Fraga GP, Catena F. Acute mesenteric ischemia: guidelines of the world Society of Emergency Surgery. World J Emerg Surg. 2017;12:38.
4. Kornhaber RA, LM ML, Baber RJ. Ongoing ethical issues concerning authorship in biomedical journals: an integrative review. Int J Nanomedicine. 2015;10:4837–46.
5. Graf C, Deakin L, Docking M, Jones J, Joshua S, McKerahan T, Ottmar M, Stevens A, Wates E, Wyatt D. John Wiley & Sons. Best practice guidelines on publishing ethics: a publisher's perspective, 2nd edition. Ann N Y Acad Sci. 2014;1334(Suppl 1):e1–e23.
6. http://www.icmje.org/recommendations/browse/roles-and-responsibilities/defining-the-role-of-authors-and-contributors.html. Accessed 1 Nov 2017.
7. Guyatt GH, Norris SL, Schulman S, Hirsh J, Eckman MH, Akl EA, Crowther M, Vandvik PO, Eikelboom JW, McDonagh MS, Lewis SZ, Gutterman DD, Cook DJ, Schünemann HJ. Methodology for the development of antithrombotic therapy and prevention of thrombosis guidelines: Antithrombotic Therapy and Prevention of Thrombosis, 9th ed: American College of Chest Physicians Evidence-Based Clinical Practice Guidelines. Chest. 2012;141:53S–70S.

Is case triaging a useful tool for emergency surgeries? A review of 106 trauma surgery cases at a level 1 trauma center in South Africa

Sharfuddin Chowdhury[1*], Andrew John Nicol[2], Mahammed Riyaad Moydien[3], Pradeep Harkison Navsaria[4] and Luis Felipe Montoya-Pelaez[5]

Abstract

Background: The optimal timing for emergency surgical interventions and implementation of protocols for trauma surgery is insufficient in the literature. The Groote Schuur emergency surgery triage (GSEST) system, based on Cape Triaging Score (CTS), is followed at Groote Schuur Hospital (GSH) for triaging emergency surgical cases including trauma cases. The study aimed to look at the effect of delay in surgery after scheduling based on the GSEST system has an impact on outcome in terms of postoperative complications and death.

Methods: Prospective audit of patients presenting to GSH trauma center following penetrating or blunt chest, abdominal, neck and peripheral vascular trauma who underwent surgery over a 4-month period was performed. Post-operative complications were graded according to Clavien-Dindo classification of surgical complications.

Results: One-hundred six patients underwent surgery during the study period. One-hundred two (96.2%) cases were related to penetrating trauma. Stab wounds comprised 71 (67%) and gunshot wounds (GSW) 31 (29.2%) cases. Of the 106 cases, 6, 47, 40, and 13 patients were booked as red, orange, yellow, and green, respectively. The median delay for green, yellow, and orange cases was within the expected time. The red patients took unexpectedly longer (median delay 48 min, IQR 35–60 min). Thirty-one (29.3%) patients developed postoperative complications. Among the booked red, orange, yellow, and green cases, postoperative complications developed in 3, 18, 9, and 1 cases, respectively. Only two (1.9%) postoperative deaths were documented during the study period. There was no statistically significant association between operative triage and post-operative complications ($p = 0.074$).

Conclusion: Surgical case categorization has been shown to be useful in prioritizing emergency trauma surgical cases in a resource constraint high-volume trauma center.

Keywords: Emergency surgery case triage, Trauma surgery, Postoperative complication, Outcome

Background

Trauma is an epidemic in South Africa [1]. The significant number of our emergency general surgical cases is injury related. These are potentially life-threatening, and urgent surgical intervention is required to reduce mortality and morbidity.

Emergency surgical cases are admitted to health institutions in an unplanned and unscheduled manner. Patients usually present with acute surgical conditions that require prompt and focused treatment to avoid increased morbidity and mortality. Currently, no specific national or provincial guidelines exist in South Africa for the categorization or triaging of emergency surgical cases. In the current climate of shrinking elective theater time and increasing surgical waiting time, the present focus is to decrease waiting times by addressing issues that have a detrimental effect on overall theater

* Correspondence: dr_smahmud@yahoo.com
[1]Consultant and head of Trauma Surgery, King Saud Medical City, 7790 Al-Imam Abdul Aziz Ibn Muhammad Ibn Saud, Ulaishah, Riyadh 12746, Kingdom of Saudi Arabia
Full list of author information is available at the end of the article

efficiency. However, emergency surgical caseloads form a significant and increasing percentage of all patients utilizing theater facilities. Finding ways to manage better this category of patients should result in more efficient utilization of available theater time without impinging on the throughput of cases on elective slates. Given this, a policy document or guideline was introduced at Groote Schuur Hospital (GSH) for use in the categorization and prioritization of emergency surgical cases before operative surgical management. At GSH, the Groote Schuur emergency surgery triage (GSEST) system is based on similar principles to the Cape Triaging Score (CTS) [2]. The color coding categories are similar, but the definitions and emphasis relating to levels of surgical acuity, and urgency for operative intervention differ. The surgical team admitting a patient after consultation with the anesthetist handles the initial categorization of the case.

The study aimed to look at the effect of delay in surgery after scheduling based on the GSEST system has an impact on outcome in terms of postoperative complications and death.

Methods

The University of Cape Town (UCT) Human Research Ethics Committee (HREC) approved the study. We conducted a descriptive, non-interventional, observational study based on the prospective analysis of data collected during 1 December 2013 to 31 March 2014. All adult (age > 13 years) acute trauma admissions presenting with penetrating or blunt chest, abdominal, neck, and peripheral vascular injury who underwent surgery were included. Burns, isolated head, orthopedic, hand, and maxillofacial trauma patients were excluded as the respective specialties managed these patients. Collected data included: patient demographic details, mechanism of injury, time of injury, Injury Severity Score (ISS), time of booking the case, triage color code, the delay from scheduling to the start of the case, reasons for the delay, and outcome regarding postoperative complications and death.

Emergency cases were scheduled according to priority as red, orange, yellow, and green for operation (Table 1). Prioritization was done by the attending trauma surgeon based on patient's hemodynamics after discussion with the anesthetist.

The red cases are an immediate priority (resuscitation with immediate operation cases). These cases usually present with hemorrhage or bleeding, requiring instant, life-saving surgical hemostasis. The orange categories are a very urgent priority (potentially life/limb threatening pathology) that should be done within 2 h. The yellow groups are an urgent priority (significant pathology) that should be done in 6 h, and the green cases are a delayed priority (minor injury/illness) that should

Table 1 Groote Schuur emergency surgery triage (GSEST) system

Icon	Case category	Parameters
Red	Immediate	Immediate life-saving operation, resuscitation simultaneous with surgical treatment, e.g., resuscitative laparotomy, ruptured aortic aneurysm threatened airway, cord prolapse, fetal bradycardia
Orange	Expedited	Operation as soon as possible after resuscitation (within 1 to 2 hours), e.g., ruptured ectopic pregnancy, leaking aortic aneurysm, cranial decompression, positive DPL in multiple traumas, threatened limb, emergent fetal concern
Yellow	Urgent	Operation within 6 h of booking, e.g., compound fractures, appendicitis, incarcerated hernia/intestinal obstruction, EUA for non-accidental injuries
Green	Emergent	Operation not immediately life or limb saving but have to be done within 24 h of booking, e.g., ORIF of simple fractures, bleeding hemorrhoids, I&D abscess
Blue	Scheduled	Semi-urgent cases, to be done within 72 h. Operation during in hours on next available slate if possible

be done within 24 h. Green cases become yellow after 24 h. Yellow cases become orange after 6 h. Booked cases are assessed on an ongoing basis and re-categorized as required. Post-operative complications were categorized according to the updated Clavien-Dindo classification of surgical complications [3, 4].

Categorical variables were evaluated using frequency tables. Associations between categorical variables were determined by contingency tables and chi-square tests of association. Numerical variables were evaluated with summary statistics (median, interquartile range, etc.). Relationships between numerical and categorical variables were determined using non-parametric tests: Mann-Whitney in instances where the categorical variable has two categories and Kruskal-Wallis otherwise. A p-value of < 0.05 was considered as statistically significant.

Results

One-hundred six patients underwent surgery during the study period with a higher male to female ratio of 14:1. The median age was 26 (IQR 22–32) years. One-hundred two (96.2%) cases were related to penetrating trauma. Stab wounds comprised 71 (67%) and gunshot wounds (GSW) 31 (29.2%) cases. On presentation 82 (77.4%), patients were admitted with ISS of greater than 15 (5–48). Trauma surgical procedures included laparotomy (48), vascular (27), subxiphoid pericardial window (13), thoracotomy (4), and sternotomy (1). There were also 13 other relatively non-urgent procedures such as debridement, removal of Foley's cath used for penetrating neck wound tamponade, skin grafting for fasciotomy wounds, etc. Of 106 cases, 6, 47, 40, and 13 cases were booked as red, orange, yellow, and green, respectively.

The median delay for green, yellow and orange cases was within expected time. The red patients took unexpectedly longer (median delay 48 min, IQR 35–60 min) to reach the theater (Table 2).

The main (49.1%) reason for the delay in starting the trauma cases was a priority of another emergency (general surgical, gynecological, etc.) booked in that category. Out of six red cases, three were delayed due to unavailability of theater or unable to open an additional theater immediately at that moment (Table 3). One red patient died who presented with a thoracic GSW was unstable on presentation and needed an emergency room thoracotomy and delay to shift to the theater was 55 min after booking.

Thirty-one (29.3%) patients developed postoperative complications (Table 4). Among the booked red, orange, yellow, and green cases, postoperative complications developed in 3, 18, 9, and 1 cases, respectively (Table 5). There was no statistically significant association between operative triage and post-operative complications ($p = 0.074$).

Discussion

Emergency surgical cases differ from elective cases that are planned. During planned or elective operation the length of surgery, hospital stay, and morbidity and mortality can be predicted or inferred. Conversely, emergency surgical cases present in an unpredicted fashion. Prompt, efficient and appropriate treatment of emergency surgical cases is a cost-effective strategy that has the potential to reduce the length of hospital stay, use of high care and intensive care facilities as well as the use of laboratory and other investigative procedures.

The concept of triage is imperative to manage multiple emergency cases with competing and diverse needs. Deficiency of a triage system leads to longer waiting times, poor clinical risk assessment, and management with subsequently increased morbidity and mortality [2]. An efficient triage system minimizes the risk to the patient and promotes effective use of available resources. The rationale and practice of triaging in mass casualty incidents are accepted worldwide [5]. Different triage systems exist for prehospital assessment and in-hospital casualty triage [6–8], yet no widely accepted methods exist for theater bookings. Triage systems should be implemented for the care of surgical emergencies [5] including trauma surgery. Early management of trauma cases is pertinent, as a delay to operative management may increase the risk of adverse outcomes [9].

Table 2 Operative triage vs. delay (min) from booking to operation

Color code	Expected time to start surgery	Number of cases	Median delay (min)	IQR
Red	Immediate	6	48	35–60
Orange	< 2 h	47	120	53–185
Yellow	< 6 h	40	213	113–300
Green	< 24 h	13	110	65–265

Table 3 Operative triage vs. Reasons for the delay

Cause	Red (N)	Orange (O)	Yellow (Y)	Green (N)	Total (N) (%)
No theater available	3	26	11	2	42 (39.6%)
Priority of other case	0	16	26	10	52 (49.1%)
Delay in shift to theater	3	5	3	1	12 (11.3%)
Total	6	47	40	13	106 (100%)

N Number of patients

Triaging of emergency surgical cases were introduced at GSH for the categorization and prioritization of emergency surgical cases at the point of contact with the surgical team before the operative surgical management of a patient. The objective is to improve communication and teamwork between anesthetic, surgical, and nursing personnel involved in the care of these patients.

Limitations

It is an observational study of a small number of trauma cases over 4-month period. The GSEST system describes the emergencies of all kinds including obstetric and gynecological. There are a few general surgical trauma diagnoses are included. It would be useful to have few more parameters perhaps in a separate column, e.g., what general surgical trauma diagnoses fit into the different category?

Future directions

Every minute is essential for the severely injured trauma patient. Delays at any stage from the scene to the operating theater may impact negatively on the outcome regarding complications and death [9]. Triaging is a crucial element for such cases. A more extensive comparative research is required before and after the

Table 4 Types of complications according to Clavien-Dindo classification

Clavien-Dindo Grading	Postoperative complications (number of patients)
I	Wound sepsis (5), Ileus (1)
II	Pneumonia (1)
IIIa	Loculated haemothorax (1)
IIIb	Empyema of chest (3)
IVa	Acute kidney injury (6), respiratory failure (9)
IVb	Multiorgan dysfunction (3)
V	Death (2)
Total	31

Table 5 Operative triage vs. complications (yes/no)

Color code	Complications	No complications	Total
Red	3	3	6
Orange	18	29	47
Yellow	9	31	40
Green	1	12	13
Total	31	75	106

introduction of GSEST system to look at the effectiveness including over- and under-triage rate, accuracy, likelihood ratios, etc.

Conclusion

Emergency trauma surgical cases vary in degree of acuity and complexity. Categorization allows the surgical and anesthetic teams to plan perioperative optimization and prioritize treatment of patients based on their clinical status and expected a progression of the disease. Assessing the South Africa's excessive rate of penetrating wounds needing an emergency operation, it is of utmost importance to create, implement, use, and disseminate national guidelines and standard for these to improve outcomes and life losses.

Acknowledgements
Research Center, King Saud Medical City, Riyadh, KSA.

Funding
Not applicable

Authors' contributions
SC, AJN, and LFMP conceived and designed the study. SC and MRM participated in the conduct of the study. SC prepared the manuscript. AJN and PHN reviewed the manuscript. All authors read and approved the final manuscript.

Competing interests
The authors declare that they have no competing interests.

Author details
[1]Consultant and head of Trauma Surgery, King Saud Medical City, 7790 Al-Imam Abdul Aziz Ibn Muhammad Ibn Saud, Ulaishah, Riyadh 12746, Kingdom of Saudi Arabia. [2]Head and Director of Trauma Centre, Groote Schuur Hospital and University of Cape Town, Cape Town, South Africa. [3]Groote Schuur Hospital and University of Cape Town, Cape Town, South Africa. [4]Deputy Director of Trauma Centre, Groote Schuur Hospital, and University of Cape Town, Cape Town, South Africa. [5]Department of Anaesthesia, Groote Schuur Hospital and University of Cape Town, Cape Town, South Africa.

References

1. Matzopoulos RG, Prinsloo M, Butchart A, et al. Estimating the South African trauma caseload. Int J Inj Control Saf Promot. 2006;13(1):49–51.
2. Wallis LA, Gottschalk SB, Wood D, et al. The cape triage score-a triage system for South Africa. S Afr Med J. 2006;96:53–6.
3. Dindo D, Demartines N, Clavien PA. Classification of surgical complications—a new proposal with evaluation in a cohort of 6336 patients and results of a survey. Ann Surg. 2004;240(2):205–13.
4. Clavien PA, Barkun J, de Oliveira ML, et al. The Clavien-Dindo classification of surgical complications—five-year experience. Ann Surg. 2009;250(2):187 96.
5. Kluger Y, Ben-Ishay O, Sartelli M, et al. World society of emergency surgery study group initiative on timing of acute care surgery classification(TACS). World J Emerg Surg. 2013;8:17. https://doi.org/10.1186/1749-7922-8-17.
6. Beveridge R, Ducharme J, Janes L, et al. Reliability of the Canadian emergency department triage and acuity scale: interrater agreement. Ann Emerg Med. 1999;34:155–9.
7. Australian College of Emergency Medicine. G24 guidelines on the implementation of the Australasian triage scale in emergency departments. Melbourne: Australian College of Emergency Medicine; 2005.
8. Manchester Triage Group. Emergency triage. Manchester: BMJ Publishing Group; 1997.
9. Chowdhury S, Navsaria PH, Edu S, et al. The effect of emergency medical services response on the outcome of trauma laparotomy at a level 1 trauma centre in South Africa. S Afr J Surg. 2016;54(4):17–21.

22

Splenic trauma: WSES classification and guidelines for adult and pediatric patients

Federico Coccolini[1*], Giulia Montori[1], Fausto Catena[2], Yoram Kluger[3], Walter Biffl[4], Ernest E. Moore[5], Viktor Reva[6], Camilla Bing[7], Miklosh Bala[8], Paola Fugazzola[1], Hany Bahouth[3], Ingo Marzi[9], George Velmahos[10], Rao Ivatury[11], Kjetil Soreide[12], Tal Horer[13,50], Richard ten Broek[14], Bruno M. Pereira[15], Gustavo P. Fraga[15], Kenji Inaba[16], Joseph Kashuk[17], Neil Parry[18], Peter T. Masiakos[19], Konstantinos S. Mylonas[19], Andrew Kirkpatrick[20], Fikri Abu-Zidan[21], Carlos Augusto Gomes[22], Simone Vasilij Benatti[23], Noel Naidoo[24], Francesco Salvetti[1], Stefano Maccatrozzo[1], Vanni Agnoletti[25], Emiliano Gamberini[25], Leonardo Solaini[1], Antonio Costanzo[1], Andrea Celotti[1], Matteo Tomasoni[1], Vladimir Khokha[26], Catherine Arvieux[27], Lena Napolitano[28], Lauri Handolin[29], Michele Pisano[1], Stefano Magnone[1], David A. Spain[30], Marc de Moya[10], Kimberly A. Davis[31], Nicola De Angelis[32], Ari Leppaniemi[33], Paula Ferrada[10], Rifat Latifi[34], David Costa Navarro[35], Yashuiro Otomo[36], Raul Coimbra[37], Ronald V. Maier[38], Frederick Moore[39], Sandro Rizoli[40], Boris Sakakushev[41], Joseph M. Galante[42], Osvaldo Chiara[43], Stefania Cimbanassi[43], Alain Chichom Mefire[44], Dieter Weber[45], Marco Ceresoli[1], Andrew B. Peitzman[46], Liban Wehlie[47], Massimo Sartelli[48], Salomone Di Saverio[49] and Luca Ansaloni[1]

Abstract

Spleen injuries are among the most frequent trauma-related injuries. At present, they are classified according to the anatomy of the injury. The optimal treatment strategy, however, should keep into consideration the hemodynamic status, the anatomic derangement, and the associated injuries. The management of splenic trauma patients aims to restore the homeostasis and the normal physiopathology especially considering the modern tools for bleeding management. Thus, the management of splenic trauma should be ultimately multidisciplinary and based on the physiology of the patient, the anatomy of the injury, and the associated lesions. Lastly, as the management of adults and children must be different, children should always be treated in dedicated pediatric trauma centers. In fact, the vast majority of pediatric patients with blunt splenic trauma can be managed non-operatively.
This paper presents the World Society of Emergency Surgery (WSES) classification of splenic trauma and the management guidelines.

Keywords: Spleen, Trauma, Adult, Pediatric, Classification, Guidelines, Embolization, Surgery, Non-operative, Conservative

Background

The management of splenic trauma has changed considerably in the last few decades especially in favor of non-operative management (NOM). NOM ranges from observation and monitoring alone to angiography/angioembolization (AG/AE) with the aim to preserve the spleen and its function, especially in children. These considerations were carried out considering the immunological function of the spleen and the high risk of immunological impairment in splenectomized patients. In contrast with liver traumatic injuries, splenic injuries can be fatal not only at the admission of the patient to the Emergency Department (ED), but also due to delayed subcapsular hematoma rupture or pseudoaneurism (PSA) rupture. Lastly, overwhelming post-splenectomy infections (OPSI) are a late cause of complications due to the lack of the immunological function of the spleen. For these reasons,

* Correspondence: federico.coccolini@gmail.com
[1]General, Emergency and Trauma Surgery, Papa Giovanni XXIII Hospital, P.zza OMS 1, 24128 Bergamo, Italy
Full list of author information is available at the end of the article

standardized guidelines in the management of splenic trauma are necessary.

The existing classification of splenic trauma considered the anatomical lesions (Table 1). However, patients' conditions may lead to an emergent transfer to the operating room (OR) without the opportunity to define the grade of the splenic lesions before the surgical exploration. This confirms the primary importance of the patient's overall clinical condition in these settings. In addition, the modern tools in bleeding management have helped in adopting a conservative approach also in severe lesions. Trauma management must be multidisciplinary and requires an assessment of both the anatomical injury and its physiologic effects. The present guidelines and classification reconsider splenic lesions in the light of the physiopathologic status of the patient associated with the anatomic grade of injury and the other associated lesions.

Notes on the use of the guidelines

The guidelines are evidence-based, with the grade of recommendation also based on the evidence. The guidelines present the diagnostic and therapeutic methods for optimal management of spleen trauma. The practice guidelines promulgated in this work do not represent a standard of practice. They are suggested plans of care, based on best available evidence and the consensus of experts, but they do not exclude other approaches as being within the standard of practice. For example, they should not be used to compel adherence to a given method of medical management, which method should be finally determined after taking account of the conditions at the relevant medical institution (staff levels, experience, equipment, etc.) and the characteristics of the individual patient. However, responsibility for the results of treatment rests with those who are directly engaged therein, and not with the consensus group.

Table 1 AAST Spleen Trauma Classification

Grade	Injury description	
I	Hematoma	Subcapsular, < 10% surface area
	Laceration	Capsular tear, < 1 cm parenchymal depth
II	Hematoma	Subcapsular, 10–50% surface area
		Intraparenchymal, < 5 cm diameter
	Laceration	1–3 cm parenchymal depth not involving a perenchymal vessel
III	Hematoma	Subcapsular, > 50% surface area or expanding
		Ruptured subcapsular or parenchymal hematoma
		Intraparenchymal hematoma > 5 cm
	Laceration	> 3 cm parenchymal depth or involving trabecular vessels
IV	Laceration	Laceration of segmental or hilar vessels producing major devascularization (> 25% of spleen)
V	Laceration	Completely shatters spleen
	Vascular	Hilar vascular injury which devascularized spleen

Methods

A computerized search was done by the bibliographer in different databanks (MEDLINE, Scopus, EMBASE) citations were included for the period between January 1980 and May 2016 using the primary search strategy: spleen, injuries, trauma, resuscitation, adult, pediatric, hemodynamic instability/stability, angioembolization, management, infection, follow-up, vaccination, and thrombo-prophylaxis combined with AND/OR. No search restrictions were imposed. The dates were selected to allow comprehensive published abstracts of clinical trials, consensus conference, comparative studies, congresses, guidelines, government publication, multicenter studies, systematic reviews, meta-analysis, large case series, original articles, and randomized controlled trials. Case reports and small cases series were excluded. Narrative review articles were also analyzed to determine other possible studies. Literature selection is reported in the flow chart (Fig. 1). The Level of evidence (LE) was evaluated using the GRADE system [1] (Table 2).

A group of experts in the field coordinated by a central coordinator was contacted to express their evidence-based opinion on several issues about the pediatric (< 15 years old) and adult splenic trauma. Splenic trauma were divided and assessed as type of injury (blunt and penetrating injury) and management (conservative and operative management). Through the Delphi process, the different issues were discussed in subsequent rounds. The central coordinator assembled the different answers derived from each round. Each version was then revised and improved. The definitive version was discussed during the WSES World Congress in May 2017 in Campinas, Brazil. The final version about which the agreement was reached resulted in present paper.

WSES classification

The WSES position paper suggested to group splenic injury into minor, moderate, and severe. This classification has not previously been clearly defined by the literature. Frequently low-grade AAST lesions (i.e., grades I–III) are considered as minor or moderate and treated with NOM. However, hemodynamically stable patients with high-grade lesions could be successfully treated non-operatively, especially exploiting the more advanced tools for bleeding management. On the other hand, "minor" lesions associated with hemodynamic instability often must be treated with

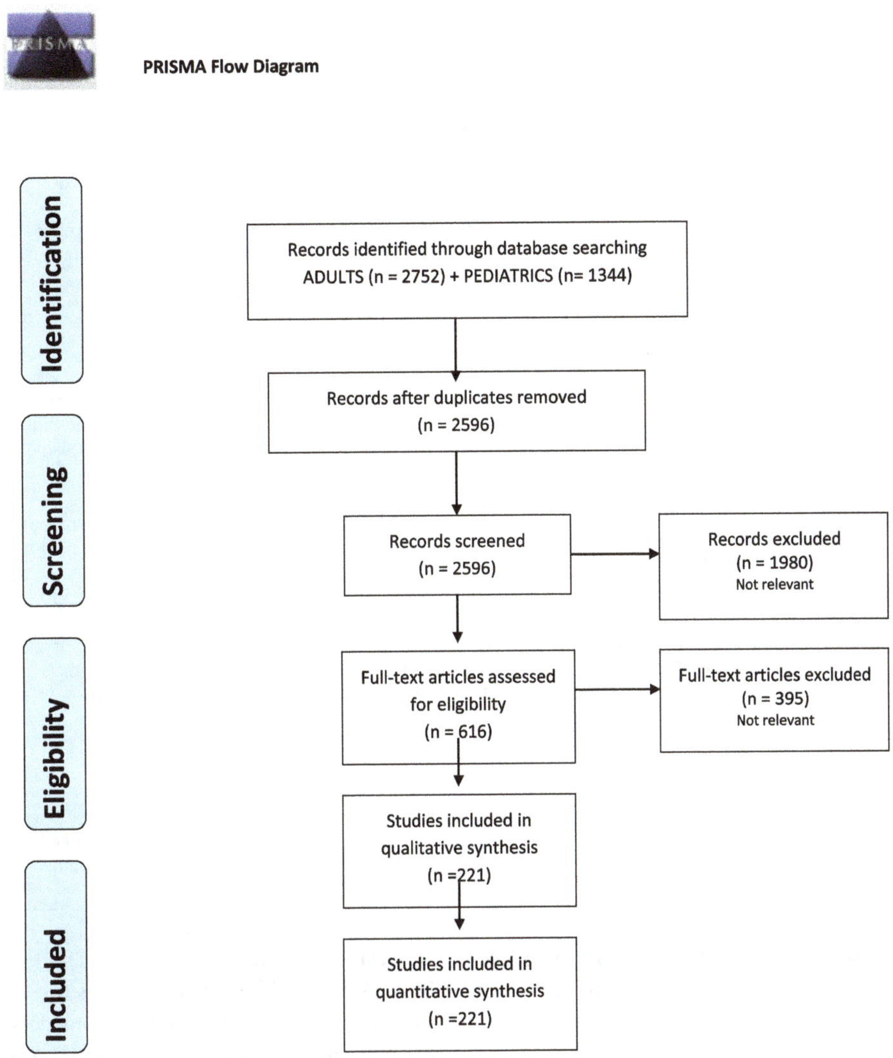

Fig. 1 PRISMA flow chart

OM. This demonstrates that the classification of spleen injuries into minor and major must consider both the anatomic AAST-OIS classification and the hemodynamic status.

The WSES classification divides spleen injuries into three classes:

- Minor (WSES class I)
- Moderate (WSES classes II and III)
- Severe (WSES class IV)

The classification considers the AAST-OIS classification and the hemodynamic status and is the same for adult and pediatric patients. Table 3 explains the classification with the different key points of treatment differentiated within adult and pediatric patients; Table 4 resumes the guidelines statements.

Minor spleen injuries:

- *WSES class I* includes hemodynamically stable AAST-OIS grade I–II blunt and penetrating lesions.

Moderate spleen injuries:

- *WSES class II* includes hemodynamically stable AAST-OIS grade III blunt and penetrating lesions.
- *WSES class III* includes hemodynamically stable AAST-OIS grade IV–V blunt and penetrating lesions.

Severe spleen injuries:

- *WSES class IV* includes hemodynamically unstable AAST-OIS grade I–V blunt and penetrating lesions.

Table 2 GRADE system to evaluate the level of evidence and recommendation

Grade of recommendation	Clarity of risk/benefit	Quality of supporting evidence	Implications
1A			
Strong recommendation, high-quality evidence	Benefits clearly outweigh risk and burdens, or vice versa	RCTs without important limitations or overwhelming evidence from observational studies	Strong recommendation, applies to most patients in most circumstances without reservation
1B			
Strong recommendation, moderate-quality evidence	Benefits clearly outweigh risk and burdens, or vice versa	RCTs with important limitations (inconsistent results, methodological flaws, indirect analyses or imprecise conclusions) or exceptionally strong evidence from observational studies	Strong recommendation, applies to most patients in most circumstances without reservation
1C			
Strong recommendation, low-quality or very low-quality evidence	Benefits clearly outweigh risk and burdens, or vice versa	Observational studies or case series	Strong recommendation but subject to change when higher quality evidence becomes available
2A			
Weak recommendation, high-quality evidence	Benefits closely balanced with risks and burden	RCTs without important limitations or overwhelming evidence from observational studies	Weak recommendation, best action may differ depending on the patient, treatment circumstances, or social values
2B			
Weak recommendation, moderate-quality evidence	Benefits closely balanced with risks and burden	RCTs with important limitations (inconsistent results, methodological flaws, indirect or imprecise) or exceptionally strong evidence from observational studies	Weak recommendation, best action may differ depending on the patient, treatment circumstances, or social values
2C			
Weak recommendation, low-quality or very low-quality evidence	Uncertainty in the estimates of benefits, risks, and burden; benefits, risk, and burden may be closely balanced	Observational studies or case series	Very weak recommendation; alternative treatments may be equally reasonable and merit consideration

Based on the present classification, WSES suggests two management algorithms for both adult and pediatric patients explained in Figs. 2 and 3.

Adult patients

Physiopathology of injuries

Some mechanisms of injuries are similar between children and adults like motor vehicle crashes and pedestrian accidents, while others like motorcycle accidents, sport injuries, gunshot or stab-related injuries, and assaults are more frequent in adults [2].

A few authors consider a normal hemodynamic status in adults when the patient does not require fluids or blood to maintain blood pressure, without signs of hypoperfusion; hemodynamic stability in adults as a counterpart is the condition in which the patient achieve a constant or an amelioration of blood pressure after fluids with a blood pressure > 90 mmHg and heart rate < 100 bpm; hemodynamic instability in adults is the condition in which the patient has an admission systolic blood pressure < 90 mmHg, or > 90 mmHg but requiring bolus infusions/transfusions and/or vasopressor drugs and/or admission base excess (BE) > −5 mmol/l and/or shock index > 1 [3, 4] and/or transfusion requirement of at least 4–6 units of packed red blood cells within the first 24 h [5]. The 9th edition of the Advanced Trauma Life Support (ATLS) definition considers as "unstable" the patient with the following: blood pressure < 90 mmHg and heart rate > 120 bpm, with evidence of skin vasoconstriction (cool, clammy, decreased capillary refill), altered level of consciousness and/or shortness of breath [5]. Moreover, transient responder patients (those showing an initial response to adequate fluid resuscitation and then signs of ongoing loss and perfusion deficits) and, more in general, those responding to therapy but not amenable of sufficient stabilization to be undergone to interventional radiology treatments, are to be considered as unstable patients. In the management of severe bleeding, the early evaluation and correction of the trauma-induced coagulopathy remains a main cornerstone. Physiologic impairment is frequently associated with aggressive resuscitation and the activation and deactivation of several procoagulant and anticoagulant factors contributes to the insurgence of trauma-induced coagulopathy. The application of massive transfusion protocols (MTP) is of paramount importance. The advanced tailored evaluation of the patient's coagulative asset is clearly demonstrated as fundamental in driving the

Table 3 WSES Spleen Trauma Classification for adult and pediatric patients

	WSES class	Mechanism of injury	AAST	Hemodynamic status[a, b]	CT scan	First-line treatment in adults	First-line treatment in pediatric
Minor	WSES I	Blunt/penetrating	I–II	Stable	Yes + local exploration in SW[d]	NOM[c] + serial clinical/laboratory/ radiological evaluation Consider angiography/ angioembolization	NOM[c] + serial clinical/laboratory/ radiological evaluation Consider angiography/ angioembolization
Moderate	WSES II	Blunt/penetrating	III	Stable			
	WSES III	Blunt/penetrating	IV–V	Stable		NOM[c] All angiography/angioembolization + serial clinical/laboratory/ radiological evaluation	
Severe	WSES IV	Blunt/penetrating	I–V	Unstable	No	OM	OM

SW stab wound, *GSW* gunshot wound

[a]*Hemodynamic instability in adults* is considered the condition in which the patient has an admission systolic blood pressure < 90 mmHg with evidence of skin vasoconstriction (cool, clammy, decreased capillary refill), altered level of consciousness and/or shortness of breath, or > 90 mmHg but requiring bolus infusions/transfusions and/or vasopressor drugs and/or admission base excess (BE) > – 5 mmol/l and/or shock index > 1 and/or transfusion requirement of at least 4–6 units of packed red blood cells within the first 24 h; moreover, transient responder patients (those showing an initial response to adequate fluid resuscitation, and then signs of ongoing loss and perfusion deficits) and more in general those responding to therapy but not amenable of sufficient stabilization to be undergone to interventional radiology treatments

[b]*Hemodynamic stability in pediatric patients* is considered systolic blood pressure of 90 mmHg plus twice the child's age in years (the lower limit is inferior to 70 mmHg plus twice the child's age in years, or inferior to 50 mmHg in some studies). Stabilized or acceptable hemodynamic status is considered in children with a positive response to fluid resuscitation: 3 boluses of 20 mL/kg of crystalloid replacement should be administered before blood replacement; positive response can be indicated by the heart rate reduction, the sensorium clearing, the return of peripheral pulses and normal skin color, an increase in blood pressure and urinary output, and an increase in warmth of extremity. Clinical judgment is fundamental in evaluating children

[c]NOM should only be attempted in centers capable of a precise diagnosis of the severity of spleen injuries and capable of intensive management (close clinical observation and hemodynamic monitoring in a high dependency/intensive care environment, including serial clinical examination and laboratory assay, with immediate access to diagnostics, interventional radiology, and surgery and immediately available access to blood and blood products or alternatively in the presence of a rapid centralization system in those patients amenable to be transferred

[d]Wound exploration near the inferior costal margin should be avoided if not strictly necessary because of the high risk to damage the intercostal vessels

Table 4 Statement summary

	Adults	Pediatrics
Diagnostic procedures	-The choice of diagnostic technique at admission must be based on the hemodynamic status of the patient (GoR 1A). -E-FAST is effective and rapid to detect free fluid (GoR 1A). -CT scan with intravenous contrast is the gold standard in hemodynamically stable or stabilized trauma patients (GoR 1A). -Doppler US and contrast-enhanced US are useful to evaluate splenic vascularization and in follow-up (GoR 1B). -Injury grade on CT scan, extent of free fluid, and the presence of PSA do not predict NOM failure or the need of OM (GoR 1B).	-The role of E-FAST in the diagnosis of pediatric spleen injury is still unclear (GoR 1A). -A positive E-FAST examination in children should be followed by an urgent CT in stable patients (GoR 1B). -Complete abdominal US may avoid the use of CT in stable patients (GoR 1B). -Contrast-enhanced CT scan is the gold standard in pediatric splenic trauma (GoR 1A).-Doppler US and contrast-enhanced US are useful to evaluate splenic vascularization (GoR 1B). -CT scan is suggested in children at risk for head and thoracic injuries, need for surgery, recurrent bleeding, and if other abdominal injuries are suspected (GoR 1A). -Injury grade on CT scan, free fluid amount, contrast blush, and the presence of pseudo-aneurysm do not predict NOM failure or the need for OM (GoR 1B).
Non-operative management • General indications		-NOM is recommended as first-line treatment for hemodynamically stable pediatric patients with blunt splenic trauma (GoR 2A). -Patients with moderate-severe blunt and all penetrating splenic injuries should be considered for transfer to dedicated pediatric trauma centers after hemodynamic stabilization (GoR2A). -NOM of spleen injuries in children should be considered only in an environment that provides capability for patient continuous monitoring, angiography, and trained surgeons, an immediately available OR and immediate access to blood and blood products or alternatively in the presence of a rapid centralization system in those patients amenable to be transferred (GoR 2A). -NOM should be attempted even in the setting of concomitant head trauma; unless the patient is unstable, this might be due to intra-abdominal bleeding (GoR 2B).
• Blunt/penetrating trauma	-Patients with hemodynamic stability and absence of other abdominal organ injuries requiring surgery should undergo an initial attempt of NOM irrespective of injury grade (GoR 2A). -NOM of moderate or severe spleen injuries should be considered only in an environment that provides capability for patient intensive monitoring, AG/AE, an immediately available OR and immediate access to blood and blood product or alternatively in the presence of a rapid centralization system and only in patients with stable or stabilized hemodynamic and absence of other internal injuries requiring surgery (GoR 2A). -NOM in splenic injuries is contraindicated in the setting of unresponsive hemodynamic instability or other indicates for laparotomy (peritonitis, hollow organ injuries, bowel evisceration, impalement) (GoR 1A). -In patients being considered for NOM, CT scan with intravenous contrast should be performed to define the anatomic spleen injury and identify associated injuries (GoR 2A). -AG/AE may be considered the first-line intervention in patients with hemodynamic stability and arterial blush on CT scan irrespective from injury grade (GoR 2B). -Strong evidence exists that age above 55 years old, high ISS, and moderate to severe splenic injuries are prognostic factors for NOM failure. These patients require more intensive monitoring and higher index of suspicion (GoR 2B). -Age above 55 years old alone, large hemoperitoneum alone, hypotension before resuscitation, GCS < 12 and low-hematocrit level at the admission, associated abdominal injuries, blush at CT scan, anticoagulation drugs, HIV disease, drug addiction, cirrhosis,	Blunt trauma -Blunt splenic injuries with hemodynamic stability and absence of other internal injuries requiring surgery, should undergo an initial attempt of NOM irrespective of injury grade (GoR 2A). -In hemodynamically stable children with isolated splenic injury splenectomy should be avoided (GoR 1A). -NOM is contraindicated in presence of peritonitis, bowel evisceration, impalement or other indications to laparotomy (GoR 2A). -The presence of contrast blush at CT scan is not an absolute indication for splenectomy or AG/AE in children (GoR 2B). Intensive care unit admission in isolated splenic injury may be required only for moderate and severe lesions (GoR 2B).

Table 4 Statement summary *(Continued)*

	and need for blood transfusions should be taken into account, but they are not absolute contraindications for NOM (GoR 2B). -In WSES class II–III spleen injuries with associated severe traumatic brain injury, NOM could be considered only if rescue therapy (OR and/or AG/AE) is rapidly available; otherwise, splenectomy should be performed (GoR 1C).	
		Penetrating trauma -No sufficient data validating NOM for penetrating spleen injury in children exist.
The role of angiography/ angioembolization (AG/AE)	-AG/AE may be performed in hemodynamically stable and rapid responder patients with moderate and severe lesions and in those with vascular injuries at CT scan (contrast blush, pseudo-aneurysms and arterio-venous fistula) (GoR 2A). -In patients with bleeding vascular injuries and in those with intraperitoneal blush, AG/AE should be performed as part of NOM only in centers where AG/AE is rapidly available. In other centers and in case of rapid hemodynamic deterioration, OM should be considered (GoR 2B). -In case of absence of blush during angiography, if blush was previously seen at CT scan, proximal angioembolization could be considered (GoR 2C). –AG/AE should be considered in all hemodynamically stable patients with WSES grade III lesions, regardless with the presence of CT blush (GoR 1B). –AG/AE could be considered in patients undergone to NOM, hemodynamically stable with sings of persistent hemorrhage regardless with the presence of CT blush once excluded extra-splenic source of bleeding (GoR 1C). –Hemodynamically stable patients with WSES grade II lesions without blush should not underwent routine AG/AE but may be considered for prophylactic proximal embolization in presence of risk factors for NOM failure (GoR 2B). –In the presence of a single vascular abnormality (contrast blush, pseudo-aneurysms, and artero-venous fistula) in minor and moderate injuries, the currently available literature is inconclusive regarding whether proximal or distal embolization should be used. In the presence of multiple splenic vascular abnormalities or in the presence of a severe lesion, proximal or combined AG/AE should be used, after confirming the presence of a permissive pancreatic vascular anatomy (GoR 1C). –In performing, AG/AE coils should be preferred to temporary agents (GoR 1C).	-The vast majority of pediatric patients do not require AG/AE for CT blush or moderate to severe injuries (GoR 1C).-AG/AE may be considered in patients undergone to NOM, hemodynamically stable with sings of persistent hemorrhage not amenable of NOM, regardless with the presence of CT blush once excluded extra-splenic source of bleeding (GoR 1C). -AG/AE may be considered for the treatment of post-traumatic splenic pseudo-aneurysms prior to patient discharge (GoR 2C). -Patients with more than 15 years old should be managed according to adults AG/AE-protocols (GoR 1C).
Operative management (OM)	-OM should be performed in patients with hemodynamic instability and/or with associated lesions like peritonitis or bowel evisceration or impalement requiring surgical exploration (GoR 2A). -OM should be performed in moderate and severe lesions even in stable patients in centers where intensive monitoring cannot be performed and/or when AG/AE is not rapidly available (GoR 2A). -Splenectomy should be performed when NOM with AG/AE failed, and patient remains hemodynamically unstable or shows a significant drop in hematocrit levels or continuous transfusion are required (GoR 2A). –During OM, salvage of at least a part of the spleen is debated and could not be suggested (GoR 2B). –Laparoscopic splenectomy in early trauma scenario in bleeding patients could not be recommended (GoR 2A).	-Patients should undergo to OM in case of hemodynamic instability, failure of conservative treatments, severe coexisting injuries necessitating intervention and peritonitis, bowel evisceration, impalement (GoR 2A). -Splenic preservation (at least partial) should be attempted whenever possible (GoR 2B).
Short- and long-term follow-up	–Clinical and laboratory observation associated to bed rest in moderate and severe lesions is the cornerstone in the first 48–72 h follow-up (GoR 1C). –CT scan repetition during the admission should be considered in patients with moderate and severe lesions or in decreasing hematocrit, in presence of vascular anomalies or underlying splenic pathology or coagulopathy, and in neurologically impaired patients (GoR 2A).	–In hemodynamic stable children without drop in hemoglobin levels for 24 h, bed rest should be suggested (GoR 2B). –The risk of pseudo-aneurysm after splenic trauma is low, and in most of cases, it resolves spontaneously (GoR 2B). –Angioembolization should be taken into consideration when a pesudoaneurysm is found (GoR 2B).

Table 4 Statement summary *(Continued)*

	–In the presence of underlying splenic pathology or coagulopathy and in neurologically impaired patients CT follow-up is to be considered after the discharge (GoR 2B). –Activity restriction may be suggested for 4–6 weeks in minor injuries and up to 2–4 months in moderate and severe injuries (GoR 2C).	–US (DUS, CEUS) follow-up seems reasonable to minimize the risk of life-threatening hemorrhage and associated complications in children (GoR 1B). –After NOM in moderate and severe injuries, the reprise of normal activity could be considered safe after at least 6 weeks (GoR 2B).
Thrombo-prophylaxis	–Mechanical prophylaxis is safe and should be considered in all patients without absolute contraindication to its use (GoR 2A). – Spleen trauma without ongoing bleeding is not an absolute contraindication to LMWH-based prophylactic anticoagulation (GoR 2A) –LMWH-based prophylactic anticoagulation should be started as soon as possible from trauma and may be safe in selected patients with blunt splenic injury undergone to NOM (GoR 2B). –In patient with oral anticoagulants the risk-benefit balance of reversal should be individualized (GoR 1C).	
Infections prophylaxis in asplenic and hyposplenic adult and pediatric patients	–Patients should receive immunization against the encapsulated bacteria (*S. pneumoniae*, *H. influenzae*, and *N. meningitidis*) (GoR 1A). –Vaccination programs should be started no sooner than 14 days after splenectomy or spleen total vascular exclusion (GoR 2C). –In patients discharged before 15 days after splenectomy or angioembolization, where the risk to miss vaccination is deemed high, the best choice is to vaccinate before discharge (GoR 1B). –Immunization against seasonal flu is recommended for patients over 6 months of age (GoR 1C). –Malaria prophylaxis is strongly recommended for travelers (GoR 2C). –Antibiotic therapy should be strongly considered in the event of any sudden onset of unexplained fever, malaise, chills or other constitutional symptoms, especially when medical review is not readily accessible (GoR 2A). –Primary care providers should be aware of the splenectomy/ angioembolization (GoR 2C).	

administration of blood products, coagulation factors, and drugs [6–9].

Diagnostic procedures:

- *The choice of diagnostic technique at admission must be based on the hemodynamic status of the patient (GoR 1A).*
- *E-FAST is effective and rapid to detect free fluid (GoR 1A).*
- *CT scan with intravenous contrast is the gold standard in hemodynamically stable or stabilized trauma patients (GoR 1A).*
- *Doppler US and contrast-enhanced US are useful to evaluate splenic vascularization and in follow-up (GoR 1B).*
- *Injury grade on CT scan, extent of free fluid, and the presence of PSA do not predict NOM failure or the need of OM (GoR 1B).*

Extended focused assessment sonography for trauma (E-FAST) and ultrasonography (US) have replaced diagnostic peritoneal lavage (DPL) management of abdominal trauma in present days [5, 10, 11]. Studies have shown a sensitivity up to 91% and a specificity up to 96% also for a small fluid amount [12, 13].

Nevertheless, 42% of false-negative have been reported [10]. This might be due to the 20% of cases in which no significant extravasation of blood is present in splenic trauma or in injuries near the diaphragm [10, 12, 13].

Contrast-enhanced US (CEUS) increases the visualization of a variety of splenic injuries and complications [12].

Doppler US (DUS) has been reported as safe and effective in evaluating PSA or blush previously found at CT scan [14].

Contrast tomography (CT) scan is considered the gold standard in trauma with a sensitivity and specificity for splenic injuries near to 96–100% [10, 15, 16]. However, Carr et al. [10] reported that CT scan can underestimate splenic injuries at ilum. CT must be rapidly available and must be performed only in hemodynamically stable patients or in those responding to fluid resuscitation [17, 18]. However, in some centers, there is the possibility to perform a fast-track CT scan that seems to permit to expand the criteria for performing CT scan in trauma patients. Delayed-phase CT helps in differentiating patients with active bleeding from those with contained vascular injuries [19]. This is important to reduce the risk of discrepancy between CT scan images

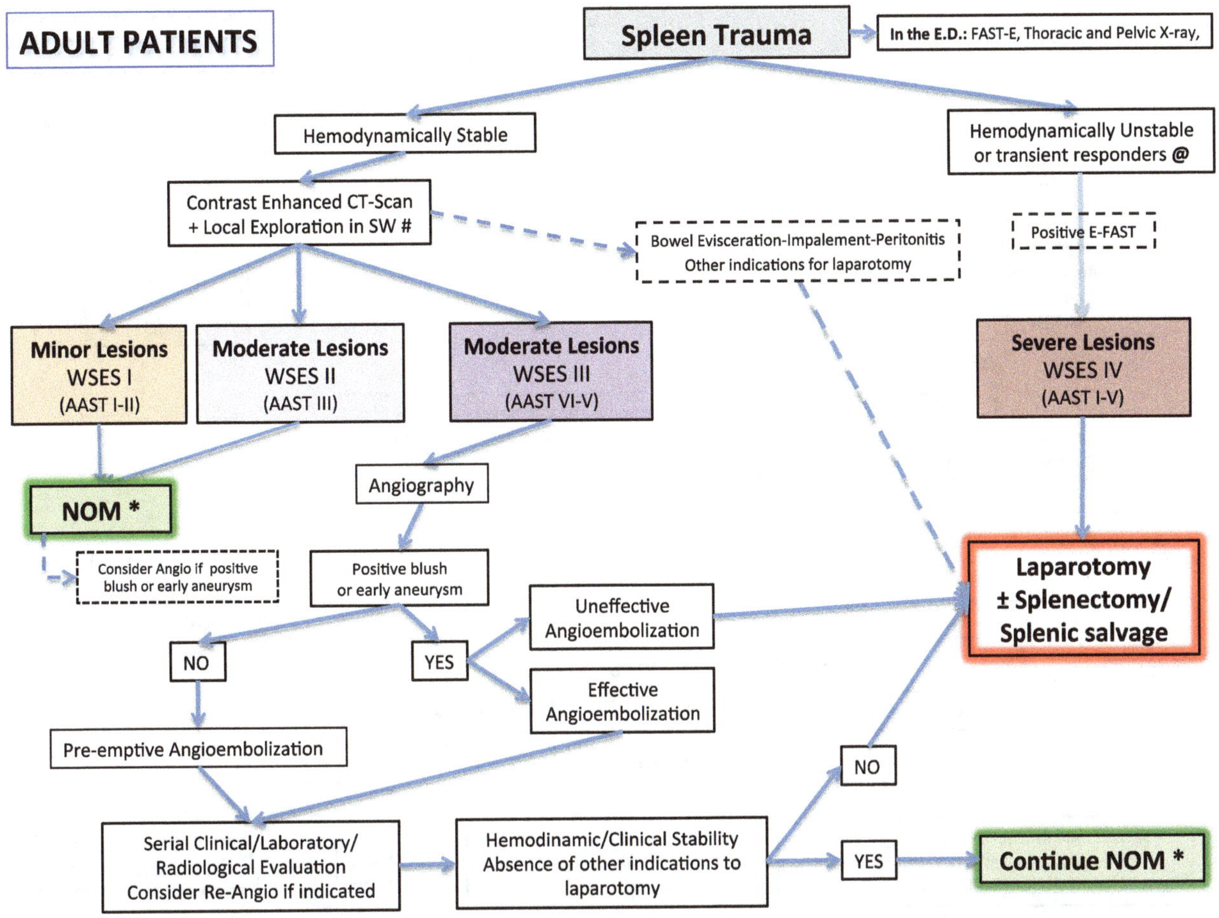

Fig. 2 Spleen Trauma Management Algorithm for Adult Patients. (*SW* stab wound, *GSW* gunshot wound. *NOM should only be attempted in centers capable of a precise diagnosis of the severity of spleen injuries and capable of intensive management (close clinical observation and hemodynamic monitoring in a high dependency/intensive care environment, including serial clinical examination and laboratory assay, with immediate access to diagnostics, interventional radiology, and surgery and immediately available access to blood and blood products or alternatively in the presence of a rapid centralization system in those patients amenable to be transferred; @ *Hemodynamic instability* is considered the condition in which the patient has an admission systolic blood pressure < 90 mmHg with evidence of skin vasoconstriction (cool, clammy, decreased capillary refill), altered level of consciousness and/or shortness of breath, or > 90 mmHg but requiring bolus infusions/transfusions and/or vasopressor drugs and/or admission base excess (BE) > – 5 mmol/l and/or shock index > 1 and/or transfusion requirement of at least 4–6 units of packed red blood cells within the first 24 h; moreover, transient responder patients (those showing an initial response to adequate fluid resuscitation, and then signs of ongoing loss and perfusion deficits) and more in general those responding to therapy but not amenable of sufficient stabilization to be undergone to interventional radiology treatments. # Wound exploration near the inferior costal margin should be avoided if not strictly necessary because of the high risk to damage the intercostal vessels)

and angio images (only 47% of patients have a confirmation of the CT findings at angio) [19]. Active contrast extravasation is a sign of active hemorrhage [20]. The use of CT helps in surgical procedure and in AG/AE to be more selective [21, 22]. Contrast blush occurs in about 17% of cases and has been demonstrated to be an important predictor of failure of NOM (more than 60% of patients with blush failed NOM). Its absence on initial CT scan in high-grade splenic injuries does not definitively exclude active bleeding and should not preclude AG/AE [15, 23, 24]. Federle et al. showed that the hemoperitoneum quantification is not related to the risk of NOM failure [20].

Non-operative management

Blunt and penetrating trauma:

- *Patients with hemodynamic stability and absence of other abdominal organ injuries requiring surgery should undergo an initial attempt of NOM irrespective of injury grade (GoR 2A).*
- *NOM of moderate or severe spleen injuries should be considered only in an environment that provides capability for patient intensive monitoring, AG/AE, an immediately available OR and immediate access to blood and blood product or alternatively in presence of a rapid centralization system and only in patients with*

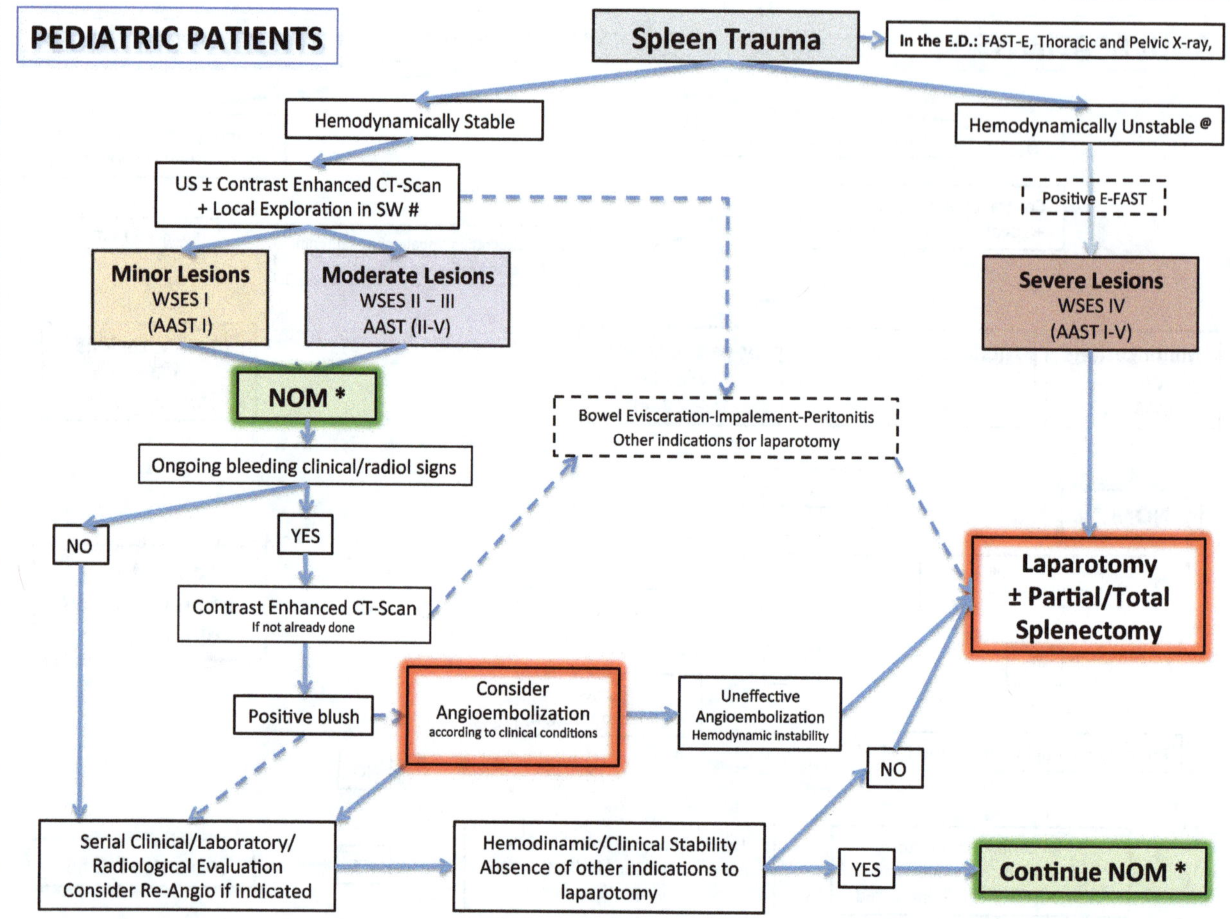

Fig. 3 Spleen Trauma Management Algorithm for Pediatrics Patients. (*SW* stab wound, *GSW* gunshot wound; *****NOM should only be attempted in centers capable of a precise diagnosis of the severity of spleen injuries and capable of intensive management (close clinical observation and hemodynamic monitoring in a high dependency/intensive care environment, including serial clinical examination and laboratory assay, with immediate access to diagnostics, interventional radiology, and surgery and immediately available access to blood and blood products or alternatively in presence of a rapid centralization system in those patients amenable to be transferred; **@** *Hemodynamic stability* is considered systolic blood pressure of 90 mmHg plus twice the child's age in years (the lower limit is inferior to 70 mmHg plus twice the child's age in years, or inferior to 50 mmHg in some studies). Stabilized or acceptable hemodynamic status is considered in children with a positive response to fluids resuscitation: 3 boluses of 20 mL/kg of crystalloid replacement should be administered before blood replacement; positive response can be indicated by the heart rate reduction, the sensorium clearing, the return of peripheral pulses and normal skin color, an increase in blood pressure and urinary output, and an increase in warmth of extremity. Clinical judgment is fundamental in evaluating children. **#** Wound exploration near the inferior costal margin should be avoided if not strictly necessary because of the high risk to damage the intercostal vessels)

stable or stabilized hemodynamic and absence of other internal injuries requiring surgery (GoR 2A).

- *NOM in splenic injuries is contraindicated in the setting of unresponsive hemodynamic instability or other indicates for laparotomy (peritonitis, hollow organ injuries, bowel evisceration, impalement) (GoR 1A).*
- *In patients being considered for NOM, CT scan with intravenous contrast should be performed to define the anatomic spleen injury and identify associated injuries (GoR 2A).*
- *AG/AE may be considered the first-line intervention in patients with hemodynamic stability and arterial blush on CT scan irrespective from injury grade (GoR 2B).*
- *Strong evidence exists that age above 55-years old, high ISS, and moderate to severe splenic injuries are prognostic factors for NOM failure. These patients require more intensive monitoring and higher index of suspicion (GoR 2B).*
- *Age above 55 years old alone, large hemoperitoneum alone, hypotension before resuscitation, GCS < 12, and low hematocrit level at the admission, associated abdominal injuries, blush at CT scan, anticoagulation drugs, HIV disease, drug addiction, cirrhosis, and need for blood transfusions should be taken into account, but they are not absolute contraindications for NOM (GoR 2B).*

- *In WSES classes II–III spleen injuries with associated severe traumatic brain injury, NOM could be considered only if rescue therapy (OR and/or AG/AE) is rapidly available; otherwise, splenectomy should be performed (GoR 1C).*

Blunt trauma

NOM is considered the gold standard for the treatment of patients with blunt splenic trauma (BST) who are hemodynamically stable after an initial resuscitation, in the absence of peritonitis and associated injuries requiring laparotomy [15, 25–28]. In high-volume centers with all facilities, the successful rate of attempted NOM is near 90% [29]. The advantages of NOM over OM were described as lower hospital costs, avoidance of non-therapeutic laparotomies, lower rates of intra-abdominal complications and of blood transfusions, lower mortality and the maintenance of the immunological function, and the prevention of OPSI [27, 30, 31]. Other guidelines have agreed the non-indication of routine laparotomy in hemodinamically stable patients with blunt splenic injury [32, 33].

NOM failure rate is reported to be between 4 and 15% [15, 29, 34–44]. Several risk factors of NOM failure have been reported [15, 29, 34–54].

In several studies, hemodynamic status at the admission has not been considered a significant prognostic indicator for NOM failure and, for this reason, should not be considered an absolute contraindication for NOM [15, 29, 36, 40, 41]. Others reported that the need for red cell transfusions in ED or during the first 24 h [40, 48], hemoglobin and hematocrit levels at admission [40], HIV disease, cirrhosis, and drug addiction [55–57] could affect the outcome after NOM.

The presence of a blush at CT scan has been considered a risk factor for NOM failure only in studies in which AG/AE was not adopted [46, 53]. In addition, the extension of hemoperitoneum at imaging alone cannot be considered an absolute contraindication for NOM [15, 19, 20, 40, 54].

In AAST-OIS injury grades above IV, the failure rate of NOM reaches 54.6% [49], while according to other studies, patients with III–V injury grades could achieve a 87% of success rate [15, 49].

Patients with higher ISS were more likely to fail NOM. According to the literature, two ISS values which were significantly associated with the failure of NOM were above 15 [40] or 25 [37]. This finding is in agreement with the increased risk of associated lesions in higher ISS.

NOM failure in case of missed concomitant abdominal injuries is reported in 1–2.5% of cases [38, 41, 47, 48, 51, 58].

GCS score below 12 alone should not be considered a contraindication for NOM as these patients can be successfully managed non-operatively with a reported overall NOM failure rate near 4.5% [15, 29, 40, 49].

The risk of NOM failure in patients older than 55 years is still debated. A few studies [15, 35, 37, 38, 41, 44, 52, 54] found older age to be a significant prognostic factor for NOM failure [15]. On the other hand, other studies [29, 39, 43, 45, 50] did not find significant differences between patients ≤ 55 and > 55 years. It has been suggested that age> 55 years could be a risk factor for NOM failure only in high AAST-OIS injury grades [36, 38, 49]. Furthermore, the failure of NOM in older patients has been found to be associated with higher mortality rates and longer length of hospital stay than patients < 55 years [44].

Some authors suggested a primary OM in the presence of hypotension in the ED, more than five red blood cell transfused, GCS < 11, high ISS, abdominal AIS > 3, age > 55, and spleen AAST-OIS injury grade > 3. However, it has also been demonstrated that NOM could be successful also in high-risk patients without an increase in complications or mortality rates related to delayed operative interventions [15, 52].

According to larger studies on patients with BST [29], in level I trauma centers, NOM success rate is higher than in level II or III centers. Nevertheless, some authors stated that this might not be associated with the failure of NOM [42, 49].

Finally, severe unstable spleen injuries could ideally benefit from a resuscitation in a hybrid OR with trauma surgeons, in order to increase the spleen salvage rate [59–61].

Penetrating trauma

Laparotomy has been the gold standard in penetrating abdominal trauma. Several studies demonstrated as the rate of negative laparotomy ranges between 9 and 14% [62, 63]. For the last 20 years, there has been an increased number of approaches with NOM for gunshot and stab injuries [64, 65].

Carlin et al. in a large series compared penetrating splenic trauma (248 patients) with blunt trauma and found that mortality was not significantly different [66]. However, when the authors compared GSW and SW versus blunt splenic trauma, they found a significant difference in mortality (24 versus 15%, $p = 0.02$). Pancreatic, diaphragmatic, and colic injuries significantly increase the rate of OM approach and mortality for septic complications. The associated pancreatic injuries require frequently spleno-pancreatectomy [66]. Demetriades et al. showed in a prospective study with 225 patients with penetrating splenic injury, the direct relationship between the degree of injury and the possibility of NOM vs. emergency laparotomy [67]. Emergency laparotomy rate was 33% in grade I lesions, and it could increase up to 84% in the grade IV; all splenectomies were in injuries with grade III or higher.

Indication to angiography and angioembolization:

- *AG/AE may be performed in hemodynamically stable and rapid responder patients with moderate and severe lesions and in those with vascular injuries at CT scan (contrast blush, pseudo-aneurysms and arterio-venous fistula) (GoR 2A).*
- *In patients with bleeding vascular injuries and in those with intraperitoneal blush, AG/AE should be performed as part of NOM only in centers where AG/AE is rapidly available. In other centers and in case of rapid hemodynamic deterioration, OM should be considered (GoR 2B).*
- *In case of absence of blush during angiography, if blush was previously seen at CT scan, proximal angioembolization could be considered (GoR 2C).*
- *AG/AE should be considered in all hemodynamically stable patients with WSES class III lesions, regardless the presence of CT blush (GoR 1B).*
- *AG/AE could be considered in patients undergone to NOM, hemodynamically stable with sings of persistent hemorrhage regardless the presence of CT blush once excluded extra-splenic source of bleeding (GoR 1C).*
- *Hemodynamically stable patients with WSES class II lesions without blush should not underwent routine AG/AE but may be considered for prophylactic proximal embolization in presence of risk factors for NOM failure (GoR 2B).*
- *In presence of a single vascular abnormality (contrast blush, pseudo-aneurysms and artero-venous fistula) in minor and moderate injuries the currently available literature is inconclusive regarding whether proximal or distal embolization should be used. In presence of multiple splenic vascular abnormalities or in presence of a severe lesion, proximal or combined AG/AE should be used, after confirming the presence of a permissive pancreatic vascular anatomy (GoR 1C).*
- *In performing AG/AE coils should be preferred to temporary agents (GoR 1C).*

The reported success rate of NOM with AG/AE ranges from 86 to 100% with a success rate of AG/AE from 73 to 100% [68–78]. In a large study, Haan et al. suggested that indications to AG/AE were pseudo-aneurysms (PSA) or active bleeding at admission CT scan, significant hemoperitoneum, and high-grade splenic injury [68–70]. More than 80% of grade IV–V splenic injuries were successfully managed non-operatively with AG/AE. A large multicenter study [76] on 10,000 patients found that AG/AE was associated with a reduced odds of splenectomy and that the earlier AG/AE was performed; the less number of patients had splenectomy. A multi-institutional study by Banerjee et al. demonstrated that level I trauma center that had AG/AE rates greater than 10% had significantly higher spleen salvage rates and fewer NOM failure, especially for AAST-OIS grade III–IV injured spleen. AG/AE was also found as an independent predictor of spleen salvage and mortality reduction [78, 79].

A few meta-analyses showed a significant improvement in NOM success following introduction of AG/AE protocols (OR 0.26, 95% CI 0.13–0.53, $p < 0.002$) [54, 80–82]. The failure rate without AG/AE is significantly higher than with AG/AE in AAST-OIS grade IV–V injuries (43.7 vs. 17.3%, $p = 0.035$, and 83.1 vs. 25.0%, $p = 0.016$, respectively) [80].

Specific CT findings can help in the therapeutic decision, and they are correlated with outcomes. As such, patients with PSA and arterovenous fistula showed higher NOM failure rates [21, 22, 53, 83–90].

NOM failure in the presence of contrast blush treated without AG/AE ranges between 67 and 82% [53, 85]. Shanmuganathan et al. reported an 83% accuracy of blush in predicting the need for AG/AE [86]. Marmery et al. showed a 4% of active bleeding vascular injuries in AAST-OIS grade I–II splenic injuries [21, 87]. Intraperitoneal splenic blush exhibited a significantly higher percentage of hemodynamic deterioration during the time required for AG/AE than intra-parenchymal bleedings ($p < 0.001$), suggesting intraperitoneal blush as an independent risk factor for OM [88].

Between 2.3 and 47% CT detected, contrast blush could not be confirmed at the subsequent angiography [89, 90]. The presence of a vascular injury is significantly associated with the splenic injury grade ($p < 0.0001$) [21]. Moreover an analysis on 143 patients with blush at CT scan suggested that an angiographic procedure without embolization increases twofold the risk of re-bleeding and NOM failure [90].

The indication for routine prophylactic AG/AE in high-grade splenic injuries is a matter of controversy [23, 68, 70, 74, 85, 91–93]. Several retrospective and prospective studies recommended the use of AG/AE in all hemodynamically stable patients with high-grade splenic injuries [23, 91–93]. NOM failure rates both with and without prophylactic AG/AE for high-grade injuries are 0–42% vs. 23–67%, respectively, [23, 68, 70, 74, 85, 91].

Controversies exist regarding which kind of lesions should be considered as "high-grade" (AAST III–V or IV–V grade) and should undergo routine AG/AE [23, 68, 91, 92]. It has been reported that NOM could fail in up to 3% of grade III lesions without blush with no AG/AE [23]. Furthermore, no outcome deterioration (in terms of NOM failure, rate of re-bleeding, complications, and mortality) was detected after excluding grade III injuries from routine AG/AE protocol [91]. Therefore, considering the AG/AE-related morbidity of 47% (versus 10% related to NOM without AG/AE) [93] and the fact that widening the selection criteria for AG/AE from grades IV–V to grades III–V may slightly decrease the overall NOM failure rate, patients with grade III lesions without blush should not undergo routine AG/AE.

To date, no randomized comparing proximal and distal embolization are available [94]. In a meta-analysis including 15 retrospective studies, proximal and distal embolization was found to be equivalent with regard to the incidence of major infarctions, infections, and major re-bleeding [95]. However, a significant higher rate of overall minor complications was found after distal AE (2.8–11.6% versus 15.9–25.2%) [95].

Several studies analyzed the morbidity related to AG/AE, to OM, and to NOM without AG/AE [23, 68, 70, 96–103]. The AG/AE major morbidity rates range from 3.7 to 28.5% including re-bleeding, total or subtotal splenic infarction, splenic abscesses, acute renal insufficiency, pseudocysts, and puncture-related complications. The rates for minor morbidities range from 23 to 61%, and they included fever, pleural effusion, coil migration, and partial splenic infarction [70, 96, 102, 103]. All studies [97, 98, 101], but one [93] reported significantly higher complication rates in patients undergone OM (increased rate of death, infectious complications, pleural drainage, acute renal failure, and pancreatitis). In particular, the incidence of infectious complications was significantly higher in the splenectomy group (observation 4.8%, AG/AE 4.2%, splenorrhaphy 10.5%, splenectomy 32.0%, $p = 0.001$) [98].

Some studies analyzed the cost of NOM and AG/AE [104]. They observed that NOM is safe and cost effective, and AG/AE is similar to surgical therapy with regard to cost.

Lastly, AG/AE does not seem to totally compromise the splenic function, and even in presence of an elevated leukocyte and platelet counts, no significant differences in immunoglobulin titers were found between splenic artery AG/AE patients and controls [91]. The spleen due to its intense vascularization could assure the necessary blood to continue its immunological function.

Operative management

Blunt trauma and penetrating:

- *OM should be performed in patients with hemodynamic instability and/or with associated lesions like peritonitis or bowel evisceration or impalement requiring surgical exploration (GoR 2A).*
- *OM should be performed in moderate and severe lesions even in stable patients in centers where intensive monitoring cannot be performed and/or when AG/AE is not rapidly available (GoR 2A).*
- *Splenectomy should be performed when NOM with AG/AE failed and patient remains hemodynamicaly unstable or shows a significant drop in hematocrit levels or continuous transfusion are required (GoR 2A).*
- *During OM, salvage of at least a part of the spleen is debated and could not be suggested (GoR 2B)*
- *Laparoscopic splenectomy in early trauma scenario in bleeding patients could not be recommended (GoR 2A).*

Operative management (OM) of splenic injuries should be performed in non-responder hemodynamic instable patients. This condition is frequently observed in high-ISS trauma, in high-grade lesions, and in patients with associated lesions. However, it can be also required in low volume trauma centers or peripheral centers where no intensive care unit or intensive monitoring can be achieve [13, 105, 106]. It has been reported that isolated splenic injury is about 42% of all abdominal trauma [107]. Multiple injuries are reported near 20–30% [107–109]. No sufficient data are available about concomitant vascular and splenic injuries. Associated hollow viscus injuries could be found in 5% of cases; the severity of splenic injury seems to be related to the incidence of hollow viscus injury (1.9, 2.4, 4.9, and 11.6% in minor, moderate, major, and massive injuries, respectively) [110].

The use of splenectomy is decreasing, and the use of splenorrhaphy is rarely adopted (35–24% and 6–1%, respectively) [108, 111]. The attempt to perform a partial splenic salvage is reported in 50–78% of cases, but when NOM fails, splenectomy is the preferred treatment [108, 111].

Laparoscopic splenectomy for trauma is reported only in some cases of hemodynamically stable low-moderate grade splenic injuries [112, 113].

The use of splenic autologous transplantation (i.e., voluntarily leaving pieces of spleen inside the abdomen), to avoid infective risk from splenectomy, has been investigated, but no reduction of morbidity or mortality has been demonstrated [114].

The reported overall hospital mortality of splenectomy in trauma is near 2%, and the incidence of postoperative bleeding after splenectomy, ranges from 1.6 to 3%, but with mortality near to 20% [115].

Spleen injuries with concomitant spinal and brain injuries

Particular attention should be posed in managing hemodynamically stable patients with blunt spinal trauma (BST) and severe traumatic brain injury (STBI).

A recent study in patients with concomitant spinal and/or brain associated to AAST-OIS grade IV–V spleen injuries reported a general survival benefit of immediate splenectomy over NOM [116]. However, in centers where AG/AE is available (having therefore a lower NOM failure rate of high-grade splenic injuries), immediate splenectomy in patients with severe brain injury does not seem to be associated with an improved survival benefit regardless the grade of injury [116]. It must be highlighted that the differences in definition of hemodynamic instability may represent a bias in this cohort of patients as a few "unstable" patients might have undergone NOM. This data strongly emphasizes the dangers related to poor patient selection for NOM in BST and STBI [34, 49].

Thrombo-prophylaxis in splenic trauma:

- *Mechanical prophylaxis is safe and should be considered in all patients without absolute contraindication to its use (GoR 2A).*
- *Spleen trauma without ongoing bleeding is not an absolute contraindication to LMWH-based prophylactic anticoagulation (GoR 2A).*
- *LMWH-based prophylactic anticoagulation should be started as soon as possible from trauma and may be safe in selected patients with blunt splenic injury undergone to NOM (GoR 2B).*
- *In patient with oral anticoagulants the risk-benefit balance of reversal should be individualized (GoR 1C).*

Trauma patients are at high risk of venous thromboembolism (VTE); the transition to a hyper-coagulation state occurs within 48 h from injury [117–119]. Without any prophylaxis, more than 50% may experience deep vein thrombosis (DVT)which substantially increases the risk of pulmonary embolism (PE) whose mortality is about 50% [117, 118]. In trauma patients surviving beyond the first 24 h, PE is the third leading cause of death. Even with chemical prophylaxis, DVT can be detected in 15% of patients. There are currently no standards for the initiation of prophylactic anticoagulation in trauma patients with blunt spleen injuries. A survey-based analysis from ASST reported a growing use of heparin according to the increasing grade of the splenic lesion, and on the contrary, an increasing use of low-molecular-weight heparin (LMWH) in low-grade lesions [120]. Heparin and LMWH can be combined with mechanical prophylaxis; however, mechanical prophylaxis alone in high-grade lesions seems to be preferred by surgeons compared with heparin. Eberle et al. [121] and Alejandro et al. [119] demonstrated no differences between VTE prophylaxis administered within and after 72 and 48 h from trauma respectively, with highest rate of failure in patients with high-grade splenic injury. Bellal et al. [122] found no difference in hemorrhagic complication and NOM failure rate in patients with early (< 48 h), intermediate (48–72 h), and late (> 72 h) VTE prophylaxis. These considerations are referred to selected patients, particularly those without significant head and spinal injuries. As a counterpart, Rostas et al. [117] show that VTE rates were over fourfold greater when LMWH was administered after 72 h from admission.

When trauma occurs in patients under anticoagulants, it is important to consider, if it is necessary, the reversal of their effects in order to avoid thrombotic complication. However, failing to resume anticoagulation in a timely fashion is associated with poor outcomes [123].

Short- and long-term follow-up in NOM (blunt and penetrating)

- *Clinical and laboratory observation associated to bed rest in moderate and severe lesions is the cornerstone in the first 48–72 h follow-up (GoR 1C).*
- *CT scan repetition during the admission should be considered in patients with moderate and severe lesions or in decreasing hematocrit, in the presence of vascular anomalies or underlying splenic pathology or coagulopathy, and in neurologically impaired patients (GoR 2A).*
- *In the presence of underlying splenic pathology or coagulopathy and in neurologically impaired patients CT follow-up is to be considered after the discharge (GoR 2B).*
- *Activity restriction may be suggested for 4–6 weeks in minor injuries and up to 2–4 months in moderate and severe injuries (GoR 2C).*

Splenic complications after blunt splenic trauma range between 0 and 7.5% with a mortality of 7–18% in adults [13]. In children, these incidences are lower [124–127]. The 19% of splenic-delayed ruptures happen within the first 48 h, more frequently between 4 and 10 days after trauma. The risk of splenectomy after discharge ranges between 3 and 146 days after injury, and the rate of readmission for splenectomy was 1.4% [128]. Savage et al. [129] showed that approximately 2% of patients discharged with a non-healed spleen required late intervention. Savage et al. [129] found an average of healing in grades I–II of 12.5 days with a complete healing after 50 days while in grades III–V, 37.2 and 75 days, respectively. In 2–2.5 months, regardless of severity of spleen injury, the 84% of patients presented a complete healing [129]. As a counterpart, Crawford et al. suggested that an early discharge is safe because late failure occurs infrequently [56, 130]. Mortality of late rupture ranges from 5 to 15% compared with 1% mortality in case of acute rupture [40, 131]. In any case, patients undergone NOM should be counseled to not remain alone or in isolated places for the first weeks after the discharge and they should be warned regarding the alert symptoms.

Radiological follow-up is used, but there are not clear information regarding the timing and type of imaging (CT vs. US); thus, imaging follow-up is usually based on clinical judgment and has been widely debated [18, 34, 40, 125, 132–134]. Management strategies that use patient education are more cost effective than to undergo imaging all patients until splenic complete healing.

In the short course (first 24–72 h), observation remains an essential part of low-grade splenic injury (AAST I–II grade); after the admission CT scan, serial abdominal examinations, and hematocrit determination every 6 h are necessary [18]. Clancy et al. [125] showed as PSA were found in patients with grade II, even months after trauma, so they recommended CT scan at 36–72 h in all injuries [129, 131, 132]. Some authors suggest to repeat CT scan only in patients with decreasing hematocrit, in AAST grades III–IV, in patients with subcapsular hematoma, or underlying splenic pathology or coagulopathy, as also in neurologically impaired patients [135].

In the intermediate-long course recent reports recommended that routine post-discharge follow-up abdominal CT is not necessary in low-grade (AAST grade I or II) injuries [132].

More than 50% of patients present a healing at CT scan after 6 weeks, and subsequent image follow-up seems to have no clinical utility [24, 135]. Complete healing of almost all grades is observed 3 months after injury. Lynch et al. [136], in a prospective study, showed that mean time to US healing in AAST grade I, II, Ill, and IV injuries was 3.1, 8.2, 12.1, and 20.7 weeks, respectively. Soffer D. et al. [14] suggest a DUS for splenic lesion follow-up. Some authors have suggested the use of magnetic resonance images [18].

The role of radiological follow-up before returning to normal activity remains controversial. According to some authors, the return to normal activity can occur 3 weeks after splenectomy, and after 2.5–3 months after NOM [126, 134, 136, 137]. Other authors suggested activity restriction of 2 weeks for mild injuries with a return to full activity after 6 weeks, and up to 4–6 months for patients with more severe injuries [120, 129].

Pediatric patients

Pediatric splenic trauma

The spleen is the most commonly injured solid organ in pediatric blunt trauma patients (25–30%) [2, 138]. The age limit for pediatric patients is considered for present guidelines to be < 15 years old. While non-operative management of splenic trauma is the mainstay in children, the available clinical guidelines are not universally applied. In urban pediatric hospitals where resources facilitate the non-operative approach, the likelihood of splenic preservation with NOM ranges from 95 to 100% [139].

The Eastern Association for the Surgery of Trauma (EAST) recommends NOM in blunt splenic trauma in all hemodynamically stable children irrespective of the AAST injury grade [140, 141]. The same guidelines recommend a "less is more" approach with respect to imaging studies during admission and follow-up, aiming to reduce the use of CT scan and radiation exposure [140, 142].

NOM seems to be more effective in children, and therefore, it is more commonly used in these patients compared to adults NOM of pediatric splenic trauma which is also associated with reduced cost and lengths of hospital stay, less need for blood transfusions, vaccinations, and antibiotic therapy, as well as higher immunity and reduced rate of infections [142–146].

Even though it is not clear why NOM outcomes are superior in children compared with adults, this phenomenon may be related to certain unique pediatric characteristics (e.g., thicker splenic capsule, higher proportion of myoepithelial cells, more efficient contraction, and retraction of the splenic arterioles [147–152]).

Clinical presentation in splenic pediatric trauma

The mechanisms of trauma are similar in children and adults. These include motor vehicle and pedestrian injuries as well as sports-related injuries, bicycle injuries, and child abuse [2].

Pediatric injuries differ from adult trauma as the elastic pediatric rib cage may cause a transmission of force into the abdominal compartment [151].

Trauma in neonates represents a rare but unique diagnostic challenge since shock and abdominal rigidity or altered mental status may be the only indications of underlying abdominal injury [2].

In adolescents, the signs of splenic trauma may include the left upper quadrant pain associated with referred left shoulder pain hypovolemic shock or generalized abdominal pain [2].

Definition of the hemodynamic status in children

According to ATLS, the normal systolic blood pressure in children is 90 mmHg plus twice the child's age in years (the lower limit is inferior to 70 mmHg plus twice the child's age in years, or inferior to 50 mmHg in some studies) [5]. Severe blood loss is defined as blood loss greater than 45% of the circulating volume and results in hemodynamic instability. Nevertheless, clinical judgment remains the most important factor in diagnosing an ongoing bleeding [153].

For fluid resuscitation, three boluses of 20 mL/kg of crystalloid replacement should be administered before blood replacement [5, 153]. Massive transfusion protocol in children should be applied with a ratio of 1:1:1 [153]. Transfusion triggers have been debated, and although, there are no class I data to support a specific numerical threshold, it is generally agreed that transfusion should be considered when hemoglobin is less than 7 g/dL [153].

Effective resuscitation is classically indicated by reduction of the heart rate, improved mental status, return of peripheral pulses and normal skin color, increase in blood pressure, and urinary output, as well as increase in extremity warmth [5].

Even though the benefit of tromboelastography (TEG) has not been confirmed in children, recent ATOMAC guidelines suggested that it may be useful in these patients as well (based on adult data) [153].

Diagnostic procedures:

- *The role of E-FAST in the diagnosis of pediatric spleen injury is still unclear (GoR 1A).*
- *A positive E-FAST examination in children should be followed by an urgent CT in stable patients (GoR 1B).*
- *Complete abdominal US may avoid the use of CT in stable patients (GoR 1B).*
- *Contrast-enhanced CT scan is the gold standard in pediatric splenic trauma (GoR 1A).*
- *Doppler US and contrast-enhanced US are useful to evaluate splenic vascularization (GoR 1B).*
- *CT scan is suggested in children at risk for head and thoracic injuries, need for surgery, recurrent bleeding, and if other abdominal injuries are suspected (GoR 1A).*
- *Injury grade on CT scan, free fluid amount, contrast blush, and the presence of pseudo-aneurysm do not predict NOM failure or the need for OM (GoR 1B).* *Thoracic X-ray* at the admission is recommended in the ATLS guidelines [2, 5].

Ultrasonography (US) is the less invasive and is considered the gold standard in trauma, according to the ATLS guidelines especially in Europe [5, 154]. The additional use of DUS or CEUS is helpful and can increase sensitivity for the evaluation of splenic flow and injuries [2]. In patients with low clinical suspicion for splenic trauma, US and CEUS may allow to avoid CT scan [2]. The routine use of CEUS can improve the search of PSA [155].

FAST (Focused Assessment with Sonography for Trauma): The role of FAST for the diagnosis of spleen injury in children is still unclear. Recent Pediatric Emergency Care Applied Research Network (PECARN) data suggest that only 13.7% of pediatric trauma patients with a suspicion of intra-abdominal injuries undergo FAST examination [156]. The sensitivity of this imaging modality in children ranges from 50 to 92%, with a comprehensive meta-analysis suggesting the sensitivity to be around 66% [157–159].

The specificity of this exam is also quite low, and therefore, in a hemodynamically stable patient, a positive FAST examination should be followed by an urgent CT. Bedside FAST may have utility in hemodynamically unstable patients to rapidly identify or rule out intraperitoneal hemorrhage when patients cannot undergo CT.

Contrast-enhanced computer tomography (CT) is the gold standard for the evaluation of blunt abdominal trauma [2, 5]. However, patients should be hemodynamically stable, as well as cooperative or sedated. Of note, surgeons should interpret CT findings cautiously before opting for OM because more than 50% of children present with grade III–IV lesions [2, 160]. Taking into account the radiation risk in children, low-dose protocols are preferred (3–6 mSv instead of 11–24 mSv) [2, 5]. APSA guidelines recommend CT scanning in children at risk for injuries that might be missed by FAST, need for surgery, recurrent bleeding, and when other abdominal injuries (such as pancreatic or hollow viscous injury) are suspected [142].

Non-operative management in splenic injury:

- *NOM is recommended as first-line treatment for hemodynamically stable pediatric patients with blunt splenic trauma (GoR 2A).*
- *Patients with moderate-severe blunt and all penetrating splenic injuries should be considered for transfer to dedicated pediatric trauma centers after hemodynamic stabilization (GoR2A).*
- *NOM of spleen injuries in children should be considered only in an environment that provides capability for patient continuous monitoring, angiography, trained surgeons, an immediately available OR and immediate access to blood and blood products or alternatively in the presence of a rapid centralization system in those patients amenable to be transferred (GoR 2A).*
- *NOM should be attempted even in the setting of concomitant head trauma; unless the patient is unstable, and this might be due to intra-abdominal bleeding (GoR 2B).*

Blunt splenic injury:

- *Blunt splenic injuries with hemodynamic stability and absence of other internal injuries requiring surgery should undergo an initial attempt of NOM irrespective of injury grade (GoR 2A).*

- *In hemodynamically stable children with isolated splenic injury splenectomy should be avoided (GoR 1A).*
- *NOM is contraindicated in the presence of peritonitis, bowel evisceration, impalement, or other indications to laparotomy (GoR 2A).*
- *The presence of contrast blush at CT scan is not an absolute indication for splenectomy or AG/AE in children (GoR 2B).*
- *Intensive care unit admission in isolated splenic injury may be required only for moderate and severe lesions (GoR 2B).*

Penetrating splenic injury:

- *No sufficient data validating NOM for penetrating spleen injury in children exist.*

NOM is successful in 95–100% of blunt pediatric trauma patients and has therefore become the gold standard of treatment in children who have sustained an isolated blunt splenic injury and are hemodynamically stable at the time of presentation [139, 161]. AG/AE at present is considered among NOM tools by several authors.

APSA trauma committee recommendations have resulted in reduced ICU stay, hospital LOS, and resource utilization, while achieving superior outcomes [142, 162, 163]. In isolated spleen injuries, ICU stay should be considered in moderate-severe lesions [153, 160].

The CT-based solid organ grading system has not only been used to triage patients but also to administer the most appropriate treatment and to predict outcomes. However, the latter remains controversial [141, 164]. The CT-based solid organ grading system has not only been used to triage patients but also to administer the most appropriate treatment and to predict outcomes. However, the latter remains controversial [154, 161, 165–167]. Therefore, CT scan should not be the only factor guiding the diagnostic process; and some authors use this argument to avoid imaging in a stable patient altogether. Surprisingly, several studies have shown that adherence to APSA guidelines is low in non-pediatric trauma centers [145, 162, 168–172]. Pediatric trauma patients treated in dedicated centers were demonstrated to have higher probability to undergo NOM than those treated in adult trauma centers [145, 162, 168–170]. Mooney et al. and Todd et al. demonstrated that children with splenic injury have a greater chance to undergo splenectomy or laparotomy in general if treated in an adult trauma center [171, 173].

NOM failure rates for pediatric splenic trauma have been shown to range from 2 to 5% [174, 175]. Of note, there is evidence suggesting that the rate of NOM failure peaks at 4 h and then declines over 36 h from admission [174]. Overall, the majority (72.5%) of NOM failures seem to occur during the first week after trauma, with 50% of them happening within the first 3–5 days [37].

Finally, there are no granular data validating NOM for penetrating spleen injury in children. However, reports on successful non-operative management of isolated penetrating spleen injuries in hemodynamically stable pediatric patients do exist [176–178].

The role of angiography/angioembolization (AG/AE):

- *The vast majority of pediatric patients do not require AG/AE for CT blush or moderate to severe injuries (GoR 1C).*
- *AG/AE may be considered in patients undergone to NOM, hemodynamically stable with sings of persistent hemorrhage not amenable of NOM, regardless the presence of CT blush once excluded extra-splenic source of bleeding (GoR 1C).*
- *AG/AE may be considered for the treatment of post-traumatic splenic pseudo-aneurysms prior to patient discharge (GoR 2C).*
- *Patients with more than 15 years old should be managed according to adults AG/AE-protocols (GoR 1C).*

The role of AG/AE in the management of pediatric splenic trauma is controversial, and its use varies widely among institutions [164, 179, 180].

Even though AG/AE appears to be a safe intervention, the vast majority of retrospective observational data show that very few pediatric patients with contrast extravasation may benefit from embolization [153, 181].

Therefore, AG/AE may only be considered in carefully selected patients, such as those with high-grade injuries, transient response to resuscitation, and/or persistent blood requirements [182]. Similarly, the role of embolization in the management of pediatric splenic pseudo-aneurysms is also unclear. Of note, PSAs often undergo spontaneous thrombosis and could resolve without any interventions [133, 144, 155, 180, 183]. Some authors proposed a distinction between adolescent of more than 13–15 years old, for which should be applied the adult protocol for AG/AE, and children of less than 13–15 years old that are more vulnerable to OPSI [184, 185]. Moreover, Skattum et al. suggested that if a patient aged less than 15 years old is found to have a PSA on admission CT, contrast-enhanced ultrasound should be performed prior to discharge. If at that time PSA is still present, embolization should be considered [184].

Mortality and major complications are rarely reported following AG/AE [180, 184, 186, 187]. Nevertheless, a post-embolization syndrome (PES), consisting of abdominal pain, nausea, ileus, and fever, seems to occur in 90% of children undergoing AG/AE. This syndrome is usually self-limited and tends to resolve spontaneously in 6 to 9 days [188]. In addition, pleural effusion (9%), pneumonia (9%), and coil migration (4.5%) can also be seen after splenic embolization [184].

Overall, AG/AE seems to preserve splenic function without lasting complications, but most children do not need this intervention [179, 189, 190].

Operative management in blunt and penetrating injuries:

- *Patients should undergo to OM in case of hemodynamic instability, failure of conservative treatments, severe coexisting injuries necessitating intervention and peritonitis, bowel evisceration, impalement (GoR 2A).*
- *Splenic preservation (at least partial) should be attempted whenever possible (GoR 2B).*

Indications for laparotomy include hemodynamic instability, ongoing blood loss, or evidence of hollow viscous injury [153, 161, 191–194]. Of note, ATOMAC guidelines recommend surgery if transfusion of 40 mL/kg of all blood products within 24 h (or more than 4 units of blood) fails to stabilize the patient hemodynamically [146, 153]. One percent (1%) of pediatric patients who undergo immediate OM are readmitted for intestinal obstruction within a year [194]. In most cases of OM, splenic partial preservation is possible. Indeed, partial (subtotal) splenectomy or splenorrhaphy are safe and viable alternatives to total splenectomy and can be performed even in high-grade injuries [193, 195–197].

Splenic trauma associated with head injuries

Head injury is an important cause of morbidity and mortality in trauma patients of all ages (50–60%). Importantly, head injuries can also result in altered mental status, which can complicate the process of clinical evaluation [198]. Especially in the setting of concurrent head injury, blood pressure and heart rate are poor markers of hemorrhagic shock in pediatric patients [153]. Nevertheless, an analysis of the National Pediatric Trauma Registry suggested that the association of altered mental status from head injury with spleen injuries should not impact the decision for observational management in pediatric patients (< 19 years old) [198].

Short- and long-term follow-up in splenic trauma (blunt and penetrating):

- *In hemodynamic stable children without drop in hemoglobin levels for 24 h, bed rest should be suggested (GoR 2B).*
- *The risk of pseudo-aneurysm after splenic trauma is low, and in most of cases, it resolves spontaneously (GoR 2B).*
- *Angioembolization should be taken into consideration when a pesudoaneurysm is found (GoR 2B).*
- *US (DUS, CEUS) follow-up seems reasonable to minimize the risk of life-threatening hemorrhage and associated complications in children (GoR 1B).*
- *After NOM in moderate and severe injuries, the reprise of normal activity could be considered safe after at least 6 weeks (GoR 2B).*

No definitive data exist regarding complication rate and short- and long-term follow-up, and no clear indications regarding the most cost-effective imaging technique (US, DUS, CEUS, CT scan). Initial APSA guidelines [142] recommended bed rest for a number of days equal to the grade of injury plus 1 day [142]. However, recent studies suggest a shorter bed rest of one night in solitary grade I–II splenic trauma and two nights for patients with more severe injuries (grade ≥ III) and stable hemoglobin level [199]. Longer admission should be considered in patients with lower hemoglobin levels on admission, higher injury grade, suspicious of other abdominal injuries (as pancreatic or small bowel injuries), blush on the CT scan, bicycle handlebar injuries, recurrent bleeding, or patients at risk for missed injuries [153, 165].

US or CEUS or DUS follow-up seems reasonable to minimize the risk of life-threatening hemorrhage and its associated complications [200]. General surgeons tend to perform routinely imaging follow-up for children differently from pediatric surgeons that only in 5% of cases suggest imaging follow-up [145, 165, 201].

The APSA guidelines [142] recommended 2–5 months of "light" activity before restart with normal activities and recommended 3 week–3 months of limited activity at home. Some authors suggested the reprise of normal activity even after 4 weeks after III–IV grade injuries. In fact, the risks of delayed splenic rupture and post-traumatic pseudocysts seem to be increase within the first 3 weeks (incidence 0.2 and 0.3%, respectively) [142, 202]. Canadian guidelines suggested a discharge at home after reprise and good toleration of oral intake, able mobilization, and analgesia with oral medications without images before discharge [160]. They reported a 32% of children that did not have any images follow-up without any complications and a restriction of activity no more than 6–8 weeks with a length of activity restriction modulated on the grade of injury [160]. The use of CEUS can improve the diagnosis of PSA that can be found in all grades of injury [155].

Patients and parents psychological involvement after trauma can be related with abdominal pain; for this reason, family and patient education post-discharge should be considered to reduce readmission rate [203].

Infection prophylaxis in asplenic and hyposplenic adult and pediatric patients:

- *Patients should receive immunization against the encapsulated bacteria (Streptococcus pneumoniae, Haemophilus influenzae, and Neisseria meningitidis) (GoR 1A).*
- *Vaccination programs should be started no sooner than 14 days after splenectomy or spleen total vascular exclusion (GoR 2C).*
- *In patients discharged before 15 days after splenectomy or angioembolization, where the risk to miss vaccination is deemed high, the best choice is to vaccinate before discharge (GoR 1B).*
- *Annual immunization against seasonal flu is recommended for all patients over 6 months of age (GoR 1C).*
- *Malaria prophylaxis is strongly recommended for travelers (GoR 2C).*
- *Antibiotic therapy should be strongly considered in the event of any sudden onset of unexplained fever, malaise, chills, or other constitutional symptoms, especially when medical review is not readily accessible (GoR 2A).*
- *Primary care providers should be aware of the splenectomy/angioembolization (GoR 2C).*

OPSI are defined as fulminant sepsis, meningitis, or pneumonia triggered mainly by *Streptococcus pneumoniae* (50% of cases) [204, 205] followed by *H. influenzae* type B and *N. meningitidis*. OPSI is a medical emergency. The risks of OPSI and associated death are highest in the first year after splenectomy, at least among young children, but remain elevated for more than 10 years and probably for life. The incidence of OPSI is 0.5–2%; the mortality rate is from 30 to 70%, and most death occurs within the first 24 h. Only prompt diagnosis and immediate treatment can reduce mortality [2, 204, 206, 207]. Asplenic/hyposplenic children younger than 5 years old have a greater overall risk of OPSI with an increased death compared with adults [204, 208]. The risk is more than 30% in neonates [2]. Evidence exist regarding the possible maintaining of the function by the embolized spleen (hyposplenic patients) however is reasonable to consider it as less effective and proceed with vaccination as well [179, 189, 190].

Vaccination against flu is recommended annually for asplenic/hyposplenic patients over 6 months of age. Prevention of influenza may decrease the risk of secondary bacterial infection, including pneumococcal infection [207, 208].

Ideally, the vaccinations against *S. pneumoniae*, *H. influenzae* type B, and *N. meningitidis* should be given at least 2 weeks before splenectomy [2]. Patients should be informed that immunization can only reduce the incidence of OPSI (vaccines so far available do not allow an exhaustive coverage neither for *S. pneumoniae*—23 of 90 serotypes are included—nor for *N. meningitidis*—5 of 6 serotypes) (Table 5).

In traumatic patients, the correct time for vaccination should be not less than 14 days after splenectomy; in fact, before 14 days, the antibody response is supposed to be suboptimal [204, 206, 209]; after that interval, the earlier the better. In asplenic/hyposplenic patients discharged before 15 days, where the risk to miss the vaccination is deemed high, the first vaccines should be given before discharge [206, 210]. The Centre for Disease Control in 2016 proposed the last updated recommendations [211]. Most episodes of severe infections occur within the first 2 years after splenectomy, and for this reason, some authors recommend at least 2 years of prophylactic antibiotics after splenectomy. However, the duration of antibiotic prophylaxis is controversial.

Community physicians should be aware of the asplenic/hyposplenic condition, in order to provide them with the most appropriate level of care.

Asplenic/hyposplenic patients should be given an antibiotic supply in the event of any sudden onset of unexplained fever, malaise, chills, or other constitutional symptoms, especially when medical review is not readily accessible. The recommended options for emergency standby in adults include the following: (a) Amoxycillin, 3 g starting dose followed by 1 g, every 8 h; (b) Levofloxacin 500 mg every 24 h or Moxifloxacin 400 mg every 24 h (for beta-lactam allergic patients).

The recommended emergency standby treatment in children is Amoxycillin 50 mg/Kg in three divided daily doses. For beta-lactam allergic patients, an alternative should be proposed by a specialist (fluoroquinolones are generally contraindicated in children, but due to the possible severity of OPSI, they might still be considered).

Antibiotic prophylaxis is necessary in patients with asplenia/hyposplenia who are bitten by dogs and other animals because of increased risk of severe sepsis (Amoxycillin/Clavulanic acid for 5 days) [205, 207, 208].

If the patient is being treated in an outpatient setting, he/she should be referred immediately to the nearest emergency department. Clinical deterioration can be rapid even after antibiotic administration. Antibiotics should be modified once blood culture results become available [208]. Failures of antibiotic prophylaxis have been reported, so patients should be warned that prophylaxis reduces but does not abolish the risk of sepsis.

Table 5 Vaccinations and antibiotic prophylaxis after splenectomy or hyposplenic status

<table>
<tr><th>Vaccination after splenectomy or in hyposplenic status</th><th>Pneumococcal</th><th>Meningococcal</th><th>H. influenzae B</th><th>Seasonal flu</th></tr>
<tr><td>Vaccination in adults and children > 24 months (unless they have already been fully vaccinated earlier in life for the bacteria considered).</td><td>1 dose of PCV13 and 1 dose of PPSV23 after at least 8 weeks.
Some authors recommend a second PPSV23 dose, after 5 years from the first one.</td><td>1 dose of Meningococcal ACWY conjugated vaccine.
A series of 2 doses of Meningococcal B vaccine at least 1 month apart.</td><td>1 dose</td><td>1 dose annually</td></tr>
<tr><td>Vaccination for children less than 24 months of age, unless already vaccinated for the bacteria considered (in those subjects, antibiotic prophylaxis is recommended for at least 1 year after splenectomy and/or until the 3rd birthday, whichever comes last).</td><td>An age-adapted PCV13 full cycle of immunization, starting from 6 weeks of life.
1 dose of PPSV 23 (minimum age 2 years) at least 8 weeks after the last PCV 13.
PPSV 23 should be re-administered only once, 3 years after the first dose.</td><td>An age-adapted, full-cycle of immunization with Meningococcal B and Meningococcal C (conjugated) vaccine if younger than 12 months or Meningococcal ACWY conjugated vaccine in > 12 months.

Before 24 months of age, only Nimerix® is licensed for use. Menveo® is licensed for use in older than 24 months.</td><td>An age-adapted, full cycle of immunization with Haemophilus type B-conjugated vaccine.</td><td>Annually (minimum age 6 months): 2 doses divided by at least 4 weeks in children aged 6 months through 8 years.
1 dose for children 9 years and older.</td></tr>
<tr><td>Antibiotic prophylaxis after splenectomy or in hyposplenic status</td><td colspan="4">Lifelong prophylactic antibiotics should be offered to patients considered at continued high risk: aged less than 6 years or greater than 50 years, or
1) Having inadequate serological response to pneumococcal vaccination, or
2) With a history of previous invasive pneumococcal disease, or
3) Splenectomized for underlying haematological malignancy particularly in the context of on-going immunosuppression

Suggested regimens:
<table><tr><td>Birth to 3rd month</td><td>AMX/CLA or AMX 10 mg/Kg BID</td></tr><tr><td>3rd month–5 years</td><td>AMX 10 mg/Kg BID</td></tr><tr><td>> 5 years and adults</td><td>AMX 250 mg BID</td></tr></table>
For penicillin allergic patients, probably TMP/SMX is the best option, but this should be discussed case-by-case, according also to the type of allergy in cause.</td></tr>
</table>

PCV13 is a tridecavalent conjugated pneumococcal vaccine, and *PPSV23* is a 23-valent polysaccaride pneumococcal vaccine. *AMX* Amoxicillin, *AMX/CLA* Amoxicillin/clavulanic, *TMP/SMX* cotrimoxazole

Due to the increased risk of severe malaria, asplenic/hyposplenic travelers to endemic areas should receive an adequate pre-departure counseling, regarding both measures aimed at reducing the exposure to mosquitos' bites and chemoprophylaxis.

Conclusions

The management of spleen trauma must be multidisciplinary and must keep into consideration the physiological and anatomical derangement together with the immunological effects. Critical and operative decisions can be taken more effectively if both anatomy of injury and its physiological effects, and the associated lesions are considered especially considering the modern tools for integrated bleeding management. The treatment algorithm must differ within adults, and children these lasts should always be treated in dedicated trauma centers.

Abbreviations

AAST: American Association for Surgery for Trauma; AG/AE: Angiography/angioembolization; AIS: Abbreviated injury score; AMX: Amoxicillin; AMX/CLA: Amoxicillin/clavulanic; APSA: American Pediatric Surgical Association; ATLS: Advanced Trauma Life Support; BE: Base excess; BST: Blunt spinal trauma; CEUS: Contrast-enhanced US; CT: Computerized tomography; DPL: Diagnostic peritoneal lavage; DUS: Doppler US; DVT: Deep venous trombosis; EAST: Eastern Association for the Surgery of Trauma; ED: Emergency Department; E-FAST: Extended focused assessment sonography for trauma; GCS: Glasgow Coma Scale; ICU: Intensive Care Unit; ISS: Injury severity score; LE: Level of evidence; LMWH: Low-molecular-weight heparin; LOS: Length of hospital stay; MTP: Massive transfusion protocols; NOM: Non-operative management; OIS: Organ Injury Scale; OM: Operative management; OPSI: Overwhelming post-splenectomy infections; OR: Operating room; PE: Pulmonary embolism; PES: Post-embolization syndrome; PSA: Pseudoaneurism; TBI: Traumatic brain injury; TEG: Thrombo-elastography; TMP/SMX: Cotrimoxazole; US: Ultrasonography; VTE: Venous thromboembolism; WSES: World Society of Emergency Surgery

Acknowledgements
Special thanks to Ms. Franca Boschini (Bibliographer, Medical Library, Papa Giovanni XXIII Hospital, Bergamo, Italy) for the precious bibliographical work.

Authors' contribution
FC, GM, FCa, YK, WB, EEM, VR, CB, MB, PF, HB, IM, GV, RI, KS, TH, RB, BMP, GPF, KI, JK, NP, KSM, PTM, AK, FAZ, CAG, SVB, NN, FS, SM, MS, VA, EG, LS, AC, AC, MT, VK, CA, LN, LH, MP, SM, DAS, MM, KAD, NDA, AL, PF, RL, DCN, YO, RC, RVM, FM, SR, BS, JMG, OC, SC, ACM, DW, MC, AH, ABP, LW, MS, SDS, and LA contributed to manuscript conception and draft, critically revised the manuscript, contributed important scientific knowledge, and gave final approval of the manuscript.

Funding
There is no funding received in this study.

Competing interests
The authors declare that they have no competing interests.

Author details
[1]General, Emergency and Trauma Surgery, Papa Giovanni XXIII Hospital, P.zza OMS 1, 24128 Bergamo, Italy. [2]Emergency and Trauma Surgery, Maggiore Hospital, Parma, Italy. [3]Division of General Surgery, Rambam Health Care Campus, Haifa, Israel. [4]Acute Care Surgery, The Queen's Medical Center, Honolulu, HI, USA. [5]Trauma Surgery, Denver Health Medical Center, Denver, CO, USA. [6]General and Emergency Surgery, Sergei Kirov Military Academy, Saint Petersburg, Russia. [7]General and Emergency Surgery Department, Empoli Hospital, Empoli, Italy. [8]General and Emergency Surgery, Hadassah Medical Center, Jerusalem, Israel. [9]Klinik für Unfall-, Hand- und Wiederherstellungschirurgie Universitätsklinikum Goethe-Universität Frankfurt, Frankfurt, Germany. [10]Trauma, Emergency Surgery, and Surgical Critical Care, Massachusetts General Hospital, Boston, MA, USA. [11]Virginia Commonwealth University, Richmond, VA, USA. [12]Department of Gastrointestinal Surgery, Stavanger University Hospital, Stavanger, Norway. [13]Department of Cardiothoracic and Vascular Surgery, Örebro University Hospital and Örebro University, Orebro, Sweden. [14]Department of Surgery, Radboud University Nijmegen Medical Center, Nijmegen, Netherlands. [15]Trauma/Acute Care Surgery and Surgical Critical Care, University of Campinas, Campinas, Brazil. [16]Division of Trauma and Critical Care, LAC+USC Medical Center, Los Angeles, CA, USA. [17]Department of Surgery, Assia Medical Group, Tel Aviv University Sackler School of Medicine, Tel Aviv, Israel. [18]General and Trauma Surgery Department, London Health Sciences Centre, Victoria Hospital, London, ON, Canada. [19]Pediatric Trauma Service, Massachusetts General Hospital, Boston, MA, USA. [20]General, Acute Care, Abdominal Wall Reconstruction, and Trauma Surgery, Foothills Medical Centre, Calgary, AB, Canada. [21]Department of Surgery, College of Medicine and Health Sciences, UAE University, Al-Ain, United Arab Emirates. [22]Universidade Federal de Juiz de Fora, Juiz de Fora, Brazil. [23]Infectivolgy Department, Papa Giovanni XXIII Hospital, Bergamo, Italy. [24]Department of Surgery, University of KwaZulu-Natal, Durban, South Africa. [25]Anesthesia Department, Bufalini Hospital, Cesena, Italy. [26]General Surgery Department, Mozir City Hospital, Mozir, Belarus. [27]Clin. Univ. de Chirurgie Digestive et de l'Urgence, CHUGA-CHU Grenoble Alpes UGA-Université Grenoble Alpes, Grenoble, France. [28]Trauma and Surgical Critical Care, University of Michigan Health System, East Medical Center Drive, Ann Arbor, MI, USA. [29]Trauma Unit, Helsinki University Hospital, Helsinki, Finland. [30]Department of Surgery, Stanford University, Stanford, CA, USA. [31]General Surgery, Trauma, and Surgical Critical Care, Yale-New Haven Hospital, New Haven, CT, USA. [32]Hopital Heri Mondor, Paris, France. [33]General Surgery Department, Mehilati Hospital, Helsinki, Finland. [34]General Surgery Department, Westchester Medical Center, Westchester, NY, USA. [35]Colorectal Surgery Unit, Trauma Care Committee, Alicante General University Hospital, Alicante, Spain. [36]Trauma and Acute Critical Care Center, Tokyo Medical and Dental University, Tokyo, Japan. [37]Department of Surgery, UC San Diego Health System, San Diego, USA. [38]Department of Surgery, University of Washington, Seattle, WA, USA. [39]Department of Surgery, Gainesville, FL, USA. [40]Trauma and Acute Care Service, St Michael's Hospital, Toronto, ON, Canada. [41]General Surgery Department, Medical University, University Hospital St George, Plovdiv, Bulgaria. [42]Division of Trauma and Acute Care Surgery, University of California, Davis Medical Center, Davis, CA, USA. [43]Trauma Team, Ospedale Niguarda, Milan, Italy. [44]Department of Surgery and Obstetric and Gynecology, University of Buea, Buea, Cameroon. [45]Department of General Surgery, Royal Perth Hospital, Perth, Australia. [46]Surgery Department, University of Pittsburgh, Pittsburgh, Pensylvania, USA. [47]General Surgery Department, Ayaan Hospital, Mogadisho, Somalia. [48]General and Emergency Surgery, Macerata Hospital, Macerata, Italy. [49]General, Emergency and Trauma Surgery Department, Maggiore Hospital, Bologna, Italy. [50]Department of Surgery, Örebro University Hospital and Örebro University, Obreo, Sweden.

References
1. Oxford Centre for Evidence-based Medicine - Levels of Evidence (March 2009) - CEBM. Available from: http://www.cebm.net/oxford-centre-evidence-based-medicine-levels-evidence-march-2009/
2. Lynn KN, Werder GM, Callaghan RM, Sullivan AN, Jafri ZH, Bloom DA. Pediatric blunt splenic trauma: a comprehensive review. Pediatr Radiol. 2009;39:904–16.
3. Mutschler M, Nienaber U, Brockamp T, Wafaisade A, Fabian T, Paffrath T, et al. Renaissance of base deficit for the initial assessment of trauma patients: a base deficit-based classification for hypovolemic shock developed on data from 16,305 patients derived from the TraumaRegister DGU®. Crit Care. 2013;17:R42.
4. Mutschler M, Nienaber U, Münzberg M, Wölfl C, Schoechl H, Paffrath T, et al. The shock index revisited—a fast guide to transfusion requirement? A retrospective analysis on 21,853 patients derived from the TraumaRegister DGU. Crit Care. 2013;17:R172.
5. American College of Surgeon's Commitee on Trauma. Advanced Trauma Life Support® (ATLS®) Student manual 9th ed.ed., American College of Surgeon, Chicago; 2012.
6. Da Luz LT, Nascimento B, Shankarakutty AK, Rizoli S, Adhikari NK. Effect of thromboelastography (TEG®) and rotational thromboelastometry (ROTEM®) on diagnosis of coagulopathy, transfusion guidance and mortality in trauma: descriptive systematic review. Crit Care. 2014;18:518.
7. Gonzalez E, Moore EE, Moore HB, Chapman MP, Chin TL, Ghasabyan A, et al. Goal-directed hemostatic resuscitation of trauma-induced coagulopathy: a pragmatic randomized clinical trial comparing a viscoelastic assay to conventional coagulation assays. Ann Surg. 2016;263:1051–9.
8. Kashuk JL, Moore EE, Sawyer M, Le T, Johnson J, Biffl WL, et al. Postinjury coagulopathy management: goal directed resuscitation via POC thrombelastography. Ann Surg. 2010;251:604–14.
9. Rossaint R, Cerny V, Coats TJ, Duranteau J, Fernández-Mondéjar E, Gordini G, et al. Key issues in advanced bleeding care in trauma. Shock. 2006;26:322–31.
10. Carr JA, Roiter C, Alzuhaili A. Correlation of operative and pathological injury grade with computed tomographic grade in the failed nonoperative management of blunt splenic trauma. Eur J Trauma Emerg Surg. 2012;38:433–8.
11. Kirkpatrick AW, Sirois M, Laupland KB, Liu D, Rowan K, Ball CG, et al. Hand-held thoracic sonography for detecting post-traumatic pneumothoraces: the extended focused assessment with sonography for trauma (EFAST). J Trauma. 2004;57:288–95.

12. Doody O, Lyburn D, Geoghegan T, Govender P, Monk PM, Torreggiani WC. Blunt trauma to the spleen: ultrasonographic findings. Clin Radiol. 2005;60: 968–76.
13. El-Matbouly M, Jabbour G, El-Menyar A, Peralta R, Abdelrahman H, Zarour A, et al. Blunt splenic trauma: assessment, management and outcomes. Surgeon. 2016;14:52–8.
14. Soffer D, Wiesel O, Schulman CI, Ben Haim M, Klausner JM, Kessler A. Doppler ultrasound for the assessment of conservatively treated blunt splenic injuries: a prospective study. Eur J Trauma Emerg Surg. 2011;37:197–202.
15. Bee TK, M a C, Miller PR, Pritchard FE, Fabian TC. Failures of splenic nonoperative management: is the glass half empty or half full? J Trauma. 2001;50:230–6.
16. Clark R, Hird K, Misur P, Ramsay D, Mendelson R. CT grading scales for splenic injury: why can't we agree? J Med Imaging Radiat Oncol. 2011;55:163–9.
17. Becker CD, Mentha G, Terrier F. Blunt abdominal trauma in adults: role of CT in the diagnosis and management of visceral injuries. Part 1: liver and spleen. Eur Radiol. 1998;8:553–62.
18. Shapiro MJ, Krausz C, Durham RM, Mazuski JE. Overuse of splenic scoring and computed tomographic scans. J Trauma. 1999;47:651–8.
19. Anderson SW, Varghese JC, Lucey BC, P a B, Hirsch EF, J a S. Blunt splenic trauma: delayed-phase CT for differentiation of active hemorrhage from contained vascular injury in patients. Radiology. 2007;243:88–95.
20. Jeffrey RB, Olcott EW. Imaging of blunt hepatic trauma. Radiol Clin N Am. 1991;29:1299–310.
21. Marmery H, Shanmuganathan K, Mirvis SE, Richard H, Sliker C, Miller LA, et al. Correlation of multidetector CT findings with splenic arteriography and surgery: prospective study in 392 patients. J Am Coll Surg. 2008;206:685–93.
22. Boscak AR, Shanmuganathan K, Mirvis SE, Fleiter TR, L a M, Sliker CW, et al. Optimizing trauma multidetector CT protocol for blunt splenic injury: need for arterial and portal venous phase scans. Radiology. 2013;268:79–88.
23. Bhullar IS, Frykberg ER, Tepas JJ, Siragusa D, Loper T, Kerwin AJ. At first blush: absence of computed tomography contrast extravasation in grade IV or V adult blunt splenic trauma should not preclude angioembolization. J Trauma Acute Care Surg. 2013;74:105-11-2.
24. Hassan R, Aziz AA, Ralib ARM, Saat A. Computed tomography of blunt spleen injury: a pictorial review. Malaysian J Med Sci. 2011;18:60–7.
25. Juyia RF, Kerr HA. Return to play after liver and spleen trauma. Sports Health. 2014;6:239–45. SAGE Publications
26. Fernandes TM, Dorigatti AE, Pereira BMT, Cruvinel Neto J, Zago TM, Fraga GP. Nonoperative management of splenic injury grade IV is safe using rigid protocol. Rev Col Bras Cir. 2013;40:323–9.
27. N a S, Bhullar I, Cheng JD, Crandall ML, Friese RS, Guillamondegui OD, et al. Selective nonoperative management of blunt splenic injury: an Eastern Association for the Surgery of Trauma practice management guideline. J Trauma Acute Care Surg. 2012;73:S294–300.
28. Velmahos GC, Toutouzas KG, Radin R, Chan L, Demetriades D. Nonoperative treatment of blunt injury to solid abdominal organs: a prospective study. Arch Surg. 2003;138:844–51.
29. Smith J, Armen S, Cook CH, Martin LC. Blunt splenic injuries: have we watched long enough? J Trauma. 2008;64:656-63-5.
30. Hafiz S, Desale S, Sava J. The impact of solid organ injury management on the US health care system. J Trauma Acute Care Surg. 2014;77:310–4.
31. Gaspar B, Negoi I, Paun S, Hostiuc S, Ganescu R, Beuran M. Selective nonoperative management of abdominal injuries in polytrauma patients: a protocol only for experienced trauma centers. Maedica. 2014;9:168–72.
32. Moore FA, Davis JW, Moore EE, Cocanour CS, West MA, McIntyre RC. Western Trauma Association (WTA) critical decisions in trauma: management of adult blunt splenic trauma. J Trauma. 2008;65:1007–11.
33. Rowell SE, Biffl WL, Brasel K, Moore EE, Albrecht RA, DeMoya M, et al. Western Trauma Association Critical Decisions in Trauma: management of adult blunt splenic trauma-2016 updates. J Trauma Acute Care Surg. 2017; 82:787–93.
34. Peitzman AB, Harbrecht BG, Rivera L, Heil B. Failure of observation of blunt splenic injury in adults: variability in practice and adverse consequences. J Am Coll Surg. 2005;201:179–87.
35. Renzulli P, Gross T, Schnüriger B, Schoepfer AM, Inderbitzin D, Exadaktylos AK, et al. Management of blunt injuries to the spleen. Br J Surg. 2010;97:1696–703.
36. J a N, Costanza M, Daley BJ, M a P, Enderson BL. Outcome of the current management of splenic injuries. J Trauma. 2001;50:835–42.
37. McIntyre LK, Schiff M, Jurkovich GJ. Failure of nonoperative management of splenic injuries: causes and consequences. Arch Surg. 2005;140:563-568-569.
38. Ong AW, Eilertson KE, Reilly EF, Geng TA, Madbak F, McNicholas A, et al. Nonoperative management of splenic injuries: significance of age. J Surg Res. 2016;201:134–40.
39. Bhullar IS, Frykberg ER, Siragusa D, Chesire D, Paul J, Tepas JJ, et al. Age does not affect outcomes of nonoperative management of blunt splenic trauma. J Am Coll Surg. 2012;214:958–64.
40. Peitzman AB, Heil B, Rivera L, Federle M, Harbrecht BG, Clancy K, et al. Blunt splenic injury in adults: multi-institutional study of the Eastern Association for the Surgery of Trauma. J Trauma-Injury Infect Crit Care. 2000;49:177–89.
41. Malhotra AK, Latifi R, Fabian TC, Ivatury RR, Dhage S, Bee TK, et al. Multiplicity of solid organ injury: influence on management and outcomes after blunt abdominal trauma. J Trauma. 2003;54:925–9.
42. Harbrecht BG, Zenati MS, Alarcon LH, Ochoa JB, Puyana JC, Schuchert VD, et al. Is outcome after blunt splenic injury in adults better in high-volume trauma centers? Am Surg. 2005;71:942-8-9.
43. Cocanour CS, Moore FA, Ware DN, Marvin RG, Duke JH. Age should not be a consideration for nonoperative management of blunt splenic injury. J Trauma-Injury Infect Crit Care. 2000;48:606–12. discussion 610–612
44. Harbrecht BG, Peitzman AB, Rivera L, Heil B, Croce M, Morris JA, et al. Contribution of age and gender to outcome of blunt splenic injury in adults: multicenter study of the eastern association for the surgery of trauma. J Trauma. 2001;51:887–95.
45. Siriratsivawong K, Zenati M, Watson GA, Harbrecht BG. Nonoperative management of blunt splenic trauma in the elderly: does age play a role? Am Surg. 2007;73:585–9. discussion 590
46. Velmahos GC, Zacharias N, Emhoff TA, Feeney JM, Hurst JM, Crookes BA, et al. Management of the most severely injured spleen: a multicenter study of the research consortium of New England centers for trauma (ReCONECT). Arch Surg. 2010;145:456–60.
47. Velmahos GC, Chan LS, Kamel E, Murray JA, Yassa N, Kahaku D, et al. Nonoperative management of splenic injuries: have we gone too far? Arch Surg. 2000;135:674–81.
48. Jeremitsky E, Kao A, Carlton C, Rodriguez A, Ong A. Does splenic embolization and grade of splenic injury impact nonoperative management in patients sustaining blunt splenic trauma? Am Surg. 2011;77:215–20.
49. G a W, Rosengart MR, Zenati MS, Tsung A, Forsythe RM, Peitzman AB, et al. Nonoperative management of severe blunt splenic injury: are we getting better? J Trauma. 2006;61:1113-1118-1119.
50. Krause KR, Howells GA, Bair HA, Glover JL, Madrazo BL, Wasvary HJ, et al. Nonoperative management of blunt splenic injury in adults 55 years and older: a twenty-year experience. Am Surg. 2000;66:636–40.
51. Sartorelli KH, Frumiento C, Rogers FB, Osler TM. Nonoperative management of hepatic, splenic, and renal injuries in adults with multiple injuries. J Trauma. 2000;49:56-61-2.
52. Albrecht RM, Schermer CR, Morris A. Nonoperative management of blunt splenic injuries: factors influencing success in age >55 years. Am Surg. 2002; 68:227-30-1.
53. Schurr MJ, Fabian TC, Gavant M, Croce MA, Kudsk KA, Minard G, et al. Management of blunt splenic trauma: computed tomographic contrast blush predicts failure of nonoperative management. J Trauma. 1995;39:507-512-513.
54. Bhangu A, Nepogodiev D, Lal N, Bowley DM. Meta-analysis of predictive factors and outcomes for failure of non-operative management of blunt splenic trauma. Injury. 2012;43:1337–46.
55. Aseervatham R, Muller M. Blunt trauma to the spleen. Aust N Z J Surg. 2000; 70:333–7.
56. Crawford RS, Tabbara M, Sheridan R, Spaniolas K, Velmahos GC. Early discharge after nonoperative management for splenic injuries: increased patient risk caused by late failure? Surgery. 2007;142:337–42.
57. Jeremitsky E, Smith RS, Ong AW. Starting the clock: defining nonoperative management of blunt splenic injury by time. Am J Surg. 2013;205:298–301.
58. Chen L-Y, Shih H-C, Wu JJ, Wen Y-S, Huang M-S, Huang C-I, et al. The role of diagnostic algorithms in the management of blunt splenic injury. J Chin Med Assoc. 2005;68:373–8.
59. Ball CG, Kirkpatrick AW, D'Amours SK. The RAPTOR: resuscitation with angiography, percutaneous techniques and operative repair. Transforming the discipline of trauma surgery. Can J Surg. 2011;54:E3–4.
60. Kirkpatrick AW, Vis C, Dubé M, Biesbroek S, Ball CG, Laberge J, et al. The evolution of a purpose designed hybrid trauma operating room from the trauma service perspective: the RAPTOR (resuscitation with angiography percutaneous treatments and operative resuscitations). Injury. 2014;45:1413–21.

61. Fehr A, Beveridge J, SD DA, Kirkpatrick AW, Ball CG. The potential benefit of a hybrid operating environment among severely injured patients with persistent hemorrhage: how often could we get it right? J Trauma Acute Care Surg. 2016;80:457–60.
62. Demetriades D, Rabinowitz B. Indications for operation in abdominal stab wounds. A prospective study of 651 patients. Ann Surg. 1987;205:129–32.
63. Velmahos GC, Demetriades D, Toutouzas KG, Sarkisyan G, Chan LS, Ishak R, et al. Selective nonoperative management in 1,856 patients with abdominal gunshot wounds: should routine laparotomy still be the standard of care? Ann Surg. 2001:234, 395-402-403.
64. Renz BM, Feliciano DV. Gunshot wounds to the right thoracoabdomen: a prospective study of nonoperative management. J Trauma. 1994;37:737–44.
65. Inaba K, Barmparas G, Foster A, Talving P, David J-S, Green D, et al. Selective nonoperative management of torso gunshot wounds: when is it safe to discharge? J Trauma. 2010;68:1301–4.
66. Carlin AM, Tyburski JG, Wilson RF, Steffes C. Factors affecting the outcome of patients with splenic trauma. Am Surg. 2002;68:232–9.
67. Berg RJ, Inaba K, Okoye O, Pasley J, Teixeira PG, Esparza M, et al. The contemporary management of penetrating splenic injury. Injury. 2014;45: 1394–400.
68. Haan JM, Bochicchio GV, Kramer N, Scalea TM. Nonoperative management of blunt splenic injury: a 5-year experience. J Trauma. 2005;58:492–8.
69. Haan J, Scott J, Boyd-Kranis RL, Ho S, Kramer M, Scalea TM. Admission angiography for blunt splenic injury: advantages and pitfalls. J Trauma. 2001;51:1161–5.
70. Haan JM, Biffl W, Knudson MM, Davis KA, Oka T, Majercik S, et al. Splenic embolization revisited: a multicenter review. J Trauma - Inj Infect Crit Care. 2004;56:542–7.
71. Tugnoli G, Bianchi E, Biscardi A, Coniglio C, Isceri S, Simonetti L, et al. Nonoperative management of blunt splenic injury in adults: there is (still) a long way to go. The results of the Bologna-Maggiore Hospital trauma center experience and development of a clinical algorithm. Surg Today. 2015;45:1210–7.
72. Bessoud B, Denys A, Calmes JM, Madoff D, Qanadli S, Schnyder P, et al. Nonoperative management of traumatic splenic injuries: is there a role for proximal splenic artery embolization? Am J Roentgenol. 2006;186:779–85.
73. Brillantino A, Iacobellis F, Robustelli U, Villamaina E, Maglione F, Colletti O, et al. Non operative management of blunt splenic trauma: a prospective evaluation of a standardized treatment protocol. Eur J Trauma Emerg Surg. 2016;42:593–8.
74. Smith HE, Biffl WL, Majercik SD, Jednacz J, Lambiase R, Cioffi WG. Splenic artery embolization: have we gone too far? J Trauma. 2006;61:541-544-546.
75. Capecci LM, Jeremitsky E, Smith RS, Philp F. Trauma centers with higher rates of angiography have a lesser incidence of splenectomy in the management of blunt splenic injury. Surgery. 2015;158:1020-4-6.
76. Zarzaur BL, Savage SA, Croce MA, Fabian TC. Trauma center angiography use in high-grade blunt splenic injuries: timing is everything. J Trauma Acute Care Surg. 2014;77:666–71.
77. Raikhlin A, Baerlocher MO, Asch MR, Myers A. Imaging and transcatheter arterial embolization for traumatic splenic injuries: review of the literature. Can J Surg. 2008;51:464–72.
78. Banerjee A, Duane TM, Wilson SP, Haney S, O'Neill PJ, Evans HL, et al. Trauma center variation in splenic artery embolization and spleen salvage: a multicenter analysis. J Trauma Acute Care Surg. 2013;75:69-74-5.
79. Rosati C, Ata A, Siskin GP, Megna D, Bonville DJ, Stain SC. Management of splenic trauma: a single institution's 8-year experience. Am J Surg. 2015;209: 308–14.
80. J a R, RB DA, Miller PR. Nonoperative management of adult blunt splenic injury with and without splenic artery embolotherapy: a meta-analysis. J Trauma Inj Infect Crit Care. 2011;71:898–903.
81. Davis KA, Fabian TC, Croce MA, Gavant ML, Flick PA, Minard G, et al. Improved success in nonoperative management of blunt splenic injuries: embolization of splenic artery pseudoaneurysms. J Trauma. 1998;44:1008-13-5.
82. Dehli T, Bagenholm A, Trasti NC, Monsen SA, Bartnes K, Bågenholm A, et al. The treatment of spleen injuries: a retrospective study. Scand J Trauma Resusc Emerg Med. 2015;23:85.
83. Shanmuganathan K, Mirvis SE, Sover ER. Value of contrast-enhanced CT in detecting active hemorrhage in patients with blunt abdominal or pelvic trauma. Am J Roentgenol. 1993;161:65–9.
84. Ryan M, Hamilton P, Chu P, Hanaghan J. Active extravasation of arterial contrast agent on post-traumatic abdominal computed tomography. Can Assoc Radiol J. 2004;55:160–9.
85. Gavant ML, Schurr M, Flick PA, Croce MA, Fabian TC, Gold RE. Predicting clinical outcome of nonsurgical management of blunt splenic injury: using CT to reveal abnormalities of splenic vasculature. Am J Roentgenol. 1997; 168:207–12.
86. Shanmuganathan K, Mirvis SE, Boyd-Kranis R, Takada T, Scalea TM. Nonsurgical management of blunt splenic injury: use of CT criteria to select patients for splenic arteriography and potential endovascular therapy. Radiology. 2000;217:75–82.
87. Marmery H, Shanmuganathan K, Alexander MT, Mirvis SE. Optimization of selection for nonoperative management of blunt splenic injury: comparison of MDCT grading systems. Am J Roentgenol. 2007;189:1421–7.
88. Fu C-Y, Wu S-C, Chen R-J, Chen Y-F, Wang Y-C, Huang H-C, et al. Evaluation of need for operative intervention in blunt splenic injury: intraperitoneal contrast extravasation has an increased probability of requiring operative intervention. World J Surg. 2010;34:2745–51.
89. Yuan K-C, Wong Y-C, Lin B-C, Kang S-C, Liu E-H, Hsu Y-P. Negative catheter angiography after vascular contrast extravasations on computed tomography in blunt torso trauma: an experience review of a clinical dilemma. Scand J Trauma Resusc Emerg Med. 2012;20:46.
90. Alarhayem AQ, Myers JG, Dent D, Lamus D, Lopera J, Liao L, et al. "blush at first sight": significance of computed tomographic and angiographic discrepancy in patients with blunt abdominal trauma. Am J Surg. 2015;210: 1104-10-1.
91. Skattum J, Naess PA, Eken T, Gaarder C. Refining the role of splenic angiographic embolization in high-grade splenic injuries. J Trauma Acute Care Surg. 2013;74:100-3-4.
92. Miller PR, Chang MC, Hoth JJ, Mowery NT, Hildreth AN, Martin RS, et al. Prospective trial of angiography and embolization for all grade III to V blunt splenic injuries: nonoperative management success rate is significantly improved. J Am Coll Surg. 2014;218:644–8.
93. Chastang L, Bège T, Prudhomme M, Simonnet AC, Herrero A, Guillon F, et al. Is non-operative management of severe blunt splenic injury safer than embolization or surgery? Results from a French prospective multicenter study. J Visc Surg. 2015;152:85–91.
94. Frandon J, Rodière M, Arvieux C, Michoud M, Vendrell A, Broux C, et al. Blunt splenic injury: outcomes of proximal versus distal and combined splenic artery embolization. Diagn Interv Imaging. 2014;95:825–31.
95. Schnüriger B, Inaba K, Konstantinidis A, Lustenberger T, Chan LS, Demetriades D. Outcomes of proximal versus distal splenic artery embolization after trauma: a systematic review and meta-analysis. J Trauma. 2011;70:252–60.
96. Ekeh AP, McCarthy MC, Woods RJ, Haley E. Complications arising from splenic embolization after blunt splenic trauma. Am J Surg. 2005;189:335–9.
97. Frandon J, Rodiere M, Arvieux C, Vendrell A, Boussat B, Sengel C, et al. Blunt splenic injury: are early adverse events related to trauma, nonoperative management, or surgery? Diagnostic Interv Radiol. 2015;21:327–33.
98. Demetriades D, Scalea TM, Degiannis E, Barmparas G, Konstantinidis A, Massahis J, et al. Blunt splenic trauma: splenectomy increases early infectious complications: a prospective multicenter study. J Trauma Acute Care Surg. 2012;72:229–34.
99. Kaseje N, Agarwal S, Burch M, Glantz A, Emhoff T, Burke P, et al. Short-term outcomes of splenectomy avoidance in trauma patients. Am J Surg. 2008; 196:213–7.
100. Freitas G, Olufajo OA, Hammouda K, Lin E, Cooper Z, Havens JM, et al. Postdischarge complications following nonoperative management of blunt splenic injury. Am J Surg. 2016;211:744–9.
101. Wei B, Hemmila MR, Arbabi S, Taheri PA, Wahl WL, et al. Angioembolization reduces operative intervention for blunt splenic injury. J Trauma - Inj Infect Crit Care. 2008;64:1472–7.
102. Ekeh AP, Khalaf S, Ilyas S, Kauffman S, Walusimbi M, McCarthy MC. Complications arising from splenic artery embolization: a review of an 11-year experience. Am J Surg. 2013;205:250–4.
103. Wu SC, Chen RJ, Yang AD, Tung CC, Lee KH. Complications associated with embolization in the treatment of blunt splenic injury. World J Surg. 2008;32: 476 82.
104. Bruce PJP, Helmer SD, Harrison PB, Sirico T, Haan JM. Nonsurgical management of blunt splenic injury: is it cost effective? Am J Surg. 2011;202:810–6.
105. Morrell DG, Chang FC, Helmer SD. Changing trends in the management of splenic injury. Am J Surg. 1995;170:686–9. discussion 690
106. Carter JW, Falco MH, Chopko MS, Flynn WJ, Wiles Iii CE, Guo WA. Do we really rely on fast for decision-making in the management of blunt abdominal trauma? Injury. 2015;46:817–21.

107. Hady HR, Łuba M, Myśliwiec P, Trochimowicz L, Łukaszewicz J, Zurawska J, et al. Surgical management in parenchymatous organ injuries due to blunt and penetrating abdominal traumas--the authors' experience. Adv Clin Exp Med. 2012;21:193–200.
108. Garber BG, Yelle JD, Fairfull-Smith R, Lorimer JW, Carson C. Management of splenic injuries in a Canadian trauma centre. Can J Surg. 1996;39:474–80.
109. Haddad SH, Yousef ZM, Al-Azzam SS, Aldawood AS, Al-Zahrani AA, Alzamel HA, et al. Profile, outcome and predictors of mortality of abdomino-pelvic trauma patients in a tertiary intensive care unit in Saudi Arabia. Injury. 2015;46:94–9.
110. Swaid F, Peleg K, Alfici R, Matter I, Olsha O, Ashkenazi I, et al. Concomitant hollow viscus injuries in patients with blunt hepatic and splenic injuries: an analysis of a National Trauma Registry database. Injury. 2014;45:1409–12.
111. Garber BG, Mmath BP, Fairfull-Smith RJ, Yelle JD. Management of adult splenic injuries in Ontario: a population-based study. Can J Surg. 2000;43:283–8.
112. Nasr WI, Collins CL, Kelly JJ. Feasibility of laparoscopic splenectomy in stable blunt trauma: a case series. J Trauma. 2004;57:887–9.
113. Hallfeldt KK, Trupka AW, Erhard J, Waldner H, Schweiberer L. Emergency laparoscopy for abdominal stab wounds. Surg Endosc. 1998;12:907–10.
114. Pisters PW, Pachter HL. Autologous splenic transplantation for splenic trauma. Ann Surg. 1994;219:225–35.
115. Qu Y, Ren S, Li C, Qian S, Liu P. Management of postoperative complications following splenectomy. Int Surg. 2013;98:55–60.
116. Alabbasi T, Nathens AB, Tien H. Blunt splenic injury and severe brain injury: a decision analysis and implications for care. Can J Surg. 2015;58:S108–17.
117. Rostas JW, Manley J, Gonzalez RP, Brevard SB, Ahmed N, Frotan MA, et al. The safety of low molecular-weight heparin after blunt liver and spleen injuries. Am J Surg. 2015;210:31–4.
118. Murphy PB, Sothilingam N, Charyk Stewart T, Batey B, Moffat B, Gray DK, et al. Very early initiation of chemical venous thromboembolism prophylaxis after blunt solid organ injury is safe. Can J Surg. 2016;59:118–22.
119. Alejandro KV, Acosta JA, Rodríguez PA. Bleeding manifestations after early use of low-molecular-weight heparins in blunt splenic injuries. Am Surg. 2003;69:1006–9.
120. Zarzaur BL, R a K, Fabian TC, Coimbra R. A survey of American Association for the Surgery of Trauma member practices in the management of blunt splenic injury. J Trauma. 2011;70:1026–31.
121. Eberle BM, Schnüriger B, Inaba K, Cestero R, Kobayashi L, Barmparas G, et al. Thromboembolic prophylaxis with low-molecular-weight heparin in patients with blunt solid abdominal organ injuries undergoing nonoperative management: current practice and outcomes. J Trauma. 2011;70:141–6. discussion 147
122. Joseph B, Pandit V, Harrison C, Lubin D, Kulvatunyou N, Zangbar B, et al. Early thromboembolic prophylaxis in patients with blunt solid abdominal organ injuries undergoing nonoperative management: is it safe? Am J Surg. 2015;209:194–8.
123. Weinberger J, Cipolle M. Optimal reversal of novel anticoagulants in trauma. Crit Care Clin. 2017;33:135–52.
124. Imbert P, Rapp C, Buffet PA. Pathological rupture of the spleen in malaria: analysis of 55 cases (1958–2008). Travel Med Infect Dis. 2009;7:147–59.
125. Clancy AA, Tiruta C, Ashman D, Ball CG, Kirkpatrick AW. The song remains the same although the instruments are changing: complications following selective non-operative management of blunt spleen trauma: a retrospective review of patients at a level I trauma centre from 1996 to 2007. J Trauma Manag Outcomes. 2012;6:4.
126. Gannon EH, Howard T. Splenic injuries in athletes: a review. Curr Sports Med Rep. 2010;9:111–4.
127. Frumiento C, Sartorelli K, Vane D. Complications of splenic injuries: expansion of the nonoperative theorem. J Pediatr Surg. 2000;35:788–91.
128. Zarzaur BL, Vashi S, Magnotti LJ, Croce MA, Fabian TC. The real risk of splenectomy after discharge home following nonoperative management of blunt splenic injury. J Trauma. 2009;66:1531–8.
129. S a S, Zarzaur BL, Magnotti LJ, J a W, Maish GO, Bee TK, et al. The evolution of blunt splenic injury: resolution and progression. J Trauma. 2008;64:1085-91-2.
130. Meguid AA, Bair HA, Howells GA, Bendick PJ, Kerr HH, Villalba MR. Prospective evaluation of criteria for the nonoperative management of blunt splenic trauma. Am Surg. 2003;69:238-42-3.
131. Riezzo I, Di Battista B, De Salvia A, Cantatore S, Neri M, Pomara C, et al. Delayed splenic rupture: dating the sub-capsular hemorrhage as a useful task to evaluate causal relationships with trauma. Forensic Sci Int. 2014;234: 64–71.
132. Haan JM, Boswell S, Stein D, Scalea TM. Follow-up abdominal CT is not necessary in low-grade splenic injury. Am Surg. 2007;73:13–8.
133. Muroya T, Ogura H, Shimizu K, Tasaki O, Kuwagata Y, Fuse T, et al. Delayed formation of splenic pseudoaneurysm following nonoperative management in blunt splenic injury: multi-institutional study in Osaka, Japan. J Trauma Acute Care Surg. 2013;75:417–20.
134. Uecker J, Pickett C, Dunn E. The role of follow-up radiographic studies in nonoperative management of spleen trauma. Am Surg. 2001;67:22–5.
135. Lyass S, Sela T, Lebensart PD, Muggia-Sullam M. Follow-up imaging studies of blunt splenic injury: do they influence management? Isr Med Assoc J. 2001;3:731–3.
136. Lynch JM, Meza MP, Newman B, Gardner MJ, Albanese CT. Computed tomography grade of splenic injury is predictive of the time required for radiographic healing. J Pediatr Surg. 1997;32:1093–6.
137. Unal E, Onur MR, Akpinar E, Ahmadov J, Karcaaltincaba M, Ozmen MN, et al. Imaging findings of splenic emergencies: a pictorial review. Insights Imaging. 2016;7:215–22.
138. Linet MS, Nyrén O, Gridley G, Adami HO, Buckland JD, McLaughlin JK, et al. Causes of death among patients surviving at least one year following splenectomy. Am J Surg. 1996;172:320–3.
139. Bairdain S, Litman HJ, Troy M, McMahon M, Almodovar H, Zurakowski D, et al. Twenty-years of splenic preservation at a level 1 pediatric trauma center. J Pediatr Surg. 2015;50:864–8.
140. Alonso M, Brathwaite C, García V, Patterson L, Scherer T, Stafford P, et al. Practice management guidelines for the nonoperative management of blunt injury to the liver and spleen. Chicago: Eastern Association for the Surgery of Trauma; 2003.
141. Moore EE, Cogbill TH, Jurkovich GJ, Shackford SR, Malangoni MA, Champion HR. Organ injury scaling: spleen and liver (1994 revision). J Trauma. 1995;38:323–4.
142. Stylianos S. Evidence-based guidelines for resource utilization in children with isolated spleen or liver injury. The APSA Trauma Committee. J Pediatr Surg. 2000;35:164–9.
143. McVay MR, Kokoska ER, Jackson RJ, Smith SD. Throwing out the "grade" book: management of isolated spleen and liver injury based on hemodynamic status. J Pediatr Surg. 2008;43:1072–6.
144. Martin K, Vanhouwelingen L, Bütter A. The significance of pseudoaneurysms in the nonoperative management of pediatric blunt splenic trauma. J Pediatr Surg. 2011;46:933–7.
145. Li D, Yanchar N. Management of pediatric blunt splenic injuries in Canada-practices and opinions. J Pediatr Surg. 2009;44:997–1004.
146. Bond SJ, Eichelberger MR, Gotschall CS, Sivit CJ, Randolph JG. Nonoperative management of blunt hepatic and splenic injury in children. Ann Surg. 1996;223:286–9.
147. Muehrcke DD, Kim SH, McCabe CJ. Pediatric splenic trauma: predicting the success of nonoperative therapy. Am J Emerg Med. 1987;5:109–12.
148. Delius RE, Frankel W, Coran AG. A comparison between operative and nonoperative management of blunt injuries to the liver and spleen in adult and pediatric patients. Surgery. 1989;106:788-92-3.
149. Lynch JM, Ford H, Gardner MJ, Weiner ES. Is early discharge following isolated splenic injury in the hemodynamically stable child possible? J Pediatr Surg. 1993;28:1403–7.
150. Konstantakos AK, Barnoski AL, Plaisier BR, Yowler CJ, Fallon WF, Malangoni MA. Optimizing the management of blunt splenic injury in adults and children. Surgery. 1999;126:805–13.
151. Upadhyaya P. Conservative management of splenic trauma: history and current trends. Pediatr Surg Int. 2003;19:617–27.
152. Rodrigues CJ, Sacchetti JC, Rodrigues AJ. Age-related changes in the elastic fiber network of the human splenic capsule. Lymphology. 1999; 32:64–9.
153. Notrica DM, Eubanks JW, Tuggle DW, Maxson RT, Letton RW, Garcia NM, et al. Nonoperative management of blunt liver and spleen injury in children: evaluation of the ATOMAC guideline using GRADE. J Trauma Acute Care Surg. 2015;79:683–93.
154. Singer G, Rieder S, Eberl R, Wegmann H, Hoellwarth ME. Comparison of two treatment eras and sonographic long-term outcome of blunt splenic injuries in children. Eur J Pediatr. 2013;172:1187–90.
155. Durkin N, Deganello A, Sellars ME, Sidhu PS, Davenport M, Makin E. Post-traumatic liver and splenic pseudoaneurysms in children: diagnosis, management, and follow-up screening using contrast enhanced ultrasound (CEUS). J Pediatr Surg. 2016;51:289–92.

156. Menaker J, Blumberg S, Wisner DH, Dayan PS, Tunik M, Garcia M, et al. Use of the focused assessment with sonography for trauma (FAST) examination and its impact on abdominal computed tomography use in hemodynamically stable children with blunt torso trauma. J Trauma Acute Care Surg. 2014;77:427–32.
157. Murphy R, Ghosh A. Towards evidence based emergency medicine: best BETs from the Manchester Royal Infirmary. The accuracy of abdominal ultrasound in paediatric trauma. Emerg Med J. 2001;18:208–9.
158. Scaife ER, Rollins MD, Barnhart DC, Downey EC, Black RE, Meyers RL, et al. The role of focused abdominal sonography for trauma (FAST) in pediatric trauma evaluation. J Pediatr Surg. 2013;48:1377–83.
159. Holmes JF, Gladman A, Chang CH. Performance of abdominal ultrasonography in pediatric blunt trauma patients: a meta-analysis. J Pediatr Surg. 2007;42:1588–94.
160. Zabolotny B, Hancock BJ, Postuma R, Wiseman N. Blunt splenic injuries in a Canadian pediatric population: the need for a management guideline. Can J Surg. 2002;45:358–62.
161. Stylianos S, Pearl R. Abdominal Trauma. In: Grosfeld JL, O'Neill J, Coran A, Fonkalsrud E, Caldamone A, editors. Pediatr Surg. 6th ed. Philadelphia: Mosby; 2006. p. 295–316.
162. Leinwand MJ, Atkinson CC, Mooney DP, Groner J, Lund D. Application of the APSA evidence-based guidelines for isolated liver or spleen injuries: a single institution experience. J Pediatr Surg. 2004;39:487–90.
163. Gutierrez IM, Zurakowski D, Chen Q, Mooney DP. Clinical practice guidelines (CPGs) reduce costs in the management of isolated splenic injuries at pediatric trauma centers. Langenbeck's Arch Surg. 2013;398:313–5.
164. Cloutier DR, Baird TB, Gormley P, McCarten KM, Bussey JG, Luks FI. Pediatric splenic injuries with a contrast blush: successful nonoperative management without angiography and embolization. J Pediatr Surg. 2004;39:969–71.
165. Al-Shanafey S, Giacomantonio M, Jackson R. Splenic injuries in children: correlation between imaging and clinical management. Pediatr Surg Int. 2001;17:365–8.
166. Ruess L, Sivit CJ, Eichelberger MR, Taylor GA, Bond SJ. Blunt hepatic and splenic trauma in children: correlation of a CT injury severity scale with clinical outcome. Pediatr Radiol. 1995;25:321–5.
167. Nance ML, Mahboubi S, Wickstrom M, Prendergast F, Stafford PW. Pattern of abdominal free fluid following isolated blunt spleen or liver injury in the pediatric patient. J Trauma. 2002;52:85–7.
168. Murphy EE, Murphy SG, Cipolle MD, Tinkoff GH. The pediatric trauma center and the inclusive trauma system: impact on splenectomy rates. J Trauma Acute Care Surg. 2015;78:930–4.
169. Sims CA, Wiebe DJ, Nance ML. Blunt solid organ injury: do adult and pediatric surgeons treat children differently? J Trauma. 2008;65:698–703.
170. Stylianos S, Egorova N, Guice KS, Arons RR, Oldham KT. Variation in treatment of pediatric spleen injury at trauma centers versus nontrauma centers: a call for dissemination of American Pediatric Surgical Association benchmarks and guidelines. J Am Coll Surg. 2006;202:247–51.
171. Mooney DP, Rothstein DH, Forbes PW. Variation in the management of pediatric splenic injuries in the United States. J Trauma Inj Infect Crit Care. 2006;61:330–3.
172. Mooney DP, Forbes PW. Variation in the management of pediatric splenic injuries in New England. J Trauma. 2004;56:328–33.
173. Todd SR, Arthur M, Newgard C, Hedges JR, Mullins RJ. Hospital factors associated with splenectomy for splenic injury: a national perspective. J Trauma. 2004;57:1065–71.
174. Holmes JH 4th, Wiebe DJ, Tataria M, Mattix KD, Mooney DP, Scaife ER, et al. The failure of nonoperative management in pediatric solid organ injury: a multi-institutional experience. J Trauma. 2005;59:1309–13.
175. Sharma OP, Oswanski MF, Singer D, Raj SS, Daoud YAH. Assessment of nonoperative management of blunt spleen and liver trauma. Am Surg. 2005;71:379–86.
176. Narci A, Solak O, Turhan-Haktanir N, Ayçiçek A, Demir Y, Ela Y, et al. The prognostic importance of trauma scoring systems in pediatric patients. Pediatr Surg Int. 2009;25:25–30.
177. Richards JR, McGahan JP, Jones CD, Zhan S, Gerscovich EO. Ultrasound detection of blunt splenic injury. Injury. 2001;32:95–103.
178. Tataria M, Nance ML, Holmes JH 4th, Miller CC 3rd, Mattix KD, Brown RL, et al. Pediatric blunt abdominal injury: age is irrelevant and delayed operation is not detrimental. J Trauma. 2007;63:608–14.
179. Gross JL, Woll NL, Hanson CA, Pohl C, Scorpio RJ, Kennedy AP Jr, et al. Embolization for pediatric blunt splenic injury is an alternative to splenectomy when observation fails. J Trauma Acute Care Surg. 2013;75:421–5.
180. Kiankhooy A, Sartorelli KH, Vane DW, Bhave AD. Angiographic embolization is safe and effective therapy for blunt abdominal solid organ injury in children. J Trauma. 2010;68:526–31.
181. Bansal S, Karrer FM, Hansen K, Partrick DA. Contrast blush in pediatric blunt splenic trauma does not warrant the routine use of angiography and embolization. Am J Surg. 2015;210:345–50.
182. Nance ML. Abdominal trauma. Fundam Pediatr Surg. New York: Springer New York; 2011. p. 135–43.
183. Yardeni D, Polley TZJ, Coran AG. Splenic artery embolization for post-traumatic splenic artery pseudoaneurysm in children. J Trauma. 2004;57:404–7.
184. Skattum J, Gaarder C, Naess PA. Splenic artery embolisation in children and adolescents—an 8 year experience. Injury. 2014;45:160–3.
185. Mayglothling JA, Haan JM, Scalea TM. Blunt splenic injuries in the adolescent trauma population: the role of angiography and embolization. J Emerg Med. 2011;41:21–8.
186. Schuster T, Leissner G. Selective angioembolization in blunt solid organ injury in children and adolescents: review of recent literature and own experiences. Eur J Pediatr Surg. 2013;23:454–63.
187. van der Vlies CH, Saltzherr TP, Wilde JCH, van Delden OM, de Haan RJ, Goslings JC. The failure rate of nonoperative management in children with splenic or liver injury with contrast blush on computed tomography: a systematic review. J Pediatr Surg. 2010;45:1044–9.
188. Ben-Ishay O, Gutierrez IM, Pennington EC, Mooney DP. Transarterial embolization in children with blunt splenic injury results in postembolization syndrome: a matched case-control study. J Trauma Acute Care Surg. 2012;73:1558–63.
189. Skattum J, Loekke RJV, Titze TL, Bechensteen AG, Aaberge IS, Osnes LT, et al. Preserved function after angioembolisation of splenic injury in children and adolescents: a case control study. Injury. 2014;45:156–9.
190. Schimmer JAG, Van Der Steeg AFW, Zuidema WP. Splenic function after angioembolization for splenic trauma in children and adults: a systematic review. Injury. 2016;47:525–30.
191. Akinkuolie AA, Lawal OO, Arowolo OA, Agbakwuru EA, Adesunkanmi ARK. Determinants of splenectomy in splenic injuries following blunt abdominal trauma. South African J Surg. 2010;48:15–9.
192. Polites SF, Zielinski MD, Zarroug AE, Wagie AE, Stylianos S, Habermann EB. Benchmarks for splenectomy in pediatric trauma: how are we doing? J Pediatr Surg. 2015;50:339–42.
193. Nwomeh BC, Nadler EP, Meza MP, Bron K, B a G, Ford HR. Contrast extravasation predicts the need for operative intervention in children with blunt splenic trauma. J Trauma. 2004;56:537–41.
194. Jen HC, Tillou A, Cryer HG, Shew SB. Disparity in management and long-term outcomes of pediatric splenic injury in California. Ann Surg. 2010;251:1162–6.
195. Mohamed AA, Mahran KM, Zaazou MM. Blunt abdominal trauma requiring laparotomy in polytraumatized patients. Saudi Med J. 2010;31:43–8.
196. Lo A, Matheson A-M, Adams D. Impact of concomitant trauma in the management of blunt splenic injuries. N Z Med J. 2004;117:U1052.
197. Resende V, Petroianu A. Functions of the splenic remnant after subtotal splenectomy for treatment of severe splenic injuries. Am J Surg. 2003;185:311–5.
198. Keller MS, Sartorelli KH, Vane DW. Associated head injury should not prevent nonoperative management of spleen or liver injury in children. J Trauma. 1996;41:471–5.
199. St Peter SD, Aguayo P, Juang D, Sharp SW, Snyder CL, Holcomb GW, et al. Follow up of prospective validation of an abbreviated bedrest protocol in the management of blunt spleen and liver injury in children. J Pediatr Surg. 2013;48:2437–41.
200. Minarik L, Slim M, Rachlin S, Brudnicki A. Diagnostic imaging in the follow-up of nonoperative management of splenic trauma in children. Pediatr Surg Int. 2002;18:429–31.
201. Huebner S, Reed MH. Analysis of the value of imaging as part of the follow-up of splenic injury in children. Pediatr Radiol. 2001;31(12):852–5.
202. Pachter HL, Guth AA, Hofstetter SR, Spencer FC. Changing patterns in the management of splenic trauma: the impact of nonoperative management. Ann Surg. 1998;227:708–9.
203. Moore HB, Vane DW. Long-term follow-up of children with nonoperative management of blunt splenic trauma. J Trauma. 2010;68:522–5.
204. Leone G, Pizzigallo E. Bacterial infections following splenectomy for malignant and nonmalignant hematologic diseases. Mediterr J Hematol Infect Dis. 2015;7

205. Skattum J, P a N, Gaarder C. Non-operative management and immune function after splenic injury. Br J Surg. 2012;99 Suppl 1:59–65.
206. Shatz DV. Vaccination practices among North American trauma surgeons in splenectomy for trauma. J Trauma. 2002;53:950–6.
207. Spelman D, Buttery J, Daley A, Isaacs D, Jennens I, Kakakios A, et al. Guidelines for the prevention of sepsis in asplenic and hyposplenic patients. Intern Med J. 2008;38:349–56.
208. Salvadori MI, Price VE. Preventing and treating infections in children with asplenia or hyposplenia. Paediatr Child Heal. 2014;19:271–4.
209. Programme Funded Pre Post Splenectomy, Immunisation Advisory Center. University of Auckland. Auckland, New Zealand http://www.immune.org.nz/sites/default/files/ProgrammeAsplenialmac20160331V01Final_0.pdf.
210. Shatz DV, Romero-Steiner S, Elie CM, Holder PF, Carlone GM. Antibody responses in postsplenectomy trauma patients receiving the 23-valent pneumococcal polysaccharide vaccine at 14 versus 28 days postoperatively. J Trauma. 2002;53:1037–42.
211. ACIP Vaccine Recommendations. Centers for disease control and prevention, recommended immunization schedules, 2016.

23

2018 WSES/SIS-E consensus conference: recommendations for the management of skin and soft-tissue infections

Massimo Sartelli[1*], Xavier Guirao[2], Timothy C. Hardcastle[3], Yoram Kluger[4], Marja. A. Boermeester[5], Kemal Raşa[6], Luca Ansaloni[7], Federico Coccolini[7], Philippe Montravers[8], Fikri M. Abu-Zidan[9], Michele Bartoletti[10], Matteo Bassetti[11], Offir Ben-Ishay[4], Walter L. Biffl[12], Osvaldo Chiara[13], Massimo Chiarugi[14], Raul Coimbra[15], Francesco Giuseppe De Rosa[16], Belinda De Simone[17], Salomone Di Saverio[18], Maddalena Giannella[10], George Gkiokas[19], Vladimir Khokha[20], Francesco M. Labricciosa[21], Ari Leppäniemi[22], Andrey Litvin[23], Ernest E. Moore[24], Ionut Negoi[25], Leonardo Pagani[26], Maddalena Peghin[11], Edoardo Picetti[27], Tadeja Pintar[28], Guntars Pupelis[29], Ines Rubio-Perez[30], Boris Sakakushev[31], Helmut Segovia-Lohse[32], Gabriele Sganga[33], Vishal Shelat[34], Michael Sugrue[35], Antonio Tarasconi[36], Cristian Tranà[1], Jan Ulrych[37], Pierluigi Viale[10] and Fausto Catena[33]

Abstract

Skin and soft-tissue infections (SSTIs) encompass a variety of pathological conditions that involve the skin and underlying subcutaneous tissue, fascia, or muscle, ranging from simple superficial infections to severe necrotizing infections. SSTIs are a frequent clinical problem in surgical departments. In order to clarify key issues in the management of SSTIs, a task force of experts met in Bertinoro, Italy, on June 28, 2018, for a specialist multidisciplinary consensus conference under the auspices of the World Society of Emergency Surgery (WSES) and the Surgical Infection Society Europe (SIS-E). The multifaceted nature of these infections has led to a collaboration among general and emergency surgeons, intensivists, and infectious disease specialists, who have shared these clinical practice recommendations.

Keywords: Soft-tissue infections, Necrotizing infection, Surgical site infection

Introduction

Skin and soft-tissue infections (SSTIs) encompass a variety of pathological conditions that involve the skin and underlying subcutaneous tissue, fascia, or muscle, ranging from simple superficial infections to severe necrotizing infections. SSTIs may affect any part of the body and are a frequent clinical problem in surgical departments [1, 2].

Successful management of patients with severe SSTIs involves prompt recognition, appropriate antibiotic therapy, timely surgical debridement or drainage, and resuscitation when required.

Several critical issues have been debated in the management of these patients. In order to clarify these major issues in the management of SSTIs, a panel of experts met in Bertinoro, Italy, on June 28, 2018, for a specialist multidisciplinary consensus conference under the auspices of the World Society of Emergency Surgery (WSES) and the Surgical Infection Society Europe (SIS-E).

During the consensus conference, 17 panelists presented the statements developed for each of the main questions regarding the diagnosis and management of SSTIs. An agreement on all the statements was reached.

The expert panel met via email to prepare and revise the consensus paper resulting from the meeting. The manuscript was successively reviewed by all members and ultimately revised as the present manuscript. This document represents the executive summary of the consensus conference which outlines clinical recommendations based on the

* Correspondence: massimosartelli@gmail.com
[1]Department of Surgery, Macerata Hospital, Macerata, Italy
Full list of author information is available at the end of the article

Grading of Recommendations Assessment, Development, and Evaluation (GRADE) hierarchy criteria summarized in Table 1 [3].

How should SSTIs be classified?

The term "skin and soft-tissue infections" describes a wide heterogeneity of clinical conditions. We recommend that the necrotizing or non-necrotizing character of the infection, the anatomical extension, the characteristics of the infection (purulent or not purulent), and the clinical condition of the patient should be always assessed independently to classify patients with soft-tissue infections (recommendation 1C).

SSTIs encompass a variety of pathological conditions involving the skin and underlying subcutaneous tissue, fascia, or muscle and ranging from simple superficial infections to severe necrotizing infections.

Various classification systems have been used to describe SSTIs including variables such as anatomic location, causative pathogen(s), rate of progression, depth of infection, and severity of clinical presentation.

In 1998, the US Food and Drug Administration (FDA) classified SSTIs into two broad categories for the purpose of clinical trials evaluating new antimicrobials for their treatment: uncomplicated and complicated. Uncomplicated SSTIs included superficial infections such as cellulitis, simple abscesses, impetigo, and furuncles and required antibiotics or surgical incision for drainage of abscess alone. In contrast, complicated SSTIs included deep soft-tissue infections such as necrotizing infections, infected ulcers, infected burns, and major abscesses which required significant surgical intervention with drainage and debridement [4].

The terms "complicated" and "uncomplicated" persist and can be useful in describing SSTIs as reported by Napolitano [5].

Uncomplicated SSTIs carry low risk for life- or limb-threatening infection unless they are improperly treated. Patients who have uncomplicated SSTIs can be treated with either empiric antibiotic therapy according to the most probable pathogen and local resistance patterns in impetigo, erysipelas, or mild cellulitis with drainage and debridement or simple surgical drainage in skin abscess.

Complicated SSTIs are associated with high risk for life-threatening infection. In patients who have complicated SSTIs, it is of paramount importance to initiate appropriate and adequate broad-spectrum initial empiric antibiotic therapy and to consider the need for surgical intervention for drainage and/or debridement.

In 2003, Eron et al. [6] classified SSTIs according to the severity of local and systemic signs and the presence or absence of comorbid conditions in patients presenting in the outpatient setting to guide the clinical management, treatment, and admission decisions. In this classification system, SSTIs were divided in four classes:

Class 1: patients with SSTI, but no signs or symptoms of systemic toxicity or co-morbidities.
Class 2: patients are either systemically unwell with stable co-morbidities or are systemically well, but have a comorbidity (e.g., diabetes, obesity) that may complicate or delay resolution.
Class 3: patients appear toxic and unwell (fever, tachycardia, tachypnoea, and/or hypotension).
Class 4: patients have sepsis syndrome and life-threatening infection; for example necrotizing fasciitis.

SSTIs may be also classified according to the anatomical tissue layers involved [7]. Superficial infections such as erysipelas, impetigo, folliculitis, furuncles, and carbuncles are located at the epidermal and dermal layer, while cellulitis is located in the dermis and subcutaneous tissue. Deep infections extend below the dermis and may involve the subcutaneous tissue, fascial planes, or muscular compartments presenting as complex abscesses, fasciitis, or myonecrosis.

Complicated SSTIs may also be classified as non-necrotizing or necrotizing infections. Necrotizing infections most commonly involve the muscular fascial layers but may also involve the dermal, subcutaneous, and muscle layers and warrant prompt, aggressive surgical debridement.

In 2014, the Infectious Diseases Society of America (IDSA) updated practice guidelines for the diagnosis and management of skin and soft-tissue infections [8]. The guidelines divided infections by purulent and non-purulent, severity (mild, moderate, and severe), and tissue necrosis (necrotizing versus non-necrotizing).

Recently, the US FDA has introduced the new definition of acute bacterial skin and skin-structure infection (ABSSSI) to more closely define complicated soft-tissue infection for the purposes of registration trials. ABSSSIs include cellulitis/erysipelas, wound infections, and major cutaneous abscesses. Thus, an ABSSSI is defined as a bacterial infection of the skin with a lesion size area of $\geq 75\ cm^2$ (lesion size measured by the area of redness, edema, or induration) [9].

In 2015, the WSES published its guidelines for management of SSTIs [10] proposing a new definition dividing SSTIs in three main groups: surgical site infections (SSIs), non-necrotizing SSTIs, and necrotizing SSTIs. SSIs are classified into two subgroups: incisional and organ and organ/space. The incisional SSIs are further divided into superficial (skin and subcutaneous tissue) and deep (deep soft-tissue muscle and fascia). Organ and organ/space infections are not truly soft-tissue infections. Non-necrotizing SSTIs including erysipelas,

Table 1 Grading of Recommendations Assessment, Development and Evaluation (GRADE) hierarchy of evidence from Guyatt et al. [3]

Grade of recommendation	Clarity of risk/benefit	Quality of supporting evidence	Implications
1A			
Strong recommendation, high-quality evidence	Benefits clearly outweigh risk and burdens, or vice versa	RCTs without important limitations or overwhelming evidence from observational studies	Strong recommendation, applies to most patients in most circumstances without reservation
1B			
Strong recommendation, moderate-quality evidence	Benefits clearly outweigh risk and burdens, or vice versa	RCTs with important limitations (inconsistent results, methodological flaws, indirect analyses, or imprecise conclusions) or exceptionally strong evidence from observational studies	Strong recommendation, applies to most patients in most circumstances without reservation
1C			
Strong recommendation, low-quality or very low-quality evidence	Benefits clearly outweigh risk and burdens, or vice versa	Observational studies or case series	Strong recommendation but subject to change when higher quality evidence becomes available
2A			
Weak recommendation, high-quality evidence	Benefits closely balanced with risks and burden	RCTs without important limitations or overwhelming evidence from observational studies	Weak recommendation, best action may differ depending on the patient, treatment circumstances, or social values
2B			
Weak recommendation, moderate-quality evidence	Benefits closely balanced with risks and burden	RCTs with important limitations (inconsistent results, methodological flaws, indirect, or imprecise) or exceptionally strong evidence from observational studies	Weak recommendation, best action may differ depending on the patient, treatment circumstances, or social values
2C			
Weak recommendation, low-quality or very low-quality evidence	Uncertainty in the estimates of benefits, risks, and burden; benefits, risk, and burden may be closely balanced	Observational studies or case series	Very weak recommendation; alternative treatments may be equally reasonable and merit consideration

impetigo, folliculitis, simple abscess, and complex abscess may be treated by antibiotics or drainage alone.

Necrotizing SSTIs (cellulitis, fasciitis, myositis, Fournier's gangrene) require surgical intervention including drainage and debridement of necrotic tissue in addition to antibiotic therapy.

Several authors and organizations have proposed classification schemes for SSTIs based on such variables as anatomic location, rate of progression, depth of extension, and clinical presentation or severity. Each has key limitations both in assisting clinical management and in providing guidance for developing new therapeutic agents.

The consensus concluded that the necrotizing or non-necrotizing character of the infection, the anatomical extension, the characteristics of the infection (purulent or non-purulent), and the clinical conditions of the patient should be always assessed independently to classify patients with soft-tissue infections.

What is new in the prevention of SSIs? What are the principles of SSI prevention?

Recent global guidelines for the prevention of SSIs can support healthcare workers to develop or strengthen infection prevention and control programs, with a focus on surgical safety, as well as antimicrobial resistance action plans. We recommend that all healthcare workers adopt these evidence-based recommendations in their clinical practice (recommendation 1C).

SSIs are the most common healthcare-associated infections among surgical patients. It is obviously important to improve patient safety by reducing the occurrence of SSIs. Preventing SSIs is a global priority. Bacteria are becoming increasingly resistant to antibiotics, making SSI prevention even more important nowadays.

SSIs are a major clinical problem in terms of morbidity, mortality, length of hospital stay, and overall direct and not-direct costs worldwide. Despite progress in prevention knowledge, SSIs remain one of the most common adverse events in hospitals. SSI prevention is complex and requires the integration of a range of measures before, during, and after surgery.

Both the World Health Organization (WHO) [11, 12] and the Centers for Disease Control and Prevention (CDC) [13] have recently published guidelines for the prevention of SSIs. The 2016 WHO Global guidelines for the prevention of surgical site infection [11, 12] are evidence-based including systematic reviews presenting additional information in support of actions to improve practice.

The guidelines include 13 recommendations for the pre-operative period, and 16 for preventing infections during and after surgery. They range from simple precautions such as ensuring that patients bathe or shower before surgery, appropriate way for surgical teams to clean their hands, guidance on when to use prophylactic antibiotics, which disinfectants to use before incision, and which sutures to use.

The proposed recommendations are as follows:

- "Strong" – Expert panel was confident that benefits outweighed risks, considered to be adaptable for implementation in most (if not all) situations, and patients should receive intervention as course of action.
- "Conditional" – Expert panel considered that benefits of intervention probably outweighed the risks; a more structured decision-making process should be undertaken, based on stakeholder consultation and involvement of patients and healthcare professionals.

Importantly, the guidelines recommend that antibiotic prophylaxis should be used to prevent infections before and during surgery only. Antibiotics should not be used after surgery, as is often done. Antibiotic prophylaxis should be administered for operative procedures that have a high rate of postoperative surgical site infection, or when foreign materials are implanted. Antibiotic prophylaxis should be administered within 120 min prior to the incision. However, administration of the first dose of antibiotics is dependent on its pharmacological characteristics. Underlying patient factors may also affect drug disposition (e.g., malnourishment, obesity, cachexia, and renal disease with protein loss may result in suboptimal antibiotic exposure through increased antibiotic clearance in the presence of normal or augmented renal function). Additional antibiotic doses should be administered intraoperatively for procedures > 2–4 h (typically where duration exceeds two half-lives of the antibiotic). There is no evidence to support the use of postoperative antibiotic prophylaxis. The key evidence-based recommendations outlined in these guidelines should be adopted by all healthcare staff that care for surgical patients throughout all stages of that patient's surgical care.

What is the best treatment of incisional SSIs? When are antibiotics needed?

Incisional SSIs require prompt and wide opening of the surgical incision. We recommend antibiotic therapy for incisional SSIs with any Systemic Inflammatory Response Syndrome criteria or signs of organ failure such as hypotension, oliguria, decreased mental alertness, or in immunocompromised patients (recommendation 1C).

SSIs are generally classified according to CDC criteria [14]. SSIs are classified as superficial incisional infection, deep incisional infection, and organ space infection. Superficial incisional infections are the most common type of SSIs. Deep incisional and organ/space are the types of SSIs that cause the most morbidity. Organ space infections are not genuine soft-tissue infections.

Incisional SSIs are the results of several factors [15]. All surgical wounds are contaminated by bacteria, but only a minority actually develops clinical infection. Colonization occurs when the bacteria begin to replicate and adhere to the wound site. If the host's immune response is not sufficient to eliminate or overcome the effects of the bacteria, infection occurs [16]. In most patients, infection does not develop because host defenses are efficient to eliminate colonizers at the surgical site; however, in some patients, host defenses fail to protect them from SSIs. It is well known that surgical trauma increases inflammatory response and counter-regulatory mechanisms. Such regulatory mechanism can decrease postoperative immune response, promoting SSIs.

The pathogens isolated from infections differ, primarily depending on the type of surgical procedure. In clean-contaminated or contaminated surgical procedures, the aerobic and anaerobic pathogens of the normal endogenous microflora of the surgically resected organ are the most frequently isolated pathogens. In clean surgical procedures, in which the gastrointestinal, gynecologic, and respiratory tracts have not been entered, *Staphylococcus aureus* from the exogenous environment or the patient's skin flora is the usual cause of infection. Nevertheless, in some specific body areas such as the groin skin could also be colonized by enteric flora. Moreover, it is possible that procedures such as hip prosthesis or vascular bypass, performed on this anatomical region, might eventually be infected by Gram-negative bacteria.

Sganga et al. [17] have recently reported that the risk factors associated with SSIs caused by *Methicillin-resistant Staphylococcus aureus* (MRSA), identified using the Delphi method were patients from long-stay care facilities, a hospitalization within the preceding 30 days, Charlson score > 5 points, chronic obstructive pulmonary disease and thoracic surgery, antibiotic therapy with beta-lactams (especially cephalosporins), and carbapenems and/or quinolones in the preceding 30 days, age 75 years or older, current duration of hospitalization > 16 days, and surgery with prosthesis implantation.

An important determinant of SSI is the integrity of host defenses. Important host factors include the following [18]: age, malnutrition status, diabetes, smoking, obesity, colonization with microorganisms, length of hospital stay or previous hospitalization, shock and hypoxemia, and hypothermia.

It is a common practice to cover surgical wounds with a dressing. The dressing acts as a physical barrier to protect the wound from contamination from the external environment until the wound becomes impermeable to microorganisms.

Postoperative care bundles recommend that surgical dressings be kept undisturbed for a minimum of 48 h after surgery unless leakage occurs. However, there are currently no specific recommendations or guidelines regarding the type of surgical dressing [19].

The diagnosis of incisional surgical site infection is clinical. Symptoms may include localized erythema, induration, warmth, and pain at the incision site. Purulent wound drainage and separation of the wound may occur. Most patients have systemic signs of infection such as fever and leukocytosis. Information on the microbiological species present in the wound is useful for determining antibiotic choice and predicting response to treatment.

An incisional SSI should be sampled if there is a clinical suspicion of infection. Lack of standardized criteria for diagnostic microbiology of SSIs present a challenge to monitor the global epidemiology of surgical site infection. Emergence of antibiotic resistance has made the management of SSIs difficult. Moreover, rapidly emerging nosocomial pathogens and the problem of multidrug resistance necessitates periodic review of isolation patterns and their sensitivity.

Adequate treatment of incisional SSIs should always include:

- Surgical incision and drainage of abscess.
- Debridement of necrotic tissue, if present.
- Appropriate wound care.
- Resuscitation to improve perfusion when sepsis is present.
- Adequate empiric antibiotic therapy when indicated.
- De-escalation when antibiogram is available.

Incisional SSIs should always be drained, irrigated, and if needed, opened and debrided. If fascial disruption is suspected, drainage should always be performed. Percutaneous drainage, wound irrigation, and negative pressure-assisted wound management are new and effective options that reduce the need for open management of wound infections. In cases where open management is needed, once the infection has cleared, the wound can be closed.

Superficial incisional SSIs that have been opened can usually be managed without antibiotics.

In patients with incisional SSIs with the presence of any systemic inflammatory response criteria or signs of organ failure such as hypotension, oliguria, decreased mental alertness, or in immunocompromised patients, empiric broad-spectrum antibiotic treatment should be started with coverage for Gram-positive cocci and/or the expected flora at the site of operation. Definitive antibiotic treatment is guided by the clinical response of the patient and, when available, results of gram stain, wound culture, and antibiogram.

What is the appropriate treatment of superficial infections (impetigo, erysipelas and cellulitis, and superficial abscesses)?

We recommend that impetigo, erysipelas, and cellulitis should be managed by antibiotics against Gram-positive bacteria (recommendation 1C).

Empiric therapy for community-acquired MRSA (CA-MRSA) should be recommended for patients at risk for CA-MRSA or who do not respond to first line therapy (recommendation 1C).

Incision and drainage is the primary treatment for simple abscesses or boils. We recommend not to use antibiotics for simple abscesses or boils (recommendation 1C).

Superficial infections encompass either superficial spreading infection and inflammation within the epidermis and dermis that may be treated with antibiotics alone or a well-circumscribed abscess that may be treated by drainage alone.

Physical examination usually reveals erythema, tenderness, and induration. The majority of superficial SSTIs are caused by Gram-positive bacteria, particularly streptococci and *S. aureus*. The three common presentations of superficial infections consist of impetigo, erysipelas, and cellulitis. They are managed by antibiotic therapy against Gram-positive bacteria.

Impetigo is a highly contagious bacterial infection of the superficial layers of the epidermis. Impetigo predominantly affects children, and it is one of the most common SSTI in children worldwide [20]. It is characterized by discrete purulent lesions nearly always caused by β-hemolytic *Streptococcus* spp. and/or *S. aureus*. Moreover, of particular concern is the rising role of CA-MRSA as impetigo's etiological agent [21–23].

Erysipelas is a fiery red, tender, painful plaque with well-demarcated edges and is commonly caused by streptococcal species, usually *Staphylococcus pyogenes. S. aureus* rarely causes erysipelas [24]. Streptococci are the primary cause of erysipelas. Most facial infections are attributed to group A *Streptococcus* (GAS), with an increasing percentage of lower extremity infections being caused by non-GAS. The role of *S. aureus*, and specifically MRSA, remains controversial [25].

Cellulitis is an acute bacterial infection of the dermis and the subcutaneous tissue that most commonly affects the lower extremities, although it can affect other areas. It causes local signs of inflammation, such as warmth, erythema, pain, lymphangitis, and frequently systemic upset with fever and raised white blood cell count [26]. As already reported in a previous paragraph, cellulitis has been recently classified as an ABSSSI together with erysipelas, SSIs, and major abscesses.

In a large European multicenter study, Garau et al. [27] analyzed a population of patients diagnosed with complicated SSTI hospitalized between December 2010 and January 2011 reporting that cellulitis was the most frequent diagnosis accounting for 59.1% of the total. Streptococci cause diffuse, rapidly spreading infection; staphylococcal cellulitis is typically more localized.

Treatment should begin promptly with agents effective against the typical Gram-positive pathogens, especially streptococci. If the cellulitis is very early and mild and no significant co-morbidities are present, oral beta-lactams might be sufficient in areas where CA-MRSA is not prevalent. Other available options are macrolides and lincosamides; however, resistance to erythromycin and clindamycin are increasing. Fluoroquinolones have been approved for the treatment of most uncomplicated cellulitis but are not adequate for treatment of MRSA infections. For more severe infections, parenteral route is the first choice.

If MRSA is suspected (both hospital acquired MRSA [HA-MRSA] and CA-MRSA), glycopeptides and newer antimicrobials are the best options [25, 28, 29]. For a simple superficial abscess or boil, incision and drainage is the primary treatment, and antibiotics are not needed. To be considered a simple abscess, induration and erythema should be limited only to a defined area of the abscess and should not extend beyond its borders. Additionally, simple abscesses do not extend into deeper tissues or have multiloculated extension. Cutaneous abscesses are typically caused by bacteria that represent the normal regional skin flora of the involved area [30].

What is the appropriate treatment of complex abscesses (perianal and perirectal, and abscesses in intravenous drug injection sites)?

Complex skin and subcutaneous abscesses are typically well circumscribed and respond to incision and drainage. We recommend antibiotic therapy if systemic signs of infection are present, in immunocompromised patients, if source control is incomplete or in cases of abscess with significant cellulitis (recommendation 1C).

We recommend empiric broad-spectrum antibiotic therapy with coverage of Gram-positive, Gram-negative, and anaerobic bacteria (recommendation 1C).

Common sites of origin of complex abscesses may be perineal or perianal, perirectal, and abscesses at intravenous drug injection sites. Complicated skin and subcutaneous abscesses are typically well circumscribed and respond to incision and drainage with adjuvant antibiotic therapy.

Perianal and perirectal abscesses originate most often from an obstructed anal crypt gland, with the resultant pus collecting in the subcutaneous tissue, intersphincteric plane, or beyond (ischiorectal space or supralevator space) where various types of anorectal abscesses form. Once diagnosed, anorectal abscesses should be promptly drained surgically. An undrained anorectal abscess can continue to expand into adjacent spaces as well as progress to generalized systemic infection. Anorectal abscess occurs more often in males than females. Most patients present between the ages of 20 to 60 with the mean age of 40 in both sexes [31].

The diagnosis of anorectal abscess is usually based on the patient's history and physical examination. The most common symptom of anorectal abscess is pain. As such, it has to be differentiated from other causes of anal pain including anal fissure, thrombosed hemorrhoids, levator spasm, sexually transmitted diseases, proctitis, and cancer. Low (intersphincteric, perianal, and ischiorectal) abscesses are usually associated with swelling, cellulites, and exquisite tenderness, but few systemic symptoms. High (submucosal, supralevator) abscesses may have few local symptoms, but significant systemic symptoms. Deeper abscesses, such as those that form in the supralevator or high ischiorectal space, may also present with pain referred to the perineum, low back, or buttocks.

The goal of surgical therapy of an abscess is to drain the abscess expeditiously, identify a fistula tract, and either proceed with primary fistulotomy to prevent recurrence or place a draining seton for future consideration.

A large abscess should be drained with multiple counter incisions rather than a long incision, which will create a step-off deformity and delay wound healing.

Complicated abscesses may involve a variety of pathogens and are frequently polymicrobial in origin.

Although most cases can be managed by incision and drainage, abscesses in injecting drug users require special considerations as compared to soft-tissue infections, which are not caused by intravenous drug abuse [32–35]. There are two main sources of organisms: the injecting drug users themselves (their oropharynx, skin, or feces), and the environment. Contamination may occur when the user prepares or injects the drug, uses shared needles, or re-uses injection paraphernalia. Manufacturing and handling of injectable drugs may be far from hygienic rules [36]. Persistent signs of systemic infection require evaluation for the presence of endocarditis. Foreign bodies, such as broken needles, should be ruled out by radiography, and duplex sonography should be performed to identify the presence of vascular complications [37]. Viral (HIV, HCV, HBV) acute or chronic infections should be always ruled out. Broad-spectrum antibiotics effective against aerobic and anaerobic organisms should be administered in patients with these infections. Broad-spectrum agents with coverage of Gram-positive, Gram-negative, and anaerobic pathogens may be required depending on the clinical setting. Given the high frequency of MRSA in some areas, this pathogen should be empirically covered if it is suspected, but no randomized studies are available for the treatment of SSTI specifically caused by CA-MRSA [1].

What is the appropriate treatment of infections developing in damaged skin (burn wounds, animal and human bites, and pressure ulcers)?

Irrigation of the wound and debridement of necrotic tissue are the most important factors in the prevention of infection and can substantially decrease the incidence of invasive wound infection. Antibiotic prophylaxis is not generally recommended (recommendation 1C).

For patients with systemic signs of infection, compromised immune status, severe comorbidities, associated severe cellulitis, severe and deep wounds, a broad-spectrum antibiotic effective against aerobic, and anaerobic organisms is always required (recommendation 1C).

Infections developing in damaged skin are a heterogeneous group that includes bite wounds (animal and human bites), burn wounds, and pressure ulcers. If managed incorrectly, these infections can develop into more complicated soft-tissue infections.

Soft-tissue infection is the most common complication of animal and human bites. The risk of infection depends on the type of bite, the site of injury, the time elapsed from the bite until presentation, host factors, and the management of the wound [38–40]. In general, 10–20% of bite wounds become infected, including 30–50% of cat bites, 5–25% of dog bites, and 20–25% of human bites, respectively [41].

The predominant pathogens in these wounds are part of the normal oral flora of the biting animal, along with human skin organisms and occasional secondary invaders (e.g., *S. aureus* and GAS). Along with *Staphylococcus* ssp. (including MRSA) and *Streptococcus* ssp. (including *S. pyogenes*), the commonly isolated pathogens include *Pasteurella* spp. (*Pasteurella multocida*, *Pasteurella canis*, *Pasteurella dagmatis*), *Capnocytophagia canimorsus*, anaerobes (*Fusobacterium* spp., *Prevotella* spp., *Bacteroides* spp., *Porphyromonas* spp.), and others. Streptococci can be isolated from 50% of human bite wounds, *S. aureus* from 40%, and *Eikenella corrodens* (a Gram-negative facultative anaerobic bacillus) from 30%. Human bites can transmit HBV, HCV, and

HIV and post-exposure prophylaxis should be considered in every case [25].

There is clinical consensus that patients may be divided into low- and high-risk groups depending on the cause, nature, and location of the injury and on patient characteristics, but no evidence-based guidelines are currently available.

Deep irrigation of the wound serves to remove foreign bodies and pathogens. Irrigation under pressure is not recommended, as it may lead to the uncontrolled spread of bacteria into deeper tissue layers. Surgical treatment is based on the removal of necrotic tissue and mechanical reduction of the burden of pathogens. Universal prophylaxis with antibiotics is not recommended. The comprehensive meta-analyses of Medeiros et al. in the Cochrane Database [42] demonstrated no evidential basis for a reduction of the infection rate by prophylactic antibiotics, except for bite wounds on the hands. Despite the poor state of the evidence, most experts recommend early antibiotic treatment for 3 to 5 days for fresh, deep wounds and wounds in certain critical bodily areas (hands, feet, areas near joints, face, genitals), for persons at elevated risk of infection, and for persons with implants, such as artificial heart valves [43–45]. Antibiotics should not be given if the patient presents 24 h or more after the bite and there are no clinical signs of infection [46].

Significant burn injuries can predispose to infectious complications. Burn wound infections are one of the most important and potentially serious complications that occur in the acute period following injury. Accurate management of the wound with early excision of the eschar can substantially decrease the incidence of invasive burn wound infection. Damage to this barrier following a burn disrupts the innate immune system and increases susceptibility to bacterial infection. Although burn wound surfaces are sterile immediately following thermal injury, these wounds may be colonized with microorganisms. If the patient's host defenses and therapeutic measures (such as excision of necrotic tissue and wound medications) are inadequate, microorganisms can colonize viable tissue, and a burn wound infection may occur.

Burn wound infections usually are polymicrobial. They can be immediately colonized by Gram-positive bacteria from the patient's endogenous skin flora or the external environment. However, they can also be rapidly colonized by Gram-negative bacteria, usually within a week of the burn injury. Bacterial cultures can aid in the selection of an appropriate antibiotic, especially in cases of bacterial drug resistance, but altered pharmacokinetic parameters in burn patients must be considered and dosing should be adjusted accordingly to maximize antibiotic efficacy [47].

Pressure ulcers are localized areas of tissue necrosis that tend to develop when soft-tissue is compressed between a bony prominence and an external surface for a prolonged period of time. The damage may be relatively minor, or it may lead to massive destruction of deeper tissues. The majority of pressure ulcers develop in areas adjacent to the ischium, sacrum, and greater trochanter. Pressure ulcers represent a frequent problem especially in frail elderly patients with chronic co-morbidities [25]. When infection occurs, it is typically polymicrobial and includes aerobes (*S. aureus*, *Enterococcus* spp., *Proteus mirabilis*, *Escherichia coli*, *Pseudomonas* spp.) and anaerobes (*Peptococcus* spp., *Bacteroides fragilis*, *Clostridium perfringens*) [25].

Combination of surgical and antibiotic interventions may be required to manage infected decubitus ulcers. Surgical debridement is necessary to remove necrotic tissue. Antibiotic therapy should be used for patients with severe pressure ulcer infections, including those with spreading cellulitis or patients with systemic signs of infection. Because such infections usually are polymicrobial, therapeutic regimens should be directed against both Gram-positive and Gram-negative facultative organisms as well as anaerobic organisms. In many cases of pressure ulcers, correct wound care management can largely prevent the occurrence of these infections.

When to administer antibiotics for MRSA in cSSTI?

We recommend to administer antibiotics directed against MRSA as an adjunct to incision and drainage based on local epidemiology (area with more than 20% of MRSA in invasive hospital isolates or high circulation of MRSA in the community), specific risk factors for MRSA, and clinical conditions (recommendation 1C).

The majority of SSTIs involving healthy skin are caused by aerobic Gram-positive cocci, specifically *S. aureus* and streptococci. Strains of *S. aureus* and GAS can produce a variety of toxins that may both potentiate their virulence and affect the soft tissues and allow invasion of the dermis. SSTIs management has recently become more complicated because of the increasing prevalence of multidrug-resistant pathogens.

Considerable variation in the resistance rates of *S. aureus* to methicillin (or oxacillin) in patients with SSTIs has been noted between continents, with the highest rates in North America (35.9%), followed by Latin America (29.4%) and Europe (22.8%) [48]. Although MRSA has been usually acquired during exposure in hospitals and other healthcare facilities, there has been a recent increase in MRSA infections presenting in the community (CA-MRSA) [49]. CA-MRSA strains are genetically and phenotypically distinct from HA-MRSA. CA-MRSA infections are becoming increasingly common.

They can have a rapid and devastating course and may produce the pathogenic Panton–Valentine leucocidin toxin (PVL), which destroys white blood cells and is an important virulence factor [50]. They may be susceptible to a wider range of anti-staphylococcal antibiotics (some are resistant only to beta-lactams). Populations at increased risk for CA-MRSA are listed below [49]:

- Children < 2 years old.
- Athletes (mainly contact-sport participants).
- Injection drug users.
- Homosexual males.
- Military personnel.
- Inmates of correctional facilities, residential homes, or shelters.
- Vets, pet owners, and pig farmers.
- Patients with post-flu-like illness and/or severe pneumonia.
- Patients with concurrent SSTI.
- History of colonization or recent infection with CA-MRSA.
- History of antibiotic consumption in the previous year, particularly quinolones, or macrolides.

MRSA poses a significant and enduring problem to the treatment of infection by such strains. Resistance is usually conferred by the acquisition of a non-native gene encoding a penicillin-binding protein (PBP2a), with significantly lower affinity for beta-lactams. This resistance allows cell-wall biosynthesis, the target of beta-lactams, to continue even in the presence of typically inhibitory concentrations of antibiotic. PBP2a is encoded by the *mecA* gene, which is carried on a distinct mobile genetic element (SCC*mec*). These genetic elements contain two required components: the *mec* gene complex and the *ccr* gene complex (which contains site-specific recombinase genes). The SCC *mec* elements have been classified into eight types (I–VIII) based on the structure and combination of *mec* and *ccr* gene complexes present. These elements also differ in what other antimicrobial resistance genes are carried on them. Types I, IV, V, VI, and VII generally do not carry other resistance genes. Types II, III, and VIII may contain one or more other resistance genes, such as *ermA* (erythromycin), *aadD* (tobramycin), and *tetK* (tetracycline). These types are also used to help distinguish CA-MRSA and HA-MRSA strains. Most HA-MRSA strains carry SCC *mec* types I, II, III, VI, and VIII; while most CA-MRSA strains carry types IV, with some carrying types V and VII [51]. If MRSA is suspected (both HA and CA-MRSA), glycopeptides and other antimicrobial options are available agents. Also, new options such as dalbavancin and tedizolid also can be administered.

What oral antibiotics can be used for the management of MRSA skin and soft-tissue infections (SSTIs)? What intravenous antibiotics can be used for the management of MRSA skin and soft-tissue infections?

For oral antibiotic coverage of MRSA in patients with SSTI, we suggest the following agents: linezolid (recommendation 1A), trimethoprim-sulfamethoxazole (TMP-SMX) (recommendation 1B), a tetracycline (doxycycline or minocycline) (recommendation 1B), or tedizolid (Recommendation 1A).

For intravenous (IV) antibiotic coverage of MRSA in patients with SSTI, we suggest the following agents: daptomycin (10 mg/kg/dose IV once daily) (recommendation 1A), IV linezolid (recommendation 1A), IV ceftaroline (recommendation 1A), IV dalbavancin (recommendation 1A), IV vancomycin (recommendation 1A), IV tigecycline (recommendation 1A), or IV tedizolid (recommendation 1A).

Seven to 14 days of therapy is recommended but should be individualized on the basis of the patient's clinical response (recommendation 1A). IV to oral switch should occur when criteria of clinical stability have been reached (recommendation 1C).

For CA-MRSA, recommended oral agents are clindamycin, although clindamycin resistance is now very common [52], tetracyclines, TMP-SMX, linezolid, tedizolid, and occasionally, fluoroquinolones. Several observational studies and one small randomized trial [53, 54] suggest that TMP-SMX, doxycycline, and minocycline are effective for such infections. If coverage for both streptococci and MRSA is desired for oral therapy, options include clindamycin alone, or the combination of either TMP-SMX or doxycycline with a beta-lactam (e.g., penicillin, cephalexin, or amoxicillin).

Glycopeptides have been for many years the microbiological agents of choice used in complicated Gram-positive infections. Fortunately, staphylococcal resistance to glycopeptides remains rare, although rising minimal inhibitory concentrations (MICs) of glycopeptides may affect the efficacy of these antibiotics [55, 56].

Increased resistance to glycopeptides has encouraged the development of new agents active against Gram-positive bacteria, particularly for severe soft-tissue infections where aggressive antimicrobial management is always recommended, such as linezolid and daptomycin. Linezolid has been considered an agent of choice in complicated skin and soft-tissue infections (cSSTIs). It has the advantages of early intravenous-to-oral switch with the oral preparation having very high bioavailability and excellent tissue penetration [57].

In 2010, an open-label study compared oral or intravenous linezolid with intravenous vancomycin for treatment of cSSTIs caused by MRSA [58]. Patients receiving linezolid had a significantly shorter length of stay and duration of intravenous therapy than those receiving vancomycin. Both agents were well tolerated. Adverse events were similar to each drug's established safety profile [58].

Recently, a Cochrane meta-analysis included all randomized controlled trials comparing linezolid with vancomycin in the treatment of SSTIs [59]. Linezolid was associated with a significantly better clinical (risk ratio [RR] = 1.09, 95% CI, 1.03–1.16) and microbiological cure rate in adults (RR = 1.08; 95% CI, 1.01–1.16). For infections caused by MRSA, linezolid was significantly more effective than vancomycin in clinical (RR = 1.09; 95% CI, 1.03–1.17) and microbiological cure rates (RR = 1.17; 95% CI, 1.04–1.32).

The daily cost of outpatient therapy was less with oral linezolid than with intravenous vancomycin. Although inpatient treatment with linezolid cost more than inpatient treatment with vancomycin per day, the median length of hospital stay was 3 days shorter with linezolid.

Daptomycin has proven efficacy in patients with Gram-positive complicated ©SSTIs, including those caused by *S. aureus* resistant to methicillin [60]. Daptomycin has been shown to achieve very good concentrations in the skin and soft tissues. In 2010, a meta-analysis compared effectiveness and toxicity of daptomycin with that of other antimicrobials for the treatment of SSTIs. Four studies were included in the analysis (three were randomized RCTs). Vancomycin and semisynthetic penicillins were used in the comparator arm. Three studies reported on patients with cSSTIs. Daptomycin tissue penetration supports its use in the treatment of cSSTIs, and it has been shown to be non-inferior to vancomycin and semisynthetic penicillins [61].

Ceftaroline is an oxyimino advanced-generation broad-spectrum cephalosporin which has in vitro activity against *S. aureus* and MRSA, both of which are associated with cSSTIs. Ceftaroline fosamil has been found to be effective in the treatment of cSSTI when compared with vancomycin plus aztreonam for the treatment of cSSTI [62–64]. Ceftaroline fosamil was also well tolerated and had a safety profile concordant with other antibiotics in the cephalosporin class.

More recently, new drugs have been approved for ABSSSI and have an important activity against MRSA, especially dalbavancin and tedizolid. Tedizolid, a novel oxazolidinone with Gram-positive activity including MRSA, is promising because it can be administered daily in oral or intravenous forms [65, 66], and dalbavancin, a second-generation lipoglycopeptide that covers MRSA, can be administered as infrequently as once weekly [67, 68].

Antibiotics recommended for MRSA infections are listed below.

Oral options:

- Minocycline100 mg q12h
- Trimethoprim and sulfamethoxazole 160/800 mg q12h
- Doxycycline 100 mg q12h
- Clindamycin 300–600 mg q8h (high resistance rate)
- Linezolid 600 mg q12h
- Tedizolid 200 mg q24 h

Intravenous options:

- Vancomycin 15 mg/kg IV q12h
- Teicoplanin LD 12 mg/kg IV q12h for 3 doses, then 6 mg/kg q12h
- Tigecycline 100 mg IV as a single dose, then 50 mg IV q12h
- Linezolid 600 mg q12h
- Daptomycin 4–6 mg/kg q24h
- Ceftaroline 600 mg q12h
- Dalbavancin 1000 mg once followed by 500 mg after 1 week or 1500 mg one dose
- Tedizolid 200 mg q24h

The decision to use intravenous or oral agents has been debated. Currently, oral therapy is recommended for mild infections and intravenous therapy for severe infections. Moderate infections may be treated via the oral route, or with one to two intravenous doses and then transitioning to oral therapy. For patients with severe infections who are able to tolerate oral therapy and in whom clinical improvement has been documented, the goal should be to transition to the oral route as soon as possible. There is evidence to suggest that this approach positively impacts length of stay as well [69].

What are necrotizing infections?

Necrotizing soft-tissue infections (NSTIs) are life-threatening, invasive, soft-tissue infections with a necrotizing component involving any or all layers of the soft-tissue compartment, from the superficial dermis and subcutaneous tissue to the deeper fascia and muscle. The latter is most commonly called "necrotizing fasciitis" [70].

The necrotizing or non-necrotizing character of the infection should be always specified when classifying patients with soft-tissue infections (recommendation 1C).

Delay in diagnosis and delay in treatment of these infections increase the risk of mortality. Because of its aggressive character, NSTIs should always be differentiated from non-necrotizing infection. Several definitions were published over the last few years, and all these definitions can be confusing. NSTIs are defined by the presence of a spreading infection in any of the layers of the soft tissues (skin, subcutaneous tissue, superficial fascia, deep fascia, or muscles) which is associated with the presence of necrosis of the layer(s) involved and hence requires surgical debridement. All NSTIs fulfill this definition and have common features in their clinical presentation and diagnosis, and most importantly, all of these infections by definition require surgical debridement. Therefore, labeling them with different terms does not serve a useful purpose and may in fact complicate management by delaying diagnosis and/or delaying surgical debridement [7, 8, 10].

How can necrotizing infections be classified?

Patients with NSTIs should be classified into the following:

- **High risk of poor outcome.**
- **Mild/moderate risk of poor outcome.**

Scores used for severity assessment of patients with necrotizing infections may be useful in the emergency room or outside the intensive care unit (ICU) and may identify patients early, who require surgical treatment and perioperative intensive care management (recommendation 1C).

Several classifications of NSTIs have been proposed; however, none are universally accepted. Necrotizing infections have been described according to their anatomical locations (i.e., Fournier gangrene) and the depth of infections: dermal and subcutaneous components (necrotizing cellulitis), fascial component (necrotizing fasciitis), and muscular components (necrotizing myositis). NSTIs may also be classified into three types defined by the bacterial pathogens initiating the infection and their typical clinical characteristics: type 1—polymicrobial, type 2—mono-microbial pathogenic β-hemolytic streptococci or CA-MRSA, and type 3—mono-microbial secondary to a variety of pathogenic bacilli. However, resolution of these nomenclature issues requires a consensus among international infectious disease physicians, surgeons, and intensivists, and probably, these various methods of classification are not clinically useful. Although many specific variations of NSTIs have been described, the initial approach to diagnosis, antimicrobial treatment, and surgical intervention is similar for all forms and identifying those infections needing immediate aggressive management is more important than determining the specific variant.

Delay in diagnosis and/or treatment of NSTIs correlates with a poor outcome, leading to multiple organ failure. Early prognostic evaluation of NSTIs is crucial to assess the severity and decide the aggressiveness of treatment. Necrotizing infections remain an important source of patient morbidity and are frequently associated with poor clinical prognosis. Any process of improving quality of care for necrotizing infections globally should focus on simple diagnostic criteria based on physical examination findings and recognition of patients needing timely critical care.

A classification of patients based on a severity assessment which could identify cases requiring surgical and critical care may be an important tool both in ICU and outside of the ICU. The Laboratory Risk Indicator for Necrotizing Fasciitis (LRINEC) score first published in 2004 [71] is based on routinely performed parameters and offers a method to identify NSTIs at early stage. With a score of 8 or higher, there is a 75% risk of a NSTI.

A systematic review of English-language literature from 2004 to 2014 to identify articles reporting use of LRINEC score and the incidence of necrotizing fasciitis was recently published [72]. After application of inclusion criteria, 16 studies with 846 patients were included. The authors concluded that the LRINEC score is a useful clinical determinant in the diagnosis and surgical treatment of patients with necrotizing fasciitis, with a statistically positive correlation between LRINEC score and a true diagnosis of necrotizing fasciitis. A second meta-analysis including English-language studies reporting the diagnostic accuracy of LRINEC score was recently published [73]. Twenty-three studies ($n = 5982$) were included. LRINEC ≥ 6 had sensitivity of 68.2% and specificity of 84.8%, while LRINEC ≥ 8 had sensitivity of 40.8% and specificity of 94.9%. The authors concluded that due to poor sensitivity, LRINEC should not be used to rule-out NSTIs.

In the setting of such aggressive infections, a feasible, low-cost method of rapidly identifying patients requiring critical care is crucial [74]. Early warning system scores utilize physiological, easy-to-measure parameters, assessing physiological parameters such as systolic blood pressure, pulse rate, respiratory rate, temperature, oxygen saturation, and level of consciousness. They are simple, non-invasive, and easy-to-repeat measurement at the bedside.

The Sepsis-3 definitions [75] suggest that patients with at least two of these three clinical variables may be prone for the poor outcome typical of sepsis: (1) low blood pressure (systolic blood pressure ≤ 100 mmHg), (2) high respiratory rate (≥ 22 breaths per minute), or (3) altered mentation (Glasgow coma scale < 15) (quick SOFA [qSOFA]). It is supposed to be useful in out-of-hospital, emergency surgery, or general hospital ward settings, and in patients with positive qSOFA, organ dysfunction should be investigated. The qSOFA score should not be regarded as a diagnostic criterion for defining sepsis. Rather, it should be regarded as a warning for patients with suspected infection who are likely to have poor outcomes. In the setting of patients with necrotizing infections, it may be useful as a warning for patient's severity assessment.

Is a multidisciplinary approach to necrotizing infections mandatory?

A multidisciplinary team is mandatory for the management of NSTIs. Depending on the time line, various specialties are involved. Specific attention should be given to the long-term management of these patients (recommendation 1C).

NSTIs rank among one of the more difficult disease processes encountered by physicians. The most critical factors for reducing mortality in NSTIs are early recognition and urgent operative debridement. Initial treatment of patients with necrotizing infections should always require coordination between the surgeons, intensivists, and infectious disease specialist. Treatment consists of radical debridement associated with broad-spectrum antimicrobial therapy and hemodynamic support.

Moreover, the magnitude of necrotic tissues that need to be radically debrided, although required to save the patient's life, often create unique and difficult challenges in terms of wound care, preservation of function, reconstruction, and cosmesis. These problems require time and a multidisciplinary approach. After an extended hospitalization, multiple dressing changes, and surgical procedures, the survivor of NSTI faces months of continued physical therapy to regain functional independence, whenever possible. Rehabilitation is an essential and integral component of recovery [76].

What is the pathophysiology of necrotizing infections

Due to the rapid progression of the inflammatory process, early treatment of necrotizing infection is always recommended (recommendation 1C).

There are two main ways by which bacteria can invade soft tissues. The most common way is through a break in the skin barrier. In case of contamination by spores of *C. perfringens*, the anaerobic environment (caused by impairment of the blood supply resulting in tissue hypoxia) is necessary for maturation and proliferation of *Clostridium* strains [77]. The second way is hematogenous spread of bacteria to the tissue; however, it is a rare condition. Local and systemic manifestations are related to specific pathophysiologic mechanisms depending upon the toxins and enzymes of involved bacteria.

Bacteria proliferate and release toxins, which cause local tissue damage and impair inflammatory responses. Some toxins produce thrombosis of larger venules and arterioles, with subsequent ischemic necrosis of all tissue layers, from the dermis to the deep muscles [77]. Systemic manifestations are also related to toxin-mediated pathophysiologic mechanisms and include fever, hypotension, tachycardia, altered mental status, and signs of organ dysfunction. In principle, these mechanisms may involve both host and pathogen factors. Host-related factors are determined by human genes that control release of cytokines and encode pro-inflammatory cytokines eliciting subsequent counter-regulatory mechanisms. Microbial virulence factors include Gram-positive and Gram-negative bacterial products. These toxins are absorbed in the bloodstream. Bacterial superantigens (pyrogenic exotoxins) directly stimulate and non-specifically activate high numbers of T cells and macrophages to produce pro-inflammatory mediators such as TNF-α, IL-1, and IL-6. The massive release of these cytokines produces an uncontrolled systemic inflammatory response that can lead to multisystem organ dysfunction and shock [77].

How can necrotizing infections be diagnosed?

Clinical signs of NSTI include pain out of proportion, edema extending beyond the erythema, and fever. A rapidly progressive soft-tissue infection should always be suspected as a necrotizing infection (recommendation 1C).

The initial differential diagnosis between a cellulitis and a necrotizing infection that requires prompt operative intervention may be difficult. Most cases of NSTI are initially diagnosed and begin as cellulitis. However, since time to operative debridement is an important determinant of outcome in necrotizing infections, timely diagnosis is essential.

Patients with NSTI usually present with severe pain which is out of proportion to the physical findings [78–82].

Typical local signs are as follows:

- Edema
- Erythema
- Severe and crescendo pain out of proportion
- Skin bullae or necrosis (at later stage)
- Swelling or tenderness
- Crepitus

Systemic signs are as follows:

- Fever
- Tachycardia
- Hypotension
- Shock

Laboratory tests are not highly sensitive or specific for NSTIs. A rapidly progressive soft-tissue infection should be treated as a necrotizing infection, from the beginning. The clinical picture may worsen very quickly, sometimes during a few hours.

In order to predict the presence of NSTI, the Laboratory Risk Indicator for Necrotizing infection (LRINEC) score was proposed [71]. LRINEC score assigns points for abnormalities in six independent variables: serum C-reactive protein level (> 150 mg/L), white blood cell (WBC) count (> 15,000/μL), hemoglobin level (< 13.5 g/dL), serum sodium level (< 135 mmol/L), serum creatinine level (> 1.6 mg/dL [142 mmol/l]), and serum glucose level (> 180 mg/dL [10 mmol/l]). With a score of 8 or higher, there is a 75% risk of a NSTI.

Subsequent evaluation of the LRINEC score has demonstrated conflicting results. Several studies have assessed the utility of LRINEC for the early diagnosis of necrotizing infections [72, 83–88].

Recent evidence has demonstrated that it lacks the sensitivity to be a useful adjunct for the diagnosis of necrotizing infections [73].

The diagnosis of necrotizing infection is primarily a clinical diagnosis. However, radiologic imaging may be able to provide useful information when the diagnosis is uncertain. A plain X-ray should not be used to rule-out necrotizing infection (recommendation 1B).

In unstable patients, ultrasound may be useful to differentiate simple cellulitis from necrotizing fasciitis (recommendation 2C).

Imaging studies should not delay surgical consultation and intervention (recommendation 1A).

Frequently, plain radiographs are normal or with increased soft-tissue thickness and opacity, unless the infection and necrosis are advanced. The characteristic finding is gas in the soft tissues, but subcutaneous gas is present only in few cases of necrotizing infection and is not present in pure aerobic infections such as those caused by *S. pyogenes*.

Additionally, subcutaneous gas may not be present in earlier stages of the disease process and only become manifest as the patient's condition deteriorates [89, 90].

Computed tomography (CT) has a higher sensitivity than plain radiography in identifying early NSTIs. Findings consistent with necrotizing infections are fat stranding, fluid and gas collections that dissect along fascial planes, and gas in the involved soft tissues. Additionally, fascial thickening and non-enhancing fascia on contrast CT suggests fascial necrosis [91].

In 2010, a case series study [92] analyzing the use of CT scanning for the diagnosis of NSTIs was published. Of 67 patients with study inclusion criteria, 58 underwent surgical exploration, and NSTIs was confirmed in 25 (43%). The remaining 42 patients had either non-necrotizing infections during surgical exploration ($n = 33$) or were treated non-operatively with successful resolution of the symptoms ($n = 9$). The sensitivity of CT to identify NSTI was 100%, specificity was 81%, positive predictive value was 76%, and negative predictive value was 100%.

Magnetic resonance imaging (MRI) has been the imaging modality of choice for necrotizing fasciitis. Patients with necrotizing fasciitis usually have a significantly greater frequency of the following MRI findings: thick (≥ 3 mm) abnormal signal intensity on fat-suppressed T2-weighted images, low signal intensity in the deep fascia on fat-suppressed T2-weighted images, a focal or diffuse non-enhancing portion in the area of abnormal signal intensity in the deep fascia, extensive involvement of the deep fascia, and involvement of three or more compartments in one extremity [93]. However, MRI may be difficult to perform under emergency conditions and is not recommended as the first-choice imaging technique.

Ultrasound has the advantage of being rapidly performed at bedside and may be helpful in differentiating simple cellulitis from necrotizing fasciitis. In a prospective observational study of 62 patients with clinically suspected necrotizing fasciitis, ultrasound had a sensitivity of 88.2%, specificity of 93.3%, positive predictive value of 95.4%, negative predictive value of 95.4%, and diagnostic accuracy of 91.9%. The authors considered the findings of diffuse subcutaneous thickening accompanied by fluid accumulation of > 4 mm in depth along the deep fascial layer predictive of necrotizing fasciitis [94].

Rapid performance of frozen-section soft-tissue biopsy, early in the evolution of a suspect lesion, may provide a definitive and life-saving diagnosis. Triple diagnostics which include an incisional biopsy over the most suspected area, a fresh frozen section and Gram staining might be an important adjunct in early stages of suspected necrotizing infections (recommendation 1C).

Early frozen-section diagnosis should be limited to those cases in which the clinical or radiographic findings are not diagnostic (recommendation 1C).

Fascial biopsy with frozen section has been suggested as a means to achieve earlier diagnosis of NSTIs [95, 96]. However, frozen-section biopsy is not very practical and requires availability and experience of the pathologists, and the time taken to carry out and analyze the sample could be used for debridement [97]. The Finger test is another adjunct method described for diagnosing NSTIs. It is performed under local anesthesia. A 2-cm incision is made down to the deep fascia. Minimal tissue resistance to finger dissection (positive Finger test), the absence of bleeding, presence of necrotic tissue, and/or murky and grayish ("dishwater") fluid following incision, all suggest the diagnosis of NSTI [98].

What is the best timing of source control?

Provide (surgical) source control in patients with NSSTI as soon as possible, but at least within the first 12 h after admission, in patients with a high suspicion for necrotizing infection. Early source control,

antimicrobial therapy, and (organ) supportive measures are the cornerstone of treatment in patients with sepsis or septic shock caused by NSSTI (recommendation 1B).

Source control for SSTIs includes drainage of infected fluids, debridement of infected soft tissues, and removal of infected devices or foreign bodies. It should also include definitive measures to correct any anatomic derangement resulting in ongoing microbial contamination and restoring optimal function. Early surgical debridement with complete removal of necrotic tissue is essential to decrease mortality and other complications in patients with NSTIs. It is the most important determinant of outcome in necrotizing infections. This was well described in a study by Bilton et al. in which patients with NSTIs, who had adequate surgical debridement (early and complete), were compared to those with either delayed or incomplete debridements. The mortality in the latter group was 38% compared to 4.2% in the group receiving early adequate surgical treatment [99].

Delay in source control in patients with NSTIs has been repeatedly associated with a greater mortality. A retrospective study including 47 patients with the diagnosis of NSTI admitted to a large academic hospital from December 2004 to December 2010 was published in 2011 [100]. Overall mortality was 17.0%. The average number of surgical debridements in patients with surgical treatment delayed > 12 h from the time of emergency department admission was significantly higher than those who had an operation within 12 h after admission (7.4 ± 2.5 versus 2.3 ± 1.2; $p < 0.001$). Delayed surgical debridement was associated with significantly higher mortality, higher incidence of septic shock and renal failure, and more surgical debridements than patients with early surgical debridements. After adjusting for possible confounding factors, the average number of surgical debridements and the presence of septic shock and acute renal failure were still significantly higher in patients in whom surgery was delayed > 12 h.

A retrospective study including 106 patients with necrotizing infections conducted in a medical ICU was published in 2009 [101]. Overall hospital mortality was 40.6%. In multivariate analysis, underlying cardiovascular disease, SAPS II, abdomino-perineal compared to limb localization, time from the first signs to diagnosis < 72 h, and time from diagnosis to surgical treatment > 14 h in patients with septic shock were independently associated with hospital mortality.

A retrospective study of 121 patients (mean age, 65.2 ± 11.6 years) with *Vibrio vulnificus*-related necrotizing infection who underwent surgical intervention between July 1998 and June 2011 was published in 2011 [102]. The patients were divided into three groups according to the time between admission and surgical treatment as follows: surgical treatment less than 12 h after admission, 12 to 24 h after admission, and more than 24 h after admission. Patients who underwent surgery less than 12 h after admission had a significantly lower mortality compared with those who had surgery either 12 to 24 h after admission (adjusted hazard ratio [HR], 0.064; 95% CI, 1.6×10^{-7} to 0.25; $p = 0.037$) or more than 24 h after admission (adjusted HR, 0.0043; 95% CI, 2.1×10^{-5} to 0.0085; $p = 0.002$). There was no difference in mortality risk between patients who underwent surgery 12 to 24 h after admission and those who had surgery more than 24 h after admission ($p = 0.8$).

We suggest to remove only devitalized/infarcted skin and spare normally perfused skin. In case where skin viability is questionable, skin preservation and reassessment at the second operation is indicated (recommendation 1C).

Once the decision to take the patient for an operation has been made, the initial incision is done in the compromised area and the wound is explored for macroscopic findings of NSTIs. Incision should take place along the involved muscular lodges. Removal of all non-viable tissue should be accomplished including muscle, fascial layers, subcutaneous tissue, and skin if they are compromised, and one should extend the incision until healthy viable tissue is seen. Removal of previously viable skin or muscle should usually not be done at the initial operation, attempting skin sparing via multiple incisions (to preserve perforators), while accounting for underlying bone, nerve, and vascular structures. Skin perfusion and viability can easily be assessed at re-exploration, and removal at that time is easy, if indicated. The wound should always be left open. Amputation of a limb does not add to the acute debridement and should be reserved for late and extreme presentations.

What is the best timing of re-exploration?

Consider to plan the first re-exploration within 12–24 h and to repeat re-exploration(s) until the patient is free of necrosis (recommendation 1C).

There is a lack of literature examining outcomes in necrotizing infections when surgical re-debridements are performed in early versus delayed intervals. Scheduled re-explorations should be done at least every 12–24 h after the initial operation or sooner if clinical local or systemic signs of worsening infection become evident, as well as with worsening laboratory parameters (particularly WBC count). Re-explorations should be repeated until the time when very little or no debridement is required.

A prospective observational study by Okoye et al. [103] showed that delayed re-debridement after initial source control in necrotizing infections results in worse survival and an increased incidence of acute kidney injury. The authors concluded that further studies to identify the optimal time interval for re-debridement are warranted.

What is the role of hyperbaric oxygen therapy (HBO) for source control in necrotizing infections?

Consider adjuvant hyperbaric oxygen therapy in patients with NSTI after prompt debridement (recommendation 2B).

Despite significant advancements in critical care management as well as improved knowledge regarding NSTIs, mortality remains relatively high. Adjunctive and less conventional treatment options have been explored in an effort to improve outcomes in this group of patients. Hyperbaric oxygen (HBO) is one of these modalities. It is a medical treatment that uses delivery of 100% oxygen at a pressure of 2–3 absolute atmospheres. Its use is motivated by the fact that oxygen delivery at these parameters achieves a much higher concentration of dissolved oxygen in blood which results in higher tissue oxygen tensions. At this higher tissue tension, beneficial effects may be seen including improved leukocyte function, inhibition of anaerobic growth, inhibition of toxin production, and enhancement of antibiotic activity.

The role of HBO as an adjunctive treatment has been debated, and no prospective randomized clinical trials have been published. In order to determine the effect of hyperbaric oxygen HBO therapy on mortality, complication rate, discharge status/location, hospital length of stay, and inflation-adjusted hospitalization cost in patients with NSTIs, a retrospective study of 45,913 patients in the Nationwide Inpatient Sample from 1988 to 2009 was published in 2012 [104]. This retrospective analysis of HBO therapy in NSTI showed that despite the higher hospitalization cost and longer length of stay, the statistically significant reduction in mortality supports the use of HBO therapy in NSTI (RR = 0.47; 95% CI, 0.30–0.74). In 2013, a review about HBO therapy for treating acute surgical and traumatic wounds was published [105]. The authors concluded that there is a lack of high-quality, valid research evidence regarding the effects of HBO therapy on wound healing.

HBO could be useful, if available, but it should not interfere with the standard treatment. Furthermore, the patient should not be transferred to carry out HBO therapy, thereby delaying standard care.

What is the role of intravenous immunoglobulin (IVIG) therapy for source control in necrotizing infections?

Consider intravenous immunoglobulin (IVIG) therapy in patients with necrotizing infections caused by GAS (recommendation 2B).

Intravenous immunoglobulin therapy has been postulated to improve outcomes in a selected population of patients with NSTIs. Most of the reported studies evaluated its use for invasive GAS infections including GAS-related NSTIs with streptococcal toxic shock syndrome (STSS).

The efficacy and safety of high-dose IVIG as adjunctive therapy in STSS were evaluated in a multicenter, randomized, double-blind, placebo-controlled trial [106]. The trial was prematurely terminated because of slow patient recruitment, and results were obtained from 21 enrolled patients (10 IVIG recipients and 11 placebo recipients). The primary end point was mortality at 28 days, and a 3.6-fold non-significant higher mortality rate was found in the placebo group. A significant decrease in the sepsis-related organ failure assessment score at days 2 ($p = 0.02$) and 3 ($p = 0.04$) was noted in the IVIG group. Furthermore, a significant increase in plasma neutralizing activity against superantigens expressed by autologous isolates was noted in the IVIG group after treatment ($p = 0.03$). Although statistical significance was not reached in the primary end point, the trial provides some supportive evidence for IVIG as an efficacious adjunctive therapy in STSS. IVIG therapy role in improving survival in STSS was also demonstrated in other prospective studies [107, 108].

In 2017, a retrospective study of adult patients with necrotizing fasciitis and vasopressor-dependent shock undergoing surgical debridement from 2010 to 2014 in 130 US hospitals was published [109]. Of 4127 cases of debrided necrotizing infection with shock at 121 centers, only 164 patients (4%) at 61 centers received IVIG. IVIG subjects were younger with lower comorbidity indices, but higher illness severity. Clindamycin and vasopressor intensity were higher among IVIG cases, as was coding for TSS and GAS. In-hospital mortality did not differ between matched IVIG and non-IVIG groups (crude mortality, 27.3 versus 23.6%; adjusted HR, 1.00 [95% CI, 0.55–1.83]; $p = 0.99$). Early IVIG (≤ 2 days) did not alter this effect ($p = 0.99$). Among patients coded for TSS, GAS, and/or *S. aureus*, IVIG use was still unusual (6.8%) and lacked benefit ($p = 0.63$). Median LOS was similar between IVIG and non-IVIG groups (26 [13–49] versus 26 [11–43]; $p = 0.84$).

Recently, a Cochrane review on intervention for NSTIs was published [110]. One trial of 100 randomized participants assessed IVIG as an adjuvant drug, given at a dose of 25 g/day, compared with placebo, given for three consecutive days. No clear difference between IVIG and placebo in terms of mortality within 30 days (RR = 1.17; 95% CI, 0.42–3.23), nor serious adverse events experienced in the ICU (RR = 0.73; 95% CI, 0.32–1.65) were observed.

What are the resuscitation principles in patients with necrotizing infection?

Supportive treatment in managing necrotizing infections must be early and aggressive to halt progression of the inflammatory process (recommendation 1A).

Early detection of sepsis and prompt aggressive treatment of the underlying organ dysfunction is an essential component for improving outcomes of critical ill patients [111]. Necrotizing infections may present with a fulminant course and may be associated with great morbidity and high case-fatality rates, especially when they occur in conjunction with TSS.

Early blood cultures, empirical antibiotic treatment, and intensive care for hemodynamic and metabolic support should be performed as soon as possible. Moreover, patients may lose fluids, proteins, and electrolytes through a large surgical wound [112]. In addition, hypotension is caused by vasodilation induced by the systemic inflammatory response syndrome to infection [113]. Fluid resuscitation and analgesia are the mainstays of support for patients with advanced sepsis usually combined with vasoactive amines associated with mechanical ventilation and other organ function supports, if needed. No ideal fluid exists: resuscitation therapy must be prompt and immediate as in any type of shock.

What are the new agents to treat necrotizing infections

AB103 (Reltecimod) is a new agent for modulation of inflammation after necrotizing infections. Further study is warranted to establish efficacy (no recommendation).

AB103 (Reltecimod) is a safe and promising new agent for modulation of inflammation after a necrotizing infections. However, further studies are warranted to establish efficacy.

AB103 (originally p2TA) is a novel synthetic CD28 mimetic octapeptide that selectively inhibits the direct binding of superantigen exotoxins to the CD28 costimulatory receptor on T-helper 1 lymphocytes [114].

Preclinical studies demonstrated that AB103 and related superantigen mimetic peptides are associated with improved survival in animal models of toxic shock and sepsis. The hypothesis is that AB103 could be administered safely in patients presenting with NSTI and would modulate the immune response to reduce the development or progression of organ failure.

To establish the safety of AB103 in patients with NSTI and evaluate the potential effects on clinically meaningful parameters related to the disease [115], a prospective, randomized, placebo-controlled, double-blinded study was performed in six academic medical centers in the USA. Participants included adults with NSTI. Of 345 patients screened, 43 were enrolled for the intent-to-treat analysis, and 40 met criteria for the modified intent-to-treat analysis; 15 patients each were included in the high-dose and low-dose treatment arms, and 10 in the placebo arm. Baseline characteristics were comparable in the treatment groups. The Sequential Organ Failure Assessment score improved from baseline in both treatment groups compared with the placebo group at 14 days (change from baseline score, − 2.8 in the high-dose, − 2 in the low-dose, and + 1.3 in the placebo groups; $p = 0.04$). AB103-treated patients had a similar number of debridements (mean [SD], 2.2[1.1] for the high-dose, 2.3[1.2] for the low-dose, and 2.8 [2.1] for the placebo groups; $p = 0.56$). There were no statistically significant differences in ICU-free and ventilator-free days or in plasma and tissue cytokine levels. No drug-related adverse events were detected. A phase 3 trial, also known as the ACCUTE trial (Reltecimod Clinical Composite Endpoint Study in Necrotizing Soft Tissue Infections), has been designed as a single pivotal study to assess the efficacy and safety of Reltecimod versus placebo in patients with necrotizing infections.

What antibiotics are recommended for empiric treatment of clinically suspected necrotizing infections?

Antibiotic treatment of necrotizing infections should be prompt and aggressive (recommendation 1B).

The initial empirical antibiotic regimen should comprise broad-spectrum drugs including anti-MRSA and anti-Gram-negative coverage (recommendation 1C).

Vancomycin treatment should be avoided in patients with renal impairment and when MRSA isolate shows a MIC for vancomycin ≥ 1.5 mg/mL (recommendation 1B).

Daptomycin or linezolid are drugs of choice for empirical anti-MRSA coverage. Alternatively, ceftaroline, telavancin, tedizolid, and dalbavacin can be used (recommendation 2C).

The choice of anti-Gram-negative treatment should be based on local prevalence of ESBL-producing *Enterobacateriaceae* and multidrug-resistant organisms (MDROs) non-fermenters (recommendation 1B).

De-escalation of antibiotic therapy should be based on clinical improvement, cultured pathogens, and results of rapid diagnostic tests where available (recommendation 1C).

Microbiologically, NSTIs have been classified as either type 1 (polymicrobial) or type 2 (mono-microbial) or type 3 (gas gangrene). Occasionally in immunocompromised patients, NSTIs may be also caused by mycotic species.

NSTIs type I is a polymicrobial infection involving aerobic and anaerobic organisms. It is usually seen in the elderly or in those with underlying illnesses [77]. Type I infection is often associated with gas in the tissue and thus is difficult to distinguish from gas gangrene. Non-clostridial anaerobic cellulitis and synergistic necrotizing cellulitis are type I variants. Both occur in patients with diabetes and typically involve the feet, with rapid extension into the leg.

NSTI type II is a mono-microbial infection. Among Gram-positive organisms, GAS remains the most common pathogen, followed by MRSA. Unlike type I infections, type II infections may occur in any age group and in persons without any underlying illness. Other pathogens include *Aeromonas hydrophila* and *V. vulnificus*. Mono-microbial necrotizing fasciitis due to Gram-negative pathogens (bacteroides and *E. coli*) have also been reported, though these infections are typically seen in immunocompromised, diabetic, obese, and postoperative patients [77].

Gas gangrene (clostridial myonecrosis), or type III NSTI, is an acute infection by clostridium or bacillus of healthy living tissue that occurs spontaneously or as a result of traumatic injury. Recurrent gas gangrene, occurring several decades after the primary infection, has also been described.

The use of antimicrobial therapy is an adjuvant treatment and must be combined with early surgical debridement. Once the diagnosis is made and blood cultures have been drawn, broad-spectrum coverage should be urgently commenced. Initial antibiotic therapy for necrotizing infections is empirical in nature because microbiological data (culture and susceptibility results) may require > 24 h before they are available for a more detailed analysis.

Since it is impossible to exclude with certainty a polymicrobial necrotizing infection, an aggressive broad-spectrum empiric antimicrobial therapy should initially be selected to cover Gram-positive, Gram-negative, and anaerobic organisms until culture-specific results and sensitivities are available. An acceptable empiric antibiotic regimen should always include antibiotics, which cover MRSA with the additional benefit of inhibiting invasive GAS virulence proteins. For the treatment of MRSA, we refer to the previous paragraphs.

For the treatment of Gram-negative bacteria, the use of piperacillin-tazobactam in the setting without high local prevalence of ESBL-producing *Enterobacateriaceae* optimizing pharmacokinetic/pharmacodynamic parameters is appropriate. Carbapenems, administered in adequate dosage, including meropenem, imipenem-cilastatin, or doripenem may be used in the settings with high local prevalence of ESBL-producing *Enterobacateriaceae*. Culture-specific results and sensitivities can direct both broadening of antimicrobial regimen if it is too narrow and a de-escalation if it is too broad particularly in critically ill patients where de-escalation strategy is one of the cornerstones of antimicrobial stewardship programs [116]. The choice of anti-Gram-negative treatment should be based on local prevalence of ESBL-producing *Enterobacateriaceae* and MDRO non-fermenters.

Should an antitoxin active drug (clindamycin or oxazolidinon) be included in the empirical regiment of clinically suspected necrotizing infection?

Either clindamycin or linezolid should be included in the empirical antibiotic regimen of NSTI (recommendation 1C).

Selection of antibiotics that inhibit toxin production may be helpful, particularly in those patients who have evidence of TSS, potentially present in patients who have streptococcal and staphylococcal infections. Protein cytotoxins play an important role in the pathogenesis of various staphylococcal infections, and toxin production should be considered when selecting an antimicrobial agent for Gram-positive pathogens. Linezolid and clindamycin play an important role because they may significantly inhibit exotoxin production from Gram-positive pathogens [117–119].

What is the optimal duration of antibiotic therapy for necrotizing infections?

In the absence of definitive clinical trials, antibiotic therapy should be administered until further debridement is no longer necessary, the patient has improved clinically, and fever has resolved for 48–72 h (recommendation 1C).

Procalcitonin monitoring may be useful to guide antimicrobial discontinuation (recommendation 2B).

There is no direct evidence about optimal duration of antibiotic therapy, and the expert panel shares that antimicrobial therapy should be administered until further debridement is no longer necessary, the patient has improved clinically, and fever has been resolved for 48–72 h.

Several controlled clinical studies have evaluated the potential of the infection biomarker procalcitonin (PCT) to improve the diagnostic work-up of patients with bacterial infections and its influence on decisions regarding antibiotic therapy [120].

In order to develop a PCT ratio indicating successful surgical intervention in patients with necrotizing infections, Friederichs et al. [121] designed a study of 38 patients treated with clinical signs of sepsis caused by a NSTI. All patients received radical surgical treatment. Serum levels of PCT and C-reactive protein were monitored postoperatively. The ratio of day 1 to day 2 was calculated. An eradication of the infectious focus was successfully performed in 84% of patients, averaging 1.9

operations (range 1–6) to achieve the elimination of the infectious source. The PCT ratio was significantly higher in the group of patients with successful surgical intervention (1.665 versus 0.9, $p < 0.001$). A ratio higher than the calculated cutoff of 1.14 indicated successful surgical treatment with a sensitivity of 83.3% and a specificity of 71.4%. The positive predictive value was 75.8%, and the negative predictive value was 80.0%.

The PCT ratio of postoperative day 1 to day 2 following major surgical procedures for necrotizing infections represented a valuable clinical tool indicating successful surgical eradication of the infectious focus and correlated with the successful elimination of the infectious source and clinical recovery.

What is the treatment of Fournier's gangrene?

Treatment of Fournier's gangrene includes prompt appropriate antibiotic therapy, hemodynamic support, and early debridement (recommendation 1C).

Early and extensive initial surgical debridement in Fournier's gangrene patients improves survival (recommendation 1C).

We suggest consideration for fecal diversion—either by colostomy, fecal tube system with or without negative pressure therapy—in cases of Fournier's gangrene with fecal contamination (recommendation 2C).

Fournier's gangrene (FG) is a severe type of NSTI involving the genital area and or perineum. It was initially described by Baurinne in 1764 and is named after Jean Alfred Fournier, a French dermatologist who in 1883 described it. Due to the complexity of fascial planes, the infection may extend up to the abdominal wall, down into the thigh areas, into the perirectal and gluteal spaces, and, occasionally, into the retroperitoneum. Advanced FG can extend through the fascial planes ascending as high as the torso and descending to the thighs. The perineal fascia, Colles' fascia, is continuous with Scarpa's fascia of the anterior abdominal wall and Buck and Dartos' fascia of the penis and scrotum. Testicular involvement is rare, and this has been attributed to their non-perineal blood supply. It has a mortality rate that approaches 20–50% in many contemporary series [122–124]. The origin of the infection is identifiable in the majority of cases and is predominantly from anorectal, genito-urinary, or local cutaneous sources [125]. The aggressive nature of the infection requires early recognition and immediate surgical intervention.

Diagnosis is based on clinical signs and physical examination. Including cutaneous manifestations, erythema, subcutaneous crepitations, patches of gangrene, a presence of potential portal of entry, foul smell, purulence and/or wound discharge, and tenderness to palpitation. Imaging, including conventional radiology, US, CT, and MRI may be used to confirm clinical suspicions and to help in identifying the extent of the soft-tissue involvement, particularly in the perirectal and retroperitoneal planes.

Fournier's Gangrene Severity Index (FGSI) is a standard score for predicting outcome in patients with FG and is obtained from a combination of physiological parameters at admission including temperature, heart rate, respiration rate, sodium, potassium, creatinine, leukocytes, hematocrit, and bicarbonate. A FGSI score above 9 has been demonstrated to be sensitive and specific as a mortality predictor in patients with Fournier's gangrene [126, 127].

Surgical debridement must be early and aggressive to halt progression of infection. Cultures of infected fluid and tissues should be obtained during the initial surgical debridement and the results used to tailor specific antibiotic management. Radical surgical debridement of the entire affected area should be performed, continuing the debridement into the healthy-looking tissue [128, 129].

In the setting of FG, diverting colostomy has been demonstrated to improve outcomes. It helps in decreasing sepsis by minimizing bacterial load in the perineal wound, thus controlling infection [130]. Diverting colostomy does not eliminate the necessity of multiple debridements, nor reduces the number of these procedures [131]. Diverting colostomy should be avoided as much as possible mainly when there are other methods to avoid wound contamination. Recently, rectal diversion devices have been marketed. They are silicone tubes designed to divert fecal matter in patients with diarrhea, local burns, or skin ulcers. The devices protect the wounds from fecal contamination and reduce, in the same way a colostomy does, both the risk of skin breakdown and repeated inoculation with colonic microbial flora. Fecal diversion tubes can be used in combination with negative pressure wound therapy (NPWT) for effective isolation of the wound from fecal contamination. Estrada et al. showed that this was an effective way for fecal diversion and constitutes an attractive alternative to colostomy [132].

What is the role of negative pressure wound therapy in soft-tissue infections and necrotizing fasciitis?

We suggest to consider negative pressure wound therapy (NPWT) for wound care after complete removal of necrosis in necrotizing infections (recommendation 1C).

The rapidly spreading infection followed by aggressive surgical intervention and repeated debridements creates challenges for wound management. NPWT refers to wound dressing systems that continuously or intermittently apply sub-atmospheric pressure to the surface of a wound. NPWT has become a popular treatment modality for the management of many acute and chronic wounds. Sub-atmospheric pressure has multiple beneficial effects on wound healing in animal models. Animal and human studies have shown that sub-atmospheric pressure improves the local wound environment through both direct and indirect effects; these effects accelerate healing and reduce the time to wound closure [133].

In the setting of necrotizing infections once the necrosis is removed, NPWT can help wound healing physiologically. The negative pressure leads to an increased blood supply, increasing tissue perfusion, reducing edema, absorbing fluids and exudates, inhibiting infection, and finally drying the wound and thus the migration of inflammatory cells into the wound. Additionally, it promotes and accelerates the formation of granulation tissue by the removal of bacterial contamination and exudates.

Although evidence of promising results with NPWT is increasing in other fields [134–143], in NSTIs, the clinical evidence of its superiority over conventional wound dressing techniques for all wound types has not been proven [144, 145].

A systematic review of PubMed and Cochrane Library databases for randomized, controlled trials (RCTs) of NPWT for the treatment of acute or chronic wounds was published in 2011, which did not find clear evidence of a beneficial effect of NPWT compared with conventional treatment [146]. However, much evidence of a positive effect of NPWT on wound in general has been published since and the 2011 systematic review is outdated.

What is the treatment of infected meshes?

Respect prevention strategies to avoid surgical site infection and prosthetic contamination (recommendation 1A).

We suggest avoidance of mesh contamination following incisional SSI by an early and adequate local source control as well as antibiotic treatment (recommendation 1C).

In chronic sinuses and infected meshes, we suggest a complete surgical removal of the mesh which remains the only way to eradicate infection (recommendation 1C).

No clear recommendations on the benefit of biologic versus synthetic mesh in potentially contaminated fields can be proposed (recommendations 1C).

Hernia repair is one of the most common surgical procedures performed globally. Mesh infection, although infrequent, is a devastating complication of mesh hernioplasties, and for this reason, a prevention strategy is essential. Currently, several types of prosthetic mesh are widely used for repairing abdominal wall defects; however, there is no single universal ideal mesh. Synthetic meshes are easy to handle and well tolerated; however, they can be potentially associated with infection when bacteria adhere to the synthetic material leading to chronic infection. Mesh infection is a challenging complication of abdominal wall defect repairs [147–149].

Polypropylene remains the most commonly used material for hernia repairs. Synthetic meshes consisting of large pore meshes are more resistant to infection than the firm, smaller pore meshes. Although biological meshes cost more than synthetic meshes and the long-term durability may be less favorable [150, 151], they can confer protective factors such as resistance to infection and high biocompatibility when implanted [148].

In order to evaluate the risk factors for mesh-related infections after surgical hernia repair, a systematic search performed in PubMed and Scopus databases was published in 2011 [152]. The crude mesh infection rate was 5%. Statistically significant risk factors were smoking (RR = 1.36 [95% CI 1.07, 1.73]; 1171 hernioplasties), American Society of Anesthesiologists (ASA) score ≥ 3 (RR = 1.40 [1.15, 1.70]; 1682 hernioplasties), and emergency operation (RR = 2.46 [1.56, 3.91]; 1561 hernioplasties). Also, mesh infections were significantly correlated with patient age (weighted mean difference [WMD] = 2.63 [0.22, 5.04]; 2364 hernioplasties), ASA score (WMD = 0.23 [0.08, 0.38]; 1682 hernioplasties), and the duration of the hernioplasty (WMD = 44.92 [25.66, 64.18]; 833 hernioplasties). A trend toward higher mesh infection rates was observed in obese patients (RR = 1.41 [0.94, 2.11]; 2243 hernioplasties) and in patients operated on by a resident (in contrast to a consultant; RR = 1.18 [0.99, 1.40]; 982 hernioplasties). Mesh infections usually resulted in mesh removal, and *Staphylococcus* spp., *Enterococcus* spp., and Gram-negative bacteria were the germs commonly isolated in the specimen.

In 2017, a retrospective review of all patients who underwent abdominal wall hernia repair from January 2004 to May 2014 at a tertiary center was published [153]. From 3470 cases of abdominal wall hernia repair, 66 cases (1.9%) of mesh infection were reported, and 48 of these patients (72.7%) required mesh explantation. Steroid or immunosuppressive drugs use (odds ratio [OR] 2.22; CI 1.16 to 3.95), urgent repair (OR 5.06; CI 2.21 to 8.60), and postoperative surgical site infection (OR 2.9; CI 1.55 to 4.10) were predictive of mesh infection. Independent predictors of mesh explantation were type of mesh (OR 3.13; CI 1.71 to 5.21), onlay position (OR 3.51; CI 1.23 to 6.12), and associated enterotomy in the same procedure (OR 5.17; CI 2.05 to 7.12).

The pathogenesis of mesh infection is a complex process involving many factors including, but not limited to, bacterial virulence, surface physicochemical properties of the prosthetic material, and alterations in host defense mechanisms. The result of this interaction is the formation of the bacterial biofilm. Embedded in self-secreted extracellular polymeric substances, biofilm can provide bacteria an effective barrier against host immune cells and antibiotics [154–156]. Early antibiotics and mechanical scrubbing or irrigation to remove the biofilm before it is consolidated are both important.

Mesh infections should be distinguished from superficial incisional SSIs. They occur in the early postoperative period and are not influenced by mesh implantation but can cause the infection of the mesh. The diagnosis of wound infection is clinical, with typical symptoms of localized inflammation and pain at the incision site. Patients with deep mesh infections may present with signs of local inflammation. However, more frequently, deep mesh infections tend to be indolent and present chronic signs and symptoms. They may be initially underestimated.

The management of mesh-site infections is challenging and always requires an individualized approach combining medical and surgical approaches. Clinical trials have demonstrated that in certain instances, non-operative strategies with conservative (non-surgical) management have been successful for salvaging a mesh [157]. If conservative treatment fails, complete surgical removal of the mesh is suggested to reduce the risk of infection recurrence or severe complications, such as visceral adhesions and fistulae. A conservative surgical approach including abscess drainage, sinus excision, or partial mesh excision can fail and may result in recurrent mesh infections.

After removing the infected mesh, the intra-operative options are (a) no implant of a new mesh, (b) re-implantation of a new synthetic light-weight, macroporous mesh, and (c) replacement of the infected synthetic by a biological mesh [158, 159]. A critical issue in the repair of contaminated abdominal wall defects is the dilemma of choosing between synthetic material, with its presumed risk of surgical site complications, and biologic material, a costly alternative with questionable durability. In 2016, Atema et al. published a systematic review and meta-analysis of the repair of potentially contaminated and contaminated abdominal wall defects [160]. Thirty-two studies published between January 1990 and June 2015 on repair of (potentially) contaminated hernias with ≥ 25 patients were reviewed. Fifteen studies solely described hernia repair with biologic mesh, 6 non-absorbable synthetic meshes, and 11 described various techniques. Studies reporting direct and prospective comparison of synthetic versus biological mesh in a cohort were not found. Surgical site complications and hernia recurrence rates were evaluated per degree of contamination and mesh type by calculating pooled proportions. In potentially contaminated hernias (CDC wound class 2), no benefit of biologic over synthetic mesh was found with comparable surgical site complication rates and a hernia recurrence rate of 9% for biologic and 9% for synthetic repair. In contaminated hernias (CDC wound class 3 and 4), most reports were on biologic mesh repair, showing high rates of surgical site complications and a hernia recurrence rate of 30%. Recurrence rates in contaminated hernias depended on whether primary fascial closure was achieved, or the repair with biologic mesh was bridging. Biologic mesh sublay repair with primary fascial closure showed lower recurrence rates than bridging repairs. Non-cross-linked biologic mesh can be used in contaminated hernia without mesh infection and subsequent need for mesh explantation. As only one study on synthetic repair of contaminated hernias was available in literature, no recommendation can be given on the use of synthetic mesh in this setting [161].

Conclusions

SSTIs encompass a variety of pathological conditions ranging from simple superficial infections to severe necrotizing infections. The multifaceted nature of these infections has led to a collaboration among general and emergency surgeons, intensivists, and infectious diseases specialists, who have shared these clinical practice recommendations.

Abbreviations

NSTIs: Necrotizing soft-tissue infections; SSIs: Surgical site infections; SSTIs: Skin and soft-tissue infections

Acknowledgements

Not applicable.

Funding

Not applicable.

Authors' contributions

MS wrote the first draft of the manuscript. All the authors reviewed the manuscript and approved the final draft.

Competing interests

In the past 5 years, MB has participated in advisory boards and/or received speaker honoraria from Achaogen, Angelini, Astellas, AstraZeneca, Bayer, Basilea, Cidara, Gilead, Melinta, Menarini, MSD, Nabriva, Paratek, Pfizer, Roche, The Medicine Company, Shionogi, Tetraphase, VenatoRX, and Vifor. All other authors declared no competing interests.

Author details
[1]Department of Surgery, Macerata Hospital, Macerata, Italy. [2]Unit of Endocrine, Head, and Neck Surgery and Unit of Surgical Infections Support, Department of General Surgery, Parc Taulí Hospital Universitari, Sabadell, Spain. [3]Trauma Service, Inkosi Albert Luthuli Central Hospital and Department of Surgery, Nelson R Mandela School of Clinical Medicine, Durban, South Africa. [4]Department of General Surgery, Division of Surgery, Rambam Health Care Campus, Haifa, Israel. [5]Department of Surgery, Academic Medical Centre, Amsterdam, Netherlands. [6]Department of Surgery, Anadolu Medical Center, Kocaali, Turkey. [7]General Surgery Department, Bufalini Hospital, Cesena, Italy. [8]Anesthesiology and Critical Care Medicine, Paris Diderot Sorbonne Cite University, Bichat-Claude Bernard University Hospital, HUPNSV, Paris, France. [9]Department of Surgery, College of Medicine and Health Sciences, UAE University, Al-Ain, United Arab Emirates. [10]Infectious Diseases Unit, Department of Medical and Surgical Sciences, Alma Mater Studiorum University of Bologna, Bologna, Italy. [11]Infectious Diseases Division, Department of Medicine University of Udine and Azienda Sanitaria Universitaria Intergrata di Udine, Udine, Italy. [12]Trauma and Acute Care Surgery, Scripps Memorial Hospital La Jolla, La Jolla, CA, USA. [13]General Surgery-Trauma Team, State University of Milano, Niguarda Hospital Milano, Milan, Italy. [14]Emergency Surgery Unit, State University of Pisa, Cisanello Hospital, Pisa, Italy. [15]Riverside University Health System Medical Center and Loma Linda University School of Medicine, Moreno Valley, CA, USA. [16]Department of Medical Sciences, Infectious Diseases, University of Turin, Turin, Italy. [17]Unit of General, Emergency and Trauma Surgery, Regional Hospital of Perpignan, Perpignan, France. [18]Department of Surgery, Addenbrooke's Hospital, Cambridge University Hospitals NHS Foundation Trust, Cambridge, UK. [19]Second Department of Surgery, Aretaieion University Hospital, National and Kapodistrian University of Athens, Athens, Greece. [20]Department of Emergency Surgery, City Hospital, Mozyr, Belarus. [21]Global Alliance for Infections in Surgery, Porto, Portugal. [22]Abdominal Center, University Hospital Meilahti, Helsinki, Finland. [23]Department of Surgical Disciplines, Immanuel Kant Baltic Federal University, Regional Clinical Hospital, Kaliningrad, Russian Federation. [24]Department of Surgery, University of Colorado, Denver Health Medical Center, Denver, CO, USA. [25]Department of Surgery, Emergency Hospital of Bucharest, Bucharest, Romania. [26]Infectious Diseases Unit, Bolzano Central Hospital, Bolzano, Italy. [27]Department of Anesthesia and Intensive Care, Azienda Ospedaliero-Universitaria Parma, Parma, Italy. [28]Department of Surgery, UMC Ljubljana, Ljubljana, Slovenia. [29]Department of General and Emergency Surgery, Riga East University Hospital 'Gailezers', Riga, Latvia. [30]General Surgery Department, Colorectal Surgery Unit, La Paz University Hospital, Madrid, Spain. [31]General Surgery Department, Medical University, University Hospital St George, Plovdiv, Bulgaria. [32]Second Department of Surgery, Hospital de Clínicas, Universidad Nacional de Asuncion, San Lorenzo, Paraguay. [33]Emergency Surgery (or Division of Emergency Surgery), Fondazione Policlinico Universitario A. Gemelli IRCCS – Università Cattolica del Sacro Cuore, Rome, Italy. [34]General Surgery, Tan Tock Seng Hospital, Singapore, Singapore. [35]Department of Surgery, Letterkenny University Hospital and Donegal Clinical Research Academy, Letterkenny, Ireland. [36]Department of Emergency Surgery, Parma Maggiore Hospital, Parma, Italy. [37]First Department of Surgery, Department of Abdominal, Thoracic Surgery and Traumatology, First Faculty of Medicine, Charles University and General University Hospital, Prague, Czech Republic.

References

1. May AK. Skin and soft tissue infections. Surg Clin North Am. 2009;89:403–20.
2. Ustin JS, Malangoni MA. Necrotizing soft-tissue infections. Crit Care Med. 2011;39:2156–62.
3. Guyatt G, Gutterman D, Baumann MH, Addrizzo-Harris D, Hylek EM, Phillips B, et al. Grading strength of recommendations and quality of evidence in clinical guidelines: report from an American College of Chest Physicians task force. Chest. 2006;129:174–81.
4. Merlino JI, Malangoni MA. Complicated skin and soft-tissue infections: diagnostic approach and empiric treatment options. Cleve Clin J Med. 2007; 74(Suppl 4):S21–8.
5. Napolitano LM. Severe soft tissue infections. Infect Dis Clin N Am. 2009;23: 571–91.
6. Eron LJ, Lipsky BA, Low DE, Nathwani D, Tice AD, Volturo GA. Expert panel on managing skin and soft tissue infections. Managing skin and soft tissue infections: expert panel recommendations on key decision points. J Antimicrob Chemother. 2003;52(Suppl 1):i3–17.
7. May AK, Stafford RE, Bulger EM, Heffernan D, Guillamondegui O, Bochicchio G, Eachempati SR. Surgical Infection Society. Surgical Infection Society. Treatment of complicated skin and soft tissue infections. Surg Infect. 2009;10:467–99.
8. Stevens DL, Bisno AL, Chambers HF, Dellinger EP, Goldstein EJ, Gorbach SL, et al. Practice guidelines for the diagnosis and management of skin and soft tissue infections: 2014 update by the Infectious Diseases Society of America. Clin Infect Dis. 2014;59:147–59.
9. US Food and Drug Administration. Guidance for industry. Acute bacterial skin and skin structure infections: developing drugs for treatment. https://www.fda.gov/downloads/Drugs/Guidances/ucm071185.pdf. Accessed on 14 Sept 2018.
10. Sartelli M, Malangoni MA, May AK, Viale P, Kao LS, Catena F, et al. World Society of Emergency Surgery (WSES) guidelines for management of skin and soft tissue infections. World J Emerg Surg. 2014;9:57.
11. Allegranzi B, Zayed B, Bischoff P, Kubilay NZ, de Jonge S, de Vries F, et al. New WHO recommendations on intraoperative and postoperative measures for surgical site infection prevention: an evidence-based global perspective. Lancet Infect Dis. 2016;16:e288–303.
12. Allegranzi B, Bischoff P, de Jonge S, Kubilay NZ, Zayed B, Gomes SM, et al. New WHO recommendations on preoperative measures for surgical site infection prevention: an evidence-based global perspective. Lancet Infect Dis. 2016;16:e276–87.
13. Berríos-Torres SI, Umscheid CA, Bratzler DW, Leas B, Stone EC, Kelz RR, et al. Centers for disease control and prevention guideline for the prevention of surgical site infection, 2017. JAMA Surg. 2017;152:784–91.
14. Horan TC, Gaynes RP, Martone WJ, Jarvis WR, Emori TG. CDC definitions of nosocomial surgical site infections, 1992: a modification of CDC definitions of surgical wound infections. Infect Control Hosp Epidemiol. 1992;13:606–8.
15. Nicks BA, Ayello EA, Woo K, Nitzki-George D, Sibbald RG. Acute wound management: revisiting the approach to assessment, irrigation, and closure considerations. Int J Emerg Med. 2010;3:399–407.
16. Ovington L. Bacterial toxins and wound healing. Ostomy Wound Manage. 2003;49(7A Suppl):8–12.
17. Sganga G, Tascini C, Sozio E, Carlini M, Chirletti P, Cortese F, et al. Focus on the prophylaxis, epidemiology and therapy of methicillin-resistant *Staphylococcus aureus* surgical site infections and a position paper on associated risk factors: the perspective of an Italian group of surgeons. World J Emerg Surg. 2016;11:267.
18. Wheadle WG. Risk factors for surgical site infection. Surg Infect. 2006;7(Suppl 1):S7–11.
19. Owens P, McHugh S, Clarke-Moloney M, Healy D, Fitzpatrick F, McCormick P, et al. Improving surgical site infection prevention practices through a multifaceted educational intervention. Ir Med J. 2015;108:78–81.
20. Romani L, Koroivueta J, Steer AC, Kama M, Kaldor JM, Wand H, et al. Scabies and impetigo prevalence and risk factors in Fiji: a national survey. PLoS Negl Trop Dis. 2015;9:e0003452.
21. Bernard P, Jarlier V, Santerre-Henriksen A. Antibiotic susceptibility of Staphylococcus aureus strains responsible for community-acquired skin infections. Ann DermatolVenereol. 2008;135:13–9.
22. Bangert S, Levy M, Hebert AA. Bacterial resistance and impetigo treatment trends: a review. Pediatr Dermatol. 2012;29:243–8.
23. Tong SY, Varrone L, Chatfield MD, Beaman M, Giffard PM. Progressive increase in community-associated methicillin-resistant Staphylococcus aureus in indigenous populations in northern Australia from 1993 to 2012. Epidemiol Infect. 2015;143:1519–23.
24. Eriksson B, Jorup-Ronstrom C, Karkkonen K, Sjoblom AC, Holm SE. Erysipelas: clinical and bacteriologic spectrum and serological aspects. Clin Infect Dis. 1996;23:1091–8.
25. Esposito S, Bassetti M, Borrè S, Bouza E, Dryden M, Fantoni M, et al. Diagnosis and management of skin and soft-tissue infections (SSTI): a literature review and consensus statement on behalf of the Italian Society of Infectious Diseases and International Society of Chemotherapy. J Chemother. 2011;23:251–62.
26. Morris AD. Cellulitis and erysipelas. BMJ Clin Evid. 2008;2008:1708.
27. Garau J, Ostermann H, Medina J, Ávila M, McBride K, Blasi F, et al. Current management of patients hospitalized with complicated skin and soft tissue

infections across Europe (2010-2011): assessment of clinical practice patterns and real-life effectiveness of antibiotics from the REACH study. Clin Microbiol Infect. 2013;19:E377–85.
28. Llera JL, Levy RC. Treatment of cutaneous abscess: a double-blind clinical study. Ann Emerg Med. 1985;14:15–9.
29. Macfie J, Harvey J. The treatment of acute superficial abscesses: a prospective clinical trial. Br J Surg. 1977;64:264–6.
30. Rossolini GM, Stefani S. Aetiology, resistance and diagnostic techniques in skin and skin structure infections. Infez Med. 2009;17(Suppl. 4):18–29.
31. Abcarian H. Anorectal infection: abscess-fistula. Clin Colon Rectal Surg. 2011; 24:14–21.
32. Binswanger IA, Kral AH, Bluthenthal RN, Rybold DJ, Edlin BR. High prevalence of abscesses and cellulitis among community-recruited injection drug users in San Francisco. Clin Infect Dis. 2000;30:579–81.
33. Lloyd-Smith E, Kerr T, Hogg RS, Li K, Montaner JS, Wood E. Prevalence and correlates of abscesses among a cohort of injection drug users. HarmReduct J. 2005;2:24.
34. Pollini RA, Gallardo M, Hasan S, Minuto J, Lozada R, Vera A, et al. High prevalence of abscesses and self-treatment among injection drug users in Tijuana, Mexico. Int J Infect Dis. 2010;14(Suppl 3):e117–22.
35. Khalil PN, Huber-Wagner S, Altheim S, Bürklein D, Siebeck M, Hallfeldt K, et al. Diagnostic and treatment options for skin and soft tissue abscesses in injecting drug users with consideration of the natural history and concomitant risk factors. Eur J Med Res. 2008;13:415–24.
36. Brett MM, Hood J, Brazier JS, Duerden BI, Hahné SJ. Soft tissue infections caused by spore-forming bacteria in injecting drug users in the United Kingdom. Epidemiol Infect. 2005;133:575–82.
37. Spijkerman IJ, van Ameijden EJ, Mientjes GH, Coutinho RA, van den Hoek A. Human immunodeficiency virus infection and other risk factors for skin abscesses and endocarditis among injection drug users. J Clin Epidemiol. 1996;49:1149–54.
38. Gilchrist J, Sacks JJ, White D, Kresnow MJ. Dog bites: still a problem? Inj Prev. 2008;14:296–301.
39. Goldstein EJC. Bite wounds and infections. Clin Infect Dis. 1992;14:633.
40. Weber DJ, Hansen AR. Infections resulting from animal bites. Infect Dis Clin North Am. 1991;5:663.
41. Abrahamian FM, Goldstein EJ. Microbiology of animal bite wound infections. Clin Microbiol Rev. 2011;24:231–46.
42. Medeiros I, Saconato H. Antibiotic prophylaxis for mammalian bites. Cochrane Database Syst Rev. 2001;2:CD001738.
43. Oehler R, Velez AP, Mizrachi M, Lamarche J, Gompf S. Bite-related and septic syndromes by cats and dogs. Lancet Infect Dis. 2009;9:439–47.
44. Jaindl M, Grünauer J, Platzer P, Endler G, Thallinger C, Leitgeb J, Kovar FM. The management of bite wounds in children—a retrospective analysis at a level I trauma centre. Injury. 2012;43:2117–21.
45. Evgeniou E, Markeson D, Iyer S, Armstrong A. The management of animal bites in the United Kingdom. Eplasty. 2013;13:e27.
46. Esposito S, Piccioli I, Semino M, Principi N. Dog and cat bite-associated infections in children. Eur J ClinMicrobiol Infect Dis. 2013;32:971–6.
47. Roberts JA, Abdul-Aziz MH, Lipman J, Mouton JW, Vinks AA, Felton TW, et al. Individualised antibiotic dosing for patients who are critically ill: challenges and potential solutions. Lancet Infect Dis. 2014;14:498–509.
48. Moet GJ, Jones RN, Biedenbach DJ, Stilwell MG, Fritsche TR. Contemporary causes of skin and soft tissue infections in North America, Latin America, and Europe: report from the SENTRY Antimicrobial Surveillance Program (1998–2004). Diagn Microbiol Infect Dis. 2007;57:7–13.
49. Nathwani D, Morgan M, Masterton RG, Dryden M, Cookson BD, French G, et al. Guidelines for UK practice for the diagnosis and management of methicillin-resistant Staphylococcus aureus (MRSA) infections presenting in the community. J Antimicrob Chemother. 2008;61:976–94.
50. Vandenesch F, Naimi T, Enright MC, Lina G, Nimmo GR, Heffernan H, et al. Community-acquired methicillin-resistant *Staphylococcus aureus* carrying Panton-Valentine leukocidin genes: worldwide emergence. Emerg Infect Dis. 2003;9:978–84.
51. Malachowa N, DeLeo FR. Mobile genetic elements of Staphylococcus aureus. Cell Mol Life Sci. 2010;67:3057–71.
52. Macmorran E, Harch S, Athan E, Lane S, Tong S, Crawford L, et al. The rise of methicillin resistant Staphylococcus aureus: now the dominant cause of skin and soft tissue infection in Central Australia. Epidemiol Infect. 2017;145:2817–26.
53. Szumowski JD, Cohen DE, Kanaya F, Mayer KH. Treatment and outcomes of infections by methicillin-resistant Staphylococcus aureus at an ambulatori clinic. Antimicrob Agents Chemother. 2007;51:423–8.
54. Cenizal MJ, Skiest D, Luber S, Bedimo R, Davis P, Fox P, et al. Prospective randomized trial of empiric therapy with trimethoprim- sulfamethoxazole or doxycycline for outpatient skin and soft tissue infections in an area of high prevalence of methicillin-resistant Staphylococcus aureus. Antimicrob Agents Chemother. 2007;51:2628–30.
55. Awad SS, Elhabash SI, Lee L, Farrow B, Berger DH. Increasing incidence of methicillin-resistant Staphylococcus aureus skin and soft-tissue infections: reconsideration of empiric antimicrobial therapy. Am J Surg. 2007;194:606–10.
56. Moise-Broder PA, Sakoulas G, Eliopoulos GM, Schentag JJ, Forrest A, Moellering RC Jr. Accessory gene regulator group II polymorphism in methicillin-resistant Staphylococcus aureus is predictive of failure of vancomycin therapy. Clin Infect Dis. 2004;38:1700–5.
57. Falagas ME, Siempos II, Vardakas KZ. Linezolid versus glycopeptide or β-lactam for treatment of Gram-positive bacterial infections: meta-analysis of randomised controlled trials. Lancet Infect Dis. 2008;8:53–66.
58. Itani KM, Dryden MS, Bhattacharyya H, Kunkel MJ, Baruch AM, Weigelt JA. Efficacy and safety of linezolid versus vancomycin for the treatment of complicated skin and soft-tissue infections proven to be due to methicillin-resistant Staphylococcus aureus. Am J Surg. 2010;199:804–16.
59. Yue J, Dong BR, Yang M, Chen X, Wu T, Liu GJ. Linezolid versus vancomycin forskin and soft tissue infections. Cochrane Database Syst Rev. 2013;7: CD008056.
60. Seaton RA. Daptomycin: rationale and role in the management of skin and soft tissue infections. J Antimicrob Chemother. 2008;62(Suppl 3):iii15–23.
61. Bliziotis IA, Plessa E, Peppas G, Falagas ME. Daptomycin versus other antimicrobial agents for the treatment of skin and soft tissue infections: a meta-analysis. Ann Pharmacother. 2010;44:97–106.
62. Corey GR, Wilcox MH, Talbot GH, Thye D, Friedland D, Baculik T, CANVAS 1 investigators. CANVAS 1: the first phase III, randomized, double-blind study evaluating ceftaroline fosamil for the treatment of patients with complicated skin and skin structure infections. J Antimicrob Chemother. 2010;65(Suppl4):iv41–51.
63. Wilcox MH, Corey GR, Talbot GH, Thye D, Friedland D, Baculik T, CANVAS 2 investigators. CANVAS 2: the second phase III, randomized, double-blind study evaluating ceftaroline fosamil for the treatment of patients with complicated skin and skin structure infections. J Antimicrob Chemother. 2010;65(Suppl 4):iv53–65.
64. Corey GR, Wilcox M, Talbot GH, Friedland HD, Baculik T, Witherell GW, et al. Integrated analysis of CANVAS 1 and 2: phase 3, multicenter, randomized, double-blind studies to evaluate the safety and efficacy of eftaroline versus vancomycin plus aztreonam in complicated skin and skin-structure infection. Clin Infect Dis. 2010;51:641–50.
65. Chahine EB, Sucher AJ, Knutsen SD. Tedizolid: a new oxazolidinone antibiotic for skin and soft tissue infections. Consult Pharm. 2015;30: 386–94.
66. McCool R, Gould IM, Eales J, Barata T, Arber M, Fleetwood K, et al. Systematic review and network meta-analysis of tedizolid for the treatment of acute bacterial skin and skin structure infections caused by MRSA. BMC Infect Dis. 2017;17:39.
67. Bassetti M, Peghin M, Carnelutti A, Righi E. The role of dalbavancin in skin and soft tissue infections. Curr Opin Infect Dis. 2018;31:141–7.
68. Agarwal R, Bartsch SM, Kelly BJ, Prewitt M, Liu Y, Chen Y, Umscheid CA. Newer glycopeptide antibiotics for treatment of complicated skin and soft tissue infections: systematic review, network meta-analysis and cost analysis. Clin Microbiol Infect. 2018;24:361–8.
69. Bassetti M, Eckmann C, Peghin M, Carnelutti A, Righi E. When to switch to an oral treatment and/or to discharge a patient with skin and soft tissue infections. Curr Opin Infect Dis. 2018;31(2):163–9.
70. Howell GM, Rosengart MR. Necrotizing soft tissue infections. Surg Infect. 2011;12:185–90.
71. Wong CH, Khin LW, Heng KS, Tan KC, Low CO. The LRINEC (laboratory risk indicator for necrotizing fasciitis) score: a tool for distinguishing necrotizing fasciitis from other soft tissue infections. Crit Care Med. 2004;32:1535.
72. Bechar J, Sepehripour S, Hardwicke J, Filobbos G. Laboratory risk indicator for necrotising fasciitis (LRINEC) score for the assessment of early necrotising fasciitis: a systematic review of the literature. Ann R Coll Surg Engl. 2017;99:341–6.
73. Fernando SM, Tran A, Cheng W, Rochwerg B, Kyeremanteng K, Seely AJE, et al. Necrotizing soft tissue infection: diagnostic accuracy of physical examination, imaging, and LRINEC score: a systematic review and meta-analysis. Ann Surg. 2018. [Epub ahead of print]

74. Marwick C, Broomhall J, McCowan C, Phillips G, Gonzalez-McQuire S, Akhras K, et al. Severity assessment of skin and soft tissue infections: cohort study of management and outcomes for hospitalized patients. J Antimicrob Chemother. 2011;66:387–97.
75. Singer M, Deutschman CS, Seymour CW, Shankar-Hari M, Annane D, Bauer M, et al. The third international consensus definitions for sepsis and septic shock (Sepsis-3). JAMA. 2016;315:801–10.
76. Hakkarainen TW, Kopari NM, Pham TN, Evans HL. Necrotizing soft tissue infections: review and current concepts in treatment, systems of care, and outcomes. Curr Probl Surg. 2014;51:344–62.
77. Stevens DL, Bryant AE. Necrotizing soft-tissue infections. N Engl J Med. 2017; 377:2253–65.
78. Wong CH, Chang HC, Pasupathy S, Khin LW, Tan JL, Low CO. Necrotizing fasciitis: clinical presentation, microbiology, and determinants of mortality. J Bone Joint Surg Am. 2003 Aug;85-A(8):1454–60.
79. Sabbaj A, Jensen B, Browning MA, Ma OJ, Newgard CD. Soft tissue infections and emergency department disposition: predicting the need for inpatient admission. Acad Emerg Med. 2009;16:1290–7.
80. Lonergan S, Rodriguez RM, Schaulis M, Navaran P. A case series of patients with black tar heroin-associated necrotizing fasciitis. J Emerg Med. 2004;26: 47–50.
81. Mongelluzzo J, Tu B, Grimes B, Ziyeh S, Fortman J, Neilson J, Rodriguez RM. Correlation of physical exam findings with fever in patients with skin and soft tissue infections. West J Emerg Med. 2017;18:398–402.
82. Carratalà J, Rosón B, Fernández-Sabé N, Shaw E, del Rio O, Rivera A, Gudiol F. Factors associated with complications and mortality in adult patients hospitalized for infectious cellulitis. Eur J Clin Microbiol Infect Dis. 2003;22: 151–7.
83. El-Menyar A, Asim M, Mudali IN, Mekkodathil A, Latifi R, Al-Thani H. The laboratory risk indicator for necrotizing fasciitis (LRINEC) scoring: the diagnostic and potential prognostic role. Scand J Trauma Resusc Emerg Med. 2017;25:28.
84. Corbin V, Vidal M, Beytout J, Laurichesse H, D'Incan M, Souteyrand P, Lesens O. Prognostic value of the LRINEC score (Laboratory Risk Indicator for Necrotizing Fasciitis) in soft tissue infections: a prospective study at Clermont-Ferrand University hospital. Ann Dermatol Venereol. 2010;137:5–11.
85. Citak M, Backhaus M, Tilkorn DJ, O'loughlin PF, Meindl R, Muhr G, Fehmer T. Necrotizing fasciitis in patients with spinal cord injury: an analysis of 25 patients. Spine (Phila Pa 1976). 2011;36:E1225–9.
86. Swain RA, Hatcher JC, Azadian BS, Soni N, De Souza B. A five-year review of necrotising fasciitis in a tertiary referral unit. Ann R Coll Surg Engl. 2013;95:57–60.
87. Colak E, Ozlem N, Kucuk GO, Aktimur R, Kesmer S. Laboratory risk indicators for necrotizing fasciitis and associations with mortality. Turk J Emerg Med. 2016;14:15–9.
88. Bozkurt O, Sen V, Demir O, Esen A. Evaluation of the utility of different scoring systems (FGSI, LRINEC and NLR) in the management of Fournier's gangrene. Int Urol Nephrol. 2015;47:243–8.
89. Malghem J, Lecouvet FE, Omoumi P, Maldague BE, Vande Berg BC. Necrotizing fasciitis: contribution and limitations of diagnostic imaging. Joint Bone Spine. 2013;80:146–54.
90. Angoules AG, Kontakis G, Drakoulakis E, Vrentzos G, Granick MS, Giannoudis PV. Necrotising fasciitis of upper and lower limb: a systematic review. Injury. 2007;38(Suppl 5):S19–26.
91. Walshaw CF, Deans H. CT findings in necrotising fasciitis—a report of four cases. Clin Radiol. 1996;51:429–32.
92. Zacharias N, Velmahos GC, Salama A, Alam HB, de Moya M, King DR, Novelline RA. Diagnosis of necrotizing soft tissue infections by computed tomography. Arch Surg. 2010;145:452–5.
93. Kim KT, Kim YJ, Won Lee J, Kim YJ, Park SW, Lim MK, Suh CH. Can necrotizing infectious fasciitis be differentiated from nonnecrotizing infectious fasciitis with MR imaging? Radiology. 2011;259:816–24.
94. Yen ZS, Wang HP, Ma HM, Chen SC, Chen WJ. Ultrasonographic screening of clinically-suspected necrotizing fasciitis. Acad Emerg Med. 2002;9:1448–51.
95. Majeski J, Majeski E. Necrotizing fasciitis: improved survival with early recognition by tissue biopsy and aggressive surgical treatment. South Med J. 1997;90:1065–8.
96. Stamenkovic I, Lew PD. Early recognition of potentially fatal necrotizing fasciitis: the use of frozen-section biopsy. N Engl J Med. 1984;310:1689–93.
97. Anaya DA, Dellinger EP. Necrotizing soft-tissue infection: diagnosis and management. Clin Infect Dis. 2007;44:705–10.
98. Andreasen TJ, Green SD, Childers BJ. Massive infectious soft-tissue injury: diagnosis and management of necrotizing fasciitis and purpura fulminans. Plast Reconstr Surg. 2001;107:1025–35.
99. Bilton BD, Zibari GB, McMillan RW, Aultman DF, Dunn G, McDonald JC. Aggressive surgical management of necrotizing fasciitis serves to decrease mortality: a retrospective study. Am Surg. 1998;64:397–400 discussion 400-1.
100. Kobayashi L, Konstantinidis A, Shackelford S, Chan LS, Talving P, Inaba K, Demetriades D. Necrotizing soft tissue infections: delayed surgical treatment is associated with increased number of surgical debridements and morbidity. J Trauma. 2011;71:1400–5.
101. Boyer A, Vargas F, Coste F, Saubusse E, Castaing Y, Gbikpi-Benissan G, et al. Influence of surgical treatment timing on mortality from necrotizing soft tissue infections requiring intensive care management. Intensive Care Med. 2009;35:847–53.
102. Chao WN, Tsai CF, Chang HR, Chan KS, Su CH, Lee YT, et al. Impact of timing of surgery on outcome of Vibrio vulnificus-related necrotizing fasciitis. Am J Surg. 2013;206:32–9.
103. Okoye O, Talving P, Lam L, Smith J, Teixeira PG, Inaba K, et al. Timing of redébridement after initial source control impacts survival in necrotizing soft tissue infection. Am Surg. 2013;79:1081–5.
104. Soh CR, Pietrobon R, Freiberger JJ, Chew ST, Rajgor D, Gandhi M, et al. Hyperbaric oxygen therapy in necrotising soft tissue infections: a study of patients in the United States nationwide inpatient sample. Intensive Care Med. 2012;38:1143–51.
105. Eskes A, Vermeulen H, Lucas C, Ubbink DT. Hyperbaric oxygen therapy for treating acute surgical and traumatic wounds. Cochrane Database Syst Rev. 2013;12:CD008059.
106. Darenberg J, Ihendyane N, Sjölin J, Aufwerber E, Haidl S, Follin P, et al. Intravenous immunoglobulin G therapy in streptococcal toxic shock syndrome: a European randomized, double-blind, placebo-controlled trial. Clin Infect Dis. 2003;37:333–40.
107. Linnér A, Darenberg J, Sjölin J, Henriques-Normark B, Norrby-Teglund A. Clinical efficacy of polyspecific intravenous immunoglobulin therapy in patients with streptococcal toxic shock syndrome: a comparative observational study. Clin Infect Dis. 2014;59:851–7.
108. Shah SS, Hall M, Srivastava R, Subramony A, Levin JE. Intravenous immunoglobulin in children with streptococcal toxic shock syndrome. Clin Infect Dis. 2009;49:1369–76.
109. Kadri SS, Swihart BJ, Bonne SL, Hohmann SF, Hennessy LV, Louras P, et al. Impact of intravenous immunoglobulin on survival in necrotizing fasciitis with vasopressor-dependent shock: a propensity score-matched analysis from 130 US hospitals. Clin Infect Dis. 2017;64:877–85.
110. Hua C, Bosc R, Sbidian E, De Prost N, Hughes C, Jabre P, et al. Interventions for necrotizing soft tissue infections in adults. Cochrane Database Syst Rev. 2018;5:CD011680.
111. Dellinger RP, Levy MM, Rhodes A, Annane D, Gerlach H, Opal SM, et al. Surviving sepsis campaign guidelines committee including the pediatric subgroup. Surviving sepsis campaign: international guidelines for management of severe sepsis and septic shock: 2012. Crit Care Med. 2013;41:580–637.
112. Smeets L, Bous A, Heymans O. Necrotizing fasciitis: case report and review of literature. Acta Chir Belg. 2007;107:29–36.
113. Angus DC, van der Poll T. Severe sepsis and septic shock. N Engl J Med. 2013;369:840–51.
114. Arad G, Levy R, Nasie I, Hillman D, Rotfogel Z, Barash U, et al. Binding of superantigen toxins into the CD28 homodimer interface is essential for induction of cytokine genes that mediate lethal shock. PLoS Biol. 2011;9: e1001149.
115. Bulger EM, Maier RV, Sperry J, Joshi M, Henry S, Moore FA, et al. A novel drug for treatment of necrotizing soft-tissue infections: a randomized clinical trial. JAMA Surg. 2014;149:528–36.
116. Tabah A, Cotta MO, Garnacho-Montero J, Schouten J, Roberts JA, Lipman J, et al. A systematic review of the definitions, determinants, and clinical outcomes of antimicrobial de-escalation in the intensive care unit. Clin Infect Dis. 2016;62:1009–17.
117. Coyle EA, Cha R, Rybak MJ. Influences of linezolid, penicillin, and clindamycin, alone and in combination, on streptococcal pyrogenic exotoxin a release. Antimicrob Agents Chemother. 2003;47:1752–5.
118. Stevens DL, Ma Y, Salmi DB, McIndoo E, Wallace RJ, Bryant AE. Impact of antibiotics on expression of virulence-associated exotoxin genes in

methicillin-sensitive and methicillin-resistant Staphylococcus aureus. J Infect Dis. 2007;195:202–11.

119. Carapetis JR, Jacoby P, Carville K, Ang SJ, Curtis N, Andrews R. Effectiveness of clindamycin and intravenous immunoglobulin, and risk of disease in contacts, in invasive group a streptococcal infections. Clin Infect Dis. 2014; 59:358–65.
120. Westwood M, Ramaekers B, Whiting P, Tomini F, Joore M, Armstrong N, et al. Procalcitonin testing to guide antibiotic therapy for the treatment of sepsis in intensive care settings and for suspected bacterial infection in emergency department settings: a systematic review and cost-effectiveness analysis. Health Technol Assess. 2015;19:v–xxv 1–236.
121. Friederichs J, Hutter M, Hierholzer C, Novotny A, Friess H, Bühren V, Hungerer S. Procalcitonin ratio as a predictor of successful surgical treatment of severe necrotizing soft tissue infections. Am J Surg. 2013; 206:368–73.
122. Ghnnam WM. Fournier's gangrene in Mansoura Egypt: a review of 74 cases. J Postgrad Med. 2008;54:106–9.
123. Ynar H, Taviloglu K, Ertekin C, Guloglu R, Zorba U, Cabioglu N, Baspinar I. Fournier's gangrene: risk factors and strategies for management. World J Surg. 2006;30:1750–4.
124. Morua AG, Lopez JA, Garcia JD, Montelongo RM, Guerra LS. Fournier's gangrene: our experience in 5 years, bibliographic review and assessment of the Fournier's gangrene severity index. Arch Esp Urol. 2009;62:532–40.
125. McCloud JM, Doucas H, Scott AD, Jameson JS. Delayed presentation of life-threatening perineal sepsis following stapled haemorrhoidectomy: a case report. Ann R Coll Surg Engl. 2007;89:301–2.
126. Yeniyol CO, Suelozgen T, Arslan M, Ayder AR. Fournier's gangrene: experience with 25 patients and use of Fournier's gangrene severity index score. Urology. 2004;64:218–22.
127. Tuncel A, Aydin O, Tekdogan U, Nalcacioglu V, Capar Y, Atan A. Fournier's gangrene: three years of experience with 20 patients and validity of the Fournier's gangrene severity index score. Eur Urol. 2006;50:838–43.
128. Corman J, Moody J, Aronson W. Fournier's gangrene in a modern surgical setting: improved survival with aggressive management. BJU Int. 1999;84:85–8.
129. Gelbard RB, Ferrada P, Yeh DD, Williams B, Loor M, Yon J, et al. Optimal timing of initial debridement for necrotizing soft tissue infection: a practice management guideline from the Eastern Association for the Surgery of Trauma. J Trauma Acute Care Surg. 2018;85:208–14.
130. Bronder CS, Cowey A, Hill J. Delayed stoma formation in Fournier's gangrene. Color Dis. 2004;6:518–20.
131. Mallikarjuna MN, Vijayakumar A, Patil VS, Shivswamy BS. Fournier's gangrene: current practices. ISRN Surg. 2012;2012:942437.
132. Estrada O, Martinez I, Del Bas M, Salvans S, Hidalgo LA. Rectal diversion without colostomy in Fournier's gangrene. Tech Coloproctol. 2009;13:157–9.
133. Orgill DP, Manders EK, Sumpio BE, Lee RC, Attinger CE, Gurtner GC, Ehrlich HP. The mechanisms of action of vacuum assisted closure: more to learn. Surgery. 2009;146:40–51.
134. Huang WS, Hsieh SC, Hsieh CS, Schoung JY, Huang T. Use of vacuum-assisted wound closure to manage limb wounds in patients suffering from acute necrotizing fasciitis. Asian J Surg. 2006;29:135–9.
135. Mulla ZD, Gibbs SG, Aronoff DM. Correlates of length of stay, cost of care, and mortality among patients hospitalized for necrotizing fasciitis. Epidemiol Infect. 2006;3:1–9.
136. Emohare O, Kowal-Vern A, Wiley D, Latenser BA. Vacuum-assisted closure use in calciphylaxis. J Burn Care Rehabil. 2004;25:161–4.
137. Fitzmaurice M, Lawson D, Friedman H. A novel approach for the application of the vacuum-assisted closure device to the difficult anatomy. J Plast Reconstr Aesthet Surg. 2006;59:1249–50.
138. Hofmann P, Friess P, Findeisen M, Tomcik P. Case report of successful therapy of necrotizing fasciitis using a device of vacuum assisted closure. Zentralbl Chir. 2006;131(suppl 1):S72–4.
139. de Geus HR, van der Klooster JM. Vacuum-assisted closure in the treatment of large skin defects due to necrotizing fasciitis. Intensive Care Med. 2005;31:601.
140. Oczenski W, Waldenberger F, Nehrer G, Kneifel W, Swoboda H, Schwarz S, Fitzgerald RD. Vacuum-assisted closure for the treatment of cervical and mediastinal necrotizing fasciitis. J Cardiothorac Vasc Anesth. 2004;18:336–8.
141. Rozeboom AL, Steenvoorde P, Hartgrink HH, Jukema GN. Necrotising fasciitis of the leg following a simple pelvic fracture: case report and literature review. J Wound Care. 2006;15:117–20.
142. Nouraei SA, Hodgson EL, Malata CM. Cervicofacial necrotising fasciitis: management with neck dissection and topical negative pressure. J Wound Care. 2003;12:147–9.
143. Oetting P, Rau B, Schlag PM. Abdominal vacuum device with open abdomen. Chirurg. 2006;77:586 588–93.
144. Ubbink DT, Westerbos SJ, Nelson EA, Vermeulen H. A systematic review of topical negative pressure therapy for acute and chronic wounds. Br J Surg. 2008;95:685–92.
145. Ubbink DT, Westerbos SJ, Evans D, Land L, Vermeulen H. Topical negative pressure for treating chronic wounds. Cochrane Database Syst Rev. 2008;3: CD001898.
146. Peinemann F, Sauerland S. Negative-pressure wound therapy: systematic review of randomized controlled trials. Dtsch Arztebl Int. 2011;108:381–9.
147. Cobb WS, Carbonell AM, Kalbaugh CL, Jones Y, Lokey JS. Infection risk of open placement of intraperitoneal composite mesh. Am Surg. 2009;75:762–7 discussion 767–8.
148. Cevasco M, Itani KM. Ventral hernia repair with synthetic, composite, and biologic mesh: characteristics, indications, and infection profile. Surg Infect. 2012;13:209–15.
149. Bachman S, Ramshaw B. Prosthetic material in ventral hernia repair: how do I choose? Surg Clin North Am. 2013;2008:101–12.
150. Rosen MJ, Krpata DM, Ermlich B, Blatnik JA. A 5-year clinical experience with single-staged repairs of infected and contaminated abdominal wall defects utilizing biologic mesh. Ann Surg. 2013;257:991–6.
151. Latifi R. Practical approaches to definitive reconstruction of complex abdominal wall defects. World J Surg. 2016;40:836–48.
152. Mavros MN, Athanasiou S, Alexiou VG, Mitsikostas PK, Peppas G, Falagas ME. Risk factors for mesh-related infections after hernia repair surgery: a meta-analysis of cohort studies. World J Surg. 2011;35:2389–98.
153. Bueno-Lledó J, Torregrosa-Gallud A, Sala-Hernandez A, Carbonell-Tatay F, Pastor PG, Diana SB, Hernández JI. Predictors of mesh infection and explantation after abdominal wall hernia repair. Am J Surg. 2017;213:50–7.
154. Costerton JW, Montanaro L, Arciola CR. Biofilm in implant infections: its production and regulation. Int J Artif Organs. 2005;28:1062–8.
155. Pérez-Köhler B, Bayon Y, Bellón JM. Mesh infection and hernia repair: a review. Surg Infect. 2016;17:124–37.
156. Kathju S, Nistico L, Melton-Kreft R, Lasko LA, Stoodley P. Direct demonstration of bacterial biofilms on prosthetic mesh after ventral herniorrhaphy. Surg Infect. 2015;16:45–53.
157. Paton BL, Novitsky YW, Zerey M, Sing RF, Kercher KW, Heniford BT. Managementof infections of polytetrafluoroethylene-based mesh. Surg Infect (Larchmt). 2007;8:337–41.
158. Montgomery A, Kallinowski F, Köckerling F. Evidence for replacement of an infected synthetic by a biological mesh in abdominal wall hernia repair. Front Surg. 2016;2:67.
159. Shubinets V, Carney MJ, Colen DL, Mirzabeigi MN, Weissler JM, Lanni MA, et al. Management of infected mesh after abdominal hernia repair: systematic review and single-institution experience. Ann Plast Surg. 2018;80:145–53.
160. Atema JJ, de Vries FE, Boermeester MA. Systematic review and meta-analysis of the repair of potentially contaminated and contaminated abdominal wall defects. Am J Surg. 2016;212:982–95 e1.
161. Atema JJ, Furnée EJ, Maeda Y, Warusavitarne J, Tanis PJ, Bemelman WA, et al. Major complex abdominal wall repair in contaminated fields with use of a non-cross-linked biologic mesh: a dual-institutional experience. World J Surg. 2017;41:1993–9.

Permissions

All chapters in this book were first published in WJES, by BioMed Central; hereby published with permission under the Creative Commons Attribution License or equivalent. Every chapter published in this book has been scrutinized by our experts. Their significance has been extensively debated. The topics covered herein carry significant findings which will fuel the growth of the discipline. They may even be implemented as practical applications or may be referred to as a beginning point for another development.

The contributors of this book come from diverse backgrounds, making this book a truly international effort. This book will bring forth new frontiers with its revolutionizing research information and detailed analysis of the nascent developments around the world.

We would like to thank all the contributing authors for lending their expertise to make the book truly unique. They have played a crucial role in the development of this book. Without their invaluable contributions this book wouldn't have been possible. They have made vital efforts to compile up to date information on the varied aspects of this subject to make this book a valuable addition to the collection of many professionals and students.

This book was conceptualized with the vision of imparting up-to-date information and advanced data in this field. To ensure the same, a matchless editorial board was set up. Every individual on the board went through rigorous rounds of assessment to prove their worth. After which they invested a large part of their time researching and compiling the most relevant data for our readers.

The editorial board has been involved in producing this book since its inception. They have spent rigorous hours researching and exploring the diverse topics which have resulted in the successful publishing of this book. They have passed on their knowledge of decades through this book. To expedite this challenging task, the publisher supported the team at every step. A small team of assistant editors was also appointed to further simplify the editing procedure and attain best results for the readers.

Apart from the editorial board, the designing team has also invested a significant amount of their time in understanding the subject and creating the most relevant covers. They scrutinized every image to scout for the most suitable representation of the subject and create an appropriate cover for the book.

The publishing team has been an ardent support to the editorial, designing and production team. Their endless efforts to recruit the best for this project, has resulted in the accomplishment of this book. They are a veteran in the field of academics and their pool of knowledge is as vast as their experience in printing. Their expertise and guidance has proved useful at every step. Their uncompromising quality standards have made this book an exceptional effort. Their encouragement from time to time has been an inspiration for everyone.

The publisher and the editorial board hope that this book will prove to be a valuable piece of knowledge for researchers, students, practitioners and scholars across the globe.

List of Contributors

Ahmer A Memon, Faisal G Siddiqui, Arshad H Abro, Ahmed H Agha and Abdul S Memon
Department of Surgery, Liaquat University of Medical & Health Sciences, Jamshoro, 71000, Pakistan

Shahzadi Lubna
Department of Gynea & Obs, Liaquat University of Medical & Health Sciences, Jamshoro, 71000, Pakistan

Robert D. Becher
Section of General Surgery, Trauma, and Surgical Critical Care, Department of Surgery, Yale School of Medicine, 330 Cedar Street, BB 310, New Haven, CT 06510, USA

Andrew B. Peitzman and Jason L. Sperry
Department of Surgery, University of Pittsburgh School of Medicine, Pittsburgh, PA, USA

Jared R. Gallaher
Department of Surgery, University of North Carolina School of Medicine, Chapel Hill, NC, USA

Lucas P. Neff
Department of Surgery, David Grant Medical Center, Travis Air Force Base, Fairfield, CA, USA

Yankai Sun, Preston R. Miller and Michael C. Chang
Department of Surgery, Wake Forest University School of Medicine, Winston-Salem, NC, USA

Hicham Elbouhaddouti, Abdesslam Bouassria, Ouadii Mouaqit, El Bachir Benjelloun, Abdelmalek Ousadden, Khalid Mazaz and Khalid Ait Taleb
Department of Surgery, School of Medicine and Pharmacy of Fez, Sidi Mohammed Ben Abdallah University, University hospital HASSAN II, BP: 1893, Km2.200, Route de Sidi Hrazem FEZ 30000, Morocco

Kerollos N Wanis, Allison M Hunter, Michael B Harington and Gary Groot
Department of Surgery, College of Medicine, University of Saskatchewan, 750 Spadina Cr. E, Saskatoon, SK S7K 3H3, Canada

Abdelkarim H Omari, Muhammad R Khammash, Ghazi R Qasaimeh and Ahmad K Shammari
Department of General Surgery and Urology, King Abdullah University Hospital, Jordan University of Science and Technology, 22110 Irbid, Jordan

Mohammad K Bani Yaseen
Department of General Surgery, Princess Basma Teaching Hospital, 22110 Irbid, Jordan

Sahel K Hammori
Department of General Surgery, Prince Rashid Military Teaching Hospital, 22110 Irbid, Jordan

Mari-Liis Kaljusto and Theis Tønnessen
Department of Cardiothoracic Surgery, Oslo University Hospital, Ullevål PB 4956 Nydalen and University of Oslo, Oslo, 0424, Norway

Osvaldo Chiara, Emanuele di Fratta, Anna Mariani, Fabrizio Sammartano and Stefania Cimbanassi
SC Trauma Team, Niguarda Trauma Center, Ospedale Niguarda Ca' Granda Milano, Milano, Italy

Bertuzzi Michaela and Lucia Prestini
SC Quality Assessment Service, Ospedale Niguarda Ca' Granda Milano, Milano, Italy

Osvaldo Chiara
Trauma Team Ospedale Niguarda, Piazza Ospedale Maggiore 3, Milano 20162, Italy

Luigi Bonavina, Alberto Aiolfi, Stefano Siboni and Emanuele Rausa
Department of Biomedical Sciences for Health, Division of General Surgery, University of Milano Medical School, IRCCS Policlinico San Donato, Via Morandi 30, 20097, San Donato Milanese, (Milano), Italy

Salomone Di Saverio
Emergency and Trauma Surgery - Maggiore Hospital, AUSL, Bologna, Italy

Arianna Birindelli
S. Orsola Malpighi University Hospital - University of Bologna, Bologna, Italy

Micheal D. Kelly
Locum Surgeon, Acute Surgical Unit, Canberra Hospital, Canberra, ACT, Australia

Kurinchi S. Gurusamy
Royal Free Campus, University College London, London, UK

Fabio Cesare Campanile
Department of Surgery, San Giovanni Decollato Andosilla Hospital, Viterbo, Italy

Walter Biffl
Queen's Medical Center, University of Hawaii, Honolulu, HI, USA

Rao Ivatury
Professor Emeritus Virginia Commonwealth University, Richmond, VA, USA

George Velmahos
Harvard Medical School - Chief of Trauma, Emergency Surgery, and Surgical Critical Care, Massachusetts General Hospital, Boston, USA

Huseyin Narci and Keziban Karabulut
Department of Emergency Medicine, Baskent Universitesi Konya Hastanesi Hocacihan mah, Saray caddesi No: 1, Selcuklu, Konya 42080, Turkey

Emin Turk and Erdal Karagulle
Department of General Surgery, Baskent University Faculty of Medicine, Ankara, Turkey

Turhan Togan
Department of Infectious Diseases and Clinical Microbiology, Baskent University Faculty of Medicine, Ankara, Turkey

Mario Testini, Germana Lissidini, Angela Gurrado, Giuseppe Massimiliano De Luca, Ilaria Fabiola Franco, Alessandro De Luca and Giuseppe Piccinni
Department of Biomedical Sciences and Human Oncology, Unit of Endocrine, Digestive and Emergency Surgery, University Medical School of Bari "Aldo Moro", Bari, Italy

Francesco Logoluso
Department of Emergency and Organ Transplantation, Unit of Endocrinology, University Medical School of Bari "Aldo Moro", Bari, Italy

Rocco Cortese
Department of Neurological and Psychiatric Sciences, Unit of Physical and Rehabilitation, University Medical School of Bari "Aldo Moro", Bari, Italy

Giuseppe Campobasso
Unit of Otorhinolaryngology; "Di Venere Hospital", Bari, Italy

Ramiro Manzano-Nunez
Clinical Research Center, Fundación Valle del Lili, Cali, Colombia

Ramiro Manzano-Nunez and Herney Andrés García-Perdomo
UROGIV Research Group, Universidad Del Valle, Cali, Colombia

Paula Ferrada
Surgical Critical Care, Virginia Commonwealth University, Richmond, VA, USA

Carlos Alberto Ordoñez Delgado
Division of Acute Care Surgery, Fundación Valle del Lili, Cali, Colombia

Jorge Esteban Foianini
Division of Surgery, Clinica Foianini, Av. Irala 468, Santa Cruz de la Sierra, Bolivia

Massimo Sartelli
Department of Surgery, Macerata Hospital, Macerata, Italy

Federico Coccolini
General Surgery Department, Papa Giovanni XXIII hospital, Bergamo, Italy

Gabrielle H van Ramshorst
Department of Surgery, Red Cross Hospital Beverwijk, Erasmus University Medical Center, Rotterdam, Netherlands

Jae Gil Lee
Department of Surgery, Yonsei University College of Medicine, Seoul, Korea

Nereo Vettoretto
Laparoscopic Surgical Unit, M. Mellini Hospital, Chiari, BS, Italy

Gianluca Guercioni
Department of Surgery, Mazzoni Hospital, Ascoli Piceno, Italy

Helmut Alfredo Segovia Lohse
II Cátedra de Clínica Quirúrgica, Hospital de Clínicas, Facultad de Ciencias Médicas, Universidad Nacional de Asuncion, San Lorenzo, Paraguay

Jakub Kenig
3rd Department of General Surgery, Jagiellonian University Collegium Medium, Krakow, Poland

Stefano Mandalà
Department of Surgery, G. Giglio Hospital Cefalù, Palermo, Italy

Hiroki Yamaguchi, Tatsuya Nakao, Noriyuki Tokunaga, Hiromasa Nakamura and Masami Takagaki
Department of Cardiovascular Surgery, New Tokyo Hospital, 1271 Wanagaya, Matsudo, Chiba 270-2232, Japan

Jean M Butte and Chad G Ball
Department of Surgery, Foothills Medical Center, University of Calgary, Calgary, AB, Canada

Morad Hameed
University of British Columbia, Vancouver, BC, Canada

Virote Chalieopanyarwong, Teeranut Boonpipattanapong and Surasak Sangkhathat
Department of Surgery, Faculty of Medicine, Prince of Songkla University, Hat Yai, Songkhla 90110, Thailand

Teeranut Boonpipattanapong and Surasak Sangkhathat
Tumor Biology Research Unit, Faculty of Medicine, Prince of Songkla University, Hat Yai, Songkhla 90110, Thailand

Paradee Prechawittayakul
Cancer Registry Unit, Songklanagarind Hospital, Faculty of Medicine, Prince of Songkla University, Hat Yai, Songkhla 90110, Thailand

Mario Testini, Antonia Girardi, Roberta Maria Isernia, Giovanni Catalano and Angela Gurrado
Unit of Endocrine, Digestive, and Emergency Surgery, Department of Biomedical Sciences and Human Oncology, University Medical School "Aldo Moro" of Bari, Bari, Italy

Angela De Palma
Department of Thoracic Surgery, University of Bari, Bari, Italy

Angela Pezzolla
Unit of Laparoscopic Surgery, Department of Emergency and Organ Transplantation, University Medical School "A. Moro" of Bari, Bari, Italy

Michael S. Bleszynski, Emilie Joos and S. Morad Hameed
Department of Surgery, University of British Columbia, Vancouver, Canada

Alexsander K. Bressan and Chad G. Ball
Department of Surgery, University of Calgary, Foothills Medical Centre, 1403 - 29 Street NW, Calgary, Alberta, Canada

M. Sugrue
Department of Surgery, Letterkenny University Hospital and Donegal Clinical Research Academy, Donegal, Ireland

R. Maier
Department of Surgery, University of Washington, Seattle, USA
Harborview Medical Center, Seattle, USA

E. E. Moore
University of Colorado, Denver, USA

M. Boermeester
Department of Surgery, Academic Medical Center, Amsterdam, Netherlands

A. W. Kirkpatrick
Department of Surgery, Critical Care Medicine and Regional Trauma Service, Foothills Medical Centre, Calgary, AB, Canada

Y. Kluger
Department of General Surgery, Division of Surgery, Rambam Health Care Campus, Haifa, Israel

L. Lawler
Department of Radiology, Mater Misericordiae University Hospital, Dublin, Ireland

S. Thomas
Department of Trauma Services, Memorial Hospital of South Bend, Indiana, USA

J. L. Vincent
Department of Intensive Care, Erasme Hospital, Université libre de bruxelles, Brussels, Belgium

L. Woods
Department of Acute Hospitals, Health Services Executive, Dublin, Ireland

Miklosh Bala
Trauma and Acute Care Surgery Unit, General Surgery Department, Hadassah Hebrew University Medical Center, Kiriat Hadassah, 91120 Jerusalem, Israel

Jeffry Kashuk
Tel Aviv University Sackler School of Medicine, Assia Medical Group, Tel Aviv, Israel

Ernest E. Moore
Department of Surgery, University of Colorado, Denver Health Medical Center, Denver, USA

Fausto Catena
Emergency Department, Maggiore University Hospital, Parma, Italy

Ari Leppaniemi
Abdominal Center, University Hospital Meilahti, Helsinki, Finland

Luca Ansaloni and, Federico Coccolini
General Surgery I, Papa Giovanni XXIII Hospital, Bergamo, Italy

Walter Biffl
Scripps Memorial Hospital La Jolla, La Jolla, USA

Andrew Peitzman
Department of Surgery, UPMC, University of Pittsburgh School of Medicine, Pittsburgh, PA, USA

Massimo Sartelli
Macerata Hospital, Ancona University, Macerata Area, Italy

Michael Sugrue
Letterkenny University Hospital and Donegal Clinical Research Academy, Letterkenny, Ireland

Gustavo P. Fraga
Division of Trauma Surgery, Hospital de Clinica, School of Medical Sciences, University of Campinas, Campinas, Brazils

Salomone Di Saverio
Department of Surgery, Maggiore Hospital, Bologna, Italy

Yoram Kluger
Department of General Surgery, Rambam Health Care Campus, Haifa, Israel

Sharfuddin Chowdhury
Consultant and head of Trauma Surgery, King Saud Medical City, 7790 Al-Imam Abdul Aziz Ibn Muhammad Ibn Saud, Ulaishah, Riyadh 12746, Kingdom of Saudi Arabia

Andrew John Nicol
Head and Director of Trauma Centre, Groote Schuur Hospital and University of Cape Town, Cape Town, South Africa

Mahammed Riyaad Moydien
Groote Schuur Hospital and University of Cape Town, Cape Town, South Africa

Pradeep Harkison Navsaria
Deputy Director of Trauma Centre, Groote Schuur Hospital, and University of Cape Town, Cape Town, South Africa

Luis Felipe Montoya-Pelaez
Department of Anaesthesia, Groote Schuur Hospital and University of Cape Town, Cape Town, South Africa

Federico Coccolini and Giulia Montori
General, Emergency and Trauma Surgery, Papa Giovanni XXIII Hospital, P.zza OMS 1, 24128 Bergamo, Italy

Fausto Catena
Emergency and Trauma Surgery, Maggiore Hospital, Parma, Italy

Yoram Kluger
Division of General Surgery, Rambam Health Care Campus, Haifa, Israel

Rifat Latifi
General Surgery Department, Westchester Medical Center, Westchester, NY, USA

David Costa Navarro
Colorectal Surgery Unit, Trauma Care Committee, Alicante General University Hospital, Alicante, Spain

Yashuiro Otomo
Trauma and Acute Critical Care Center, Tokyo Medical and Dental University, Tokyo, Japan

Liban Wehlie
General Surgery Department, Ayaan Hospital, Mogadisho, Somalia

Massimo Sartelli
General and Emergency Surgery, Macerata Hospital, Macerata, Italy

Salomone Di Saverio
General, Emergency and Trauma Surgery Department, Maggiore Hospital, Bologna, Italy

Massimo Sartelli
Department of Surgery, Macerata Hospital, Macerata, Italy

Xavier Guirao
Unit of Endocrine, Head, and Neck Surgery and Unit of Surgical Infections Support, Department of General Surgery, Parc Taulí Hospital Universitari, Sabadell, Spain

Timothy C. Hardcastle
Trauma Service, Inkosi Albert Luthuli Central Hospital and Department of Surgery, Nelson R Mandela School of Clinical Medicine, Durban, South Africa

Index

R

S

T

U

V

www.ingramcontent.com/pod-product-compliance
Lightning Source LLC
LaVergne TN
LVHW080702210926
848485LV00003B/404